Pocket Drug Guide

Pocket Drug Guide

Constantine J. Gean, M.D.

Gerald F. S. Hiatt, Ph.D.

Frederick H. Meyers, M.D.

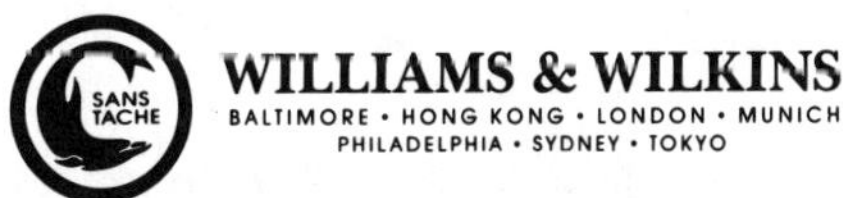

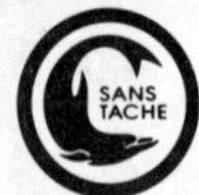

Editor: John P. Butler
Associate Editor: Linda Napora
Copy Editor: Shelly Hyatt-Blankman
Design: Dan Pfisterer
Production: Barbara Felton

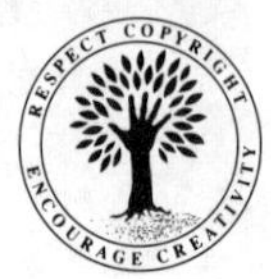

The authors have made every effort to assure that the recommended doses and dose schedules are accurate and in agreement with current good medical practice. However, medical research and other sources of new information are constantly changing drug therapy and doses. The physician is advised to verify doses and schedules in the manufacturer's product information insert prior to the administration of a drug. This is particularly important when new or infrequently used drugs are given. It remains the responsibility of the individual physician to determine the suitability for his particular patient of any dosage regimen recommended or other information offered in this book.

Printed in the United States of America

Library of Congress Cataloging-in-Publication Data

Gean, Constantine J.
Pocket drug guide.
Includes index.
1. Drugs — Handbooks, manuals, etc. I. Hiatt, Gerald F. S. II. Meyers, Frederick H. III. Title.
(DNLM: 1. Drugs — handbooks. QV 39 G292p)
RM301.12.G43 1989 615'.1 88-27886
ISBN 0-683-03440-5

6 7 8 9 10

This work is dedicated
to the memory
of June and George Hiatt.

Preface

Central to the organization of this book is the concept that drugs with mechanistically similar effects can be grouped into classes. The practitioner is encouraged by the marketing efforts of industry (and, less importantly, by investigators interested in evaluating one new drug) to conclude that he must independently evaluate thousands of individual drugs and that each drug requires a separate analysis. However, as this handbook demonstrates, drugs can be classified into a manageable number of groups. Most newly marketed drugs are not truly new, and can be fitted into familiar groups. Once a familiar group is appropriately assigned, much of the therapist's previous training and experience can be applied. From time to time (unfortunately with decreasing frequency) a genuinely new drug effect is identified. These discoveries have had a revolutionary impact on medicine since World War II, and they will be recognized and applied more appropriately if their failure to fit into an existing group is recognized. When differences exist between drugs in a large category, that is, when subclasses are necessary for understanding, the charts in this book include such subclasses. However, it is rarely necessary to go deeply into a chart's subclassifications to provide the distinctions that are needed to demonstrate virtuosity in the use of drugs and to assure the currency of the information therein obtained. Of course, if you and your patient are to benefit maximally from our organizing efforts, it is necessary that you show the same active interest in therapy that you do in diagnosis, and that you actively follow the patient's response, modifying therapy as needed.

This book will present the majority of drugs used by the modern physician in a format facilitating an appreciation of the different drug classes and the similarity of drugs within any one class. We hope this will aid the physician in making intelligent, logical therapeutic decisions. The book has been designed to be a true "reference guide" source by making it small enough to be kept at hand always.

Acknowledgments

No project the size of this book can be done in isolation. The authors would like to express their gratitude to the talented and thoughtful people who aided us with insight and helpful comments.

Special thanks to Karen Quon for her untiring efforts. Additional thanks to Carmelita and Edith Cruz and Conrad and Lillian Camden.

Our gratitude is also extended to Doctors John L. Gean, Geoffrey Gean, Sheldon Amsel, Frank Calia, Michael Fisher, J. J. Gunning, John Kastor, Robert Peters, James Quinlan, and Mario Zarate, whose helpful comments and assistance helped the goal of writing this book become a reality.

Contents

Section 1: CARDIOVASCULAR SYSTEM AGENTS
Table of Contents

THIAZIDE DIURETICS AND RELATED AGENTS

GROUP REMARKS: Moderately potent diuretics, "first-line" use. **SIDE EFFECTS:** Mainly due to potassium depletion (routine serum K^+ levels NOT useful EXCEPT patients at risk for hypokalemia): weakness, dizziness, cramps, anorexia, nausea, drowsiness, paresthesias, jaundice, increased digitalis toxicity and hypokalemic hypochloremic alkalosis (cirrhotics esp. susceptible). Effects most intense early in therapy. Glucose tolerance impaired (caution in diabetics). Dilutional hyponatremia (discontinue treatment & restrict fluids). Increased serum uric acid and serum lithium via inhibition of excretion. Increased ammonia serum levels (caution with liver disease). Photosensitivity, allergic skin rashes. **CAUTIONS:** Use with caution in: renal insufficiency, concurrent digitalis, gout, diabetes, cirrhosis, concurrent corticosteroids or history of sulfa drug allergy. Rare side effects: hypocalcemia, hypomagnesemia, blood dyscrasias. **RECOMMENDATIONS:** Add KCl supplement or switch to K^+-sparing diuretic if serum $K^+ < 3$ mEq/l. **NOTE:** All (EXCEPT metazolone) ineffective if GFR $<$ 25 cc/min or if BUN/serum creatinine $>$ 2x normal. Probably not useful if GFR $<$ 50 cc/min.

DRUG	1st DOSE (PO)	DOSE RANGE	DOSE FORMS	SIDE EFFECTS & REMARKS
BENDROFLUMETHIAZIDE (Naturetin)	HTN: 5-20 mg/d. Edema: 10 mg bid.	HTN: 2.5-15 mg/d. Edema: 2.5-5 mg/d.	PO (Tab's): 2.5, 5, 10 mg	Nadolol combination (Corzide) may offer increased bio-availability.
BENZTHIAZIDE (Aquatag) (Exna) (Aquapres) (Proaqua)(Marazine) (Urazide)	HTN: 50-100 mg/d Edema: 50-200 mg/d.	HTN: 50-200 mg/d. Edema: 50-150 mg/d.	PO (Tab's): 25, 50 mg	Split doses if $\geq$ 100 mg/d.
CHLORTHALIDONE (Hygroton)	HTN: 25 mg/d. Edema: 50-100 mg/d.	HTN: 25-100 mg/d. Edema: 50-200 mg/d.	PO (Tab's): 25, 50, 100 mg	Duration of action: 48-72 h, qod dosing possible.
CHLOROTHIAZIDE (Diuril)	HTN/Edema: 250 mg bid.	HTN: 250-2000 mg/d. Edema: 500-2000 mg/d.	PO (Tab's): 250, 500 mg	IV dose (Chlorothiazide sodium) same as PO dose.
CYCLOTHIAZIDE (Anhydron) (Fluidil)	HTN: 2 mg/d. Edema: 1 mg/d.	HTN: 2-6 mg/d. Edema: 1-2 mg qod.	PO (Tab's): 2 mg	
HYDROCHLOROTHIAZIDE (HCTZ) (Esidrex) (Hydrodiuril) (Oretec) (Hydromal) (Thiuretic) (Diaqua) (Hydrochlor) (Hydro-Z-50) (Dydrozide-50) (Hyperetic) (Lexor)	HTN/Edema: 25 mg bid.	HTN: 25-100 mg/d. Edema: 25-200 mg/d.	PO (Tab's): 25, 50, 100 mg	
HYDROFLUMETHIAZIDE (Saluron) (Diucardin)	HTN: 50 mg bid. Edema: 25 mg/d.	HTN: 50-100 mg/d. Edema: 25-200 mg/d.	PO (Tab's): 50 mg	
METHYCLOTHIAZIDE (Aquatensin) (Enduron)	HTN/Edema: 2.5 mg/d.	HTN: 2.5-5 mg/d. Edema: 2.5-10 mg/d.	PO (Tab's): 2.5, 5 mg	
METOLAZONE (Zaroxolyn)	HTN: 2.5-5 mg/d. Edema: 5-20 mg bid.	Same as 1st dose.	PO (T's): 2.5, 5, 10 mg	Not a usual antihypertensive agent. Some efficacy in renal failure refractory to Lasix. Toxicity: abdominal bloating, palpitations, chest pain, chills. Prominent hypokalemia.
POLYTHIAZIDE (Renese)	HTN/Edema: 1-2 mg/d.	HTN/Edema: 1-4 mg/d.	PO (Tab's): 1, 2, 4 mg	
QUINETHAZONE (Hydromox)	HTN/Edema: 50 mg/d.	HTN/Edema: 50-200 mg/d.	PO (Tab's): 50 mg	

POTENT ("LOOP") DIURETICS

GROUP REMARKS: "Loop diuretics" more potent than the thiazides. **SIDE EFFECTS**: Dehydration, hypochloremia, nausea, vomiting, diarrhea, hyponatremia, pre-renal azotemia, hypomagnesemia. Diuretic treatment can precipitate encephalopathy in cirrhotics. ATN can develop without excess dehydration (esp. with pre-existing renal failure): Hyperuricemia, hemoconcentration (possible increased risk of thrombosis). Potent diuretics can produce marked hypokalemia: contraction alkalosis, tinnitus, temporary or permanent deafness. Pre-load reduction can markedly decrease BP in dehydrated patients (esp. with IV dosing). **CAUTIONS**: May increase serum lithium levels. History of hyperuricemia or gout necessitates careful monitoring. Caution in advanced cirrhosis (encephalopathy). Hypokalemia & hypomagnesemia can precipitate digitalis arrhythmias. **RECOMMENDATIONS:** Closely monitor body weight, BUN, creatinine, electrolyte status, Ca^{++}, & Mg^{++} (esp. early in therapy). Consider increasing patient's Na^+ intake to counter increased loss. When possible use: low doses, careful adjustment and intermittent schedules. Discontinue if patient develops azotemia, oliguria, severe electrolyte depletion or severe watery diarrhea. **CONTRAINDICATIONS:** Anuria, hypotension, dehydration, severe hyponatremia.

DRUG	INDICATIONS & DOSAGE	SIDE EFFECTS & REMARKS	
FUROSEMIDE (Lasix)	<u>**Peripheral Edema**</u>: **PO**: 20-80 mg/d qAM initially (increase by 20-40 mg q6-8h if no response); 20-600 mg/d maintenance as1-2 doses. **IV, IM**: 20-40 mg/d initially (increase by 20 mg q2h PRN); 20-120 mg/d maintenance as 1-2 doses. <u>**Acute Pulmonary Edema**</u>: **IV**: 40 mg (infuse over 1-2 min); 80 mg at 1 h if no response. <u>**Renal Failure**</u>: **PO**: 80 mg/d qAM initially; 80-400 mg/d maintenance as1-4 doses. **IV**: 60-100 mg/d initially; 100-2000 mg/d maintenance as1-8 doses. <u>**Hypertension**</u>: **PO**: 40 mg bid. <u>**Hypercalcemia**</u>: **PO**: 120 mg/d as 1-2 doses. **IV**: 80-100 mg/d (adminst. q1-2h in saline); maximum 160-3200 mg/d.	Net diuresis is approx. 0.25 isotonic for Na^+. Effective even with GFR < 15 cc/min. Member of sulfanilamide class (allergic potential). Peripheral edema may imply bowel wall edema, hence decreased PO absorption. Can convert non-oliguric renal failure to oliguric (nausea, vomiting, diarrhea, jaundice, dehydration - may worsen renal failure). May increase serum ammonia levels. Rare: Erythema multiforma, agranulocytosis, thrombocytopenia, pancreatitis, allergic nephritis. **CAUTION**: Ototoxicity assoc'd with high doses and rapid infusion (is additive with aminoglycosides). **RECOMMEND**: IV infusion < 4 mg/min. Avoid evening doses (nighttime voiding). Monitor BUN, creatinine, HCO_3^-, electrolytes & body weight. Intermittent dosing with low doses if possible. **CONTRAINDICATIONS**: Anuric patients, azotemia secondary to dehydration. <u>**Pediatric Edema**</u>: **PO**: 2 mg/kg initially (can increase by 1 mg/kg q6-8h); 2-6 mg/kg/d maintenance as 2-6 doses. <u>**Pediatric Pulmonary Edema**</u>: **IM, IV**: 1 mg/kg initially (repeat after 2 h, or more); 1-6 mg/kg/d maintenance as 2-4 doses.	<u>**DOSE FORMS**</u>: PO (Tab's): 20, 40, 80 mg IV ampules: 10 mg/ml
ETHACRYNIC ACID (Ethacrynate) (Edecrin)	<u>**Edema**</u>: **PO**: 50mg/d qAM initially;100-400 mg/d maintenance as 1-2 doses. (50 mg on day 1, may increase 25-50 qd). **IV**: 50 mg/d as 1 dose. <u>**Pediatric Edema**</u>: **PO**: 25 mg/d qAM; 2-3 mg/kg/d maintenance. <u>**DOSE FORMS**</u>: PO (Tab): 25, 50 mg	Group remarks, also GI side effects with high doses given > 1-3 months. Hyperglycemia with > 200 mg/dose (esp. with hepatic disease & hypokalemia). Useful as independent agent or adjunct to others (esp in renal failure - see "furosemide"). Hypoprotenemia may decrease response. IV form prone to thrombophlebitis. **RECOMMEND**: Adjust dose for gradual body weight loss (1-2 kg/d).	
BUMETANIDE (Bumex)	<u>**Edema**</u>: **PO**: 0.5 mg/d qAM initially; 0.5-10 mg/d maint. **IV**: 0.5 mg q2-3h; 0.5-10 mg/d maintenance. <u>**DOSE FORMS**</u>: PO (Tab's): 0.5, 1 mg	Group remarks. Adminst. IV q 2-3h, until response. Sulfonamide derivative with low allergic potential (use in patients allergic to furosemide). Rare: Transient LFT elevation.	

POTASSIUM-SPARING DIURETICS

GENERAL REMARKS: Usefulness of these agents lies in combination with other, more potent, diuretics (counter potassium loss produced by others). Hypotensive effect additive with other diuretics. **SIDE EFFECTS:** Hyperkalemia, additive with other diuretics in this class, risk increased with pre-existing renal impairment. Hyperchloremic acidosis. Dehydration, hypochloremia, nausea, vomiting, diarrhea, hyponatremia, pre-renal azotemia, hypomagnesemia. Diuretic treatment can precipitate encephalopathy in cirrhotics. Acute tubular necrosis can develop without excess dehydration (esp. with pre-existing renal failure). Hyperuricemia, hemoconcentration (possible increased risk of thrombosis). **CAUTIONS:** May increase serum lithium levels. History of hyperuricemia or gout necessitates careful monitoring of patient. Caution in advanced cirrhosis (encephalopathy). Hypokalemia & hypomagnesemia can precipitate digitalis arrhythmias. **RECOMMENDATIONS:** Used with other diuretics in cases at risk of hypokalemia (e.g., digitalized patients.). Carefully monitor serum potassium while adjusting dosage. Closely monitor body weight, BUN, creatinine, electrolyte status, Ca^{++}, & Mg^{++} (esp. early in therapy). Consider increasing patient's Na^{+} intake to counter increased loss. When possible use: low doses, careful adjustment, intermittent schedules. Discontinue if patient develops azotemia, oliguria, severe electrolyte depletion or watery diarrhea. **CONTRAINDICATIONS:** Anuria, hypotension, dehydration, severe hyponatremia.

DRUG	INDICATIONS & DOSAGE	SIDE EFFECTS & REMARKS	
SPIRONOLACTONE (Aldactone) (Spiractone) (in Aldactazide, with hydrochorthiazide)	<u>Edema</u>: **PO:** 25-100 mg/d initially; 25-200 mg/d maint. as 1-2 doses (continue initial dose for 5 d, if needed). <u>Hypokalemia</u>: **PO:** 25 mg/d initially; 25-100 mg/d maintenance as 1-2 doses.	Indicated for edema secondary to increased aldosterone (cirrhosis, CHF, nephrotic syndrome). Onset delayed 3-5 d. Gynecomastia, decreased libido, menstrual irregularties, post-menopausal bleeding. **CAUTIONS:** Renal or hepatic disease. **RECOMMEND:** Add prednisone (15-20 mg/d) to edema treatment if no response to Spironolactone + another diuretic. Use may require decreasing dose of concurrent ganglionic blocker by 50%. **CONTRAINDICATIONS:** Rapidly deteriorating renal function.	
	<u>Diagnosis of Primary Aldosteronism</u>: **PO:** 400 mg/d (administer 3-4 wk; test positive if K^{+} then normal). <u>Pediatric</u>: **PO:** 1 mg/kg/d initially; 1.0-3.3 mg/kg/d maintenance as 2-4 doses.		<u>**DOSE FORMS:**</u> PO (Tab's): 25, 50, 100 mg
TRIAMTERENE (Dyrenium) (in Dyazide, with hydrochorthiazide)	<u>Edema</u>: **PO:** 100 mg bid initially; 100-300 mg qd or qod maintenance (maximum 300 mg/d).	Elevation of BUN (prevented with qod dosing). Use with NSAIAs may accelerate renal failure. Megaloblastic anemia possible (taper to discontinue - abrupt discontinuence may precipitate rebound kaliuresis). **RECOMMEND:** Take after meals to decrease nausea. **CAUTION:** May predispose to renal stones (discontinue). **CONTRAINDICATIONS:** Severe kidney, liver disease.	<u>**DOSE FORMS:**</u> PO (Tab's): 50, 100 mg
AMILORIDE (Midamor)	<u>Antikaleuretic</u>: **PO:** 5 mg/d initially; 5-20 mg/d (single dose) maintenance.	Hyperkalemia (K^{+} > 55 mEq/l) in 10% when used alone; when used in combination with another diuretic, hyperkalemia in 1-2% patients. Hyperkalemia worse with renal failure. Increased intraocular pressure, dyspnea, headaches (3%). **CONTRAINDICATIONS:** Serum K^{+} > 5.5 mEq/l.	<u>**DOSE FORMS:**</u> PO (Tab's): 5 mg

OSMOTIC DIURETICS

DRUG	INDICATIONS & DOSAGE	SIDE EFFECTS & REMARKS
MANNITOL (Resectisol) (Osmitrol)	<u>**Test Dose**</u>: **IV:** 0.2 gm/kg or 12.5 gm as 15-20% sln over 3-5 min. Positive test if > 30 cc/h urine for 3h (can repeat once in 3h if negative). <u>**Oliguric Acute Renal Failure**</u>: **IV:** 50-100 gm (15-20% sln) over 30-60 min. <u>**Increased Intracranial (ICP) or Intraocular (IOP) Pressure**</u>: **IV:** 1.5-2 gm/kg (15-20% sln) over 30-60 min. (Many other dosing schemes available.)	**SIDE EFFECTS:** Dehydration, hyperosmolarity, nausea, vomiting, fever, hypokalemia, circulatory overload (pulmonary edema, CHF, signs of water intoxication). CNS effects, chest pain, nephrosis, increased lithium excretion. **NOTE:** Diuresis ocurrs in 1-3 h, decreased ICP at 15 min (duration = 3-8 h), decreased IOP in 30 min (duration= 3-8 h). Oral use induces osmotic diarrhea. IV extravasation may cause necrosis. **CAUTION:** Rebound increased ICP 12 h after dosing. Over-diuresis may dehydrate and worsen renal failure. Normally excreted renally, caution with pre-existing renal impairment or with rapid injection. Urine output <40 cc/h may imply dehydration. **RECOMMEND:** Monitor urine output, electrolyte/fluid balance. Maintain fluid balance > 1 liter/d, hold urine output at 100-500 cc/h. **CONTRAINDICATIONS:** Anuria. Patients not responsive to test dose. Pulmonary edema, CHF, active intracranial bleeding. Discontinue if: progressive azotemia, oliguria, CHF develop.
	<u>**Barbiturate OD**</u>: **IV:** 0.5 gm/kg bolus, then 1 liter 10% sln over 1h. Repeat q2h, maintain positive fluid balance = 1-2 liter/h. <u>**Uricemia**</u>: **IV:** 50 gm/m^2 over 24 h.	
UREA (Ureaphil)	<u>**Increased ICP, IOP**</u>: **IV:** 0.5-1.5 gm/kg over 1.5-2 h. <u>**Oral Diuretic**</u>: **PO:** 20 gm, 2-5 times/d. <u>**Hyponatremia (SIADH)**</u>: **IV:** 80 gm given as 30% sln over 6 h. **PO:** 30 gm q8h (3 doses total). <u>**Sickle Cell Crisis**</u>: **IV:** 6 gm/kg as 15% sln at 4.5 cc/kg/h over 12-16 h. **PO:** 1-2.3 gm/kg/d in 3-4 doses.	**SIDE EFFECTS:** Circulatory overload (pulmonary edema, CHF, signs of water intoxication), dehydration, electrolyte depletion. Rebound increased ICP 12 h after dosing (worse than mannitol). Nausea, vomiting, headache, syncope, dizziness, confusion, cardiotoxicity, hypotension, hyperthermia, thrombophlebitis, hemolysis. Extravasation may cause necrosis. May increase prothrombin time. **CAUTION:** Increased ammonia in cirrhotics. AVOID in increased IOP due to inflammation. BUN increases; discontinue or reduce dose if BUN > 75 gm/dl. **RECOMMEND:** Do NOT exceed 1.5 gm/kg or 120 gm IV in 24 h. Dilute in 5-10% dextrose to minimize hemolysis; infusion < 4 ml/min (30% sln.). **CONTRAINDICATIONS:** Severe renal impairment, dehydration, liver failure, active intracranial bleeding.

beta-BLOCKERS

GROUP REMARKS: Recommended over thiazides for initial treatment of hypertension with high plasma renin. All (exceptions noted): "quinidine-like" membrane stabilizing effect, extensive first-pass liver metabolism, negatively inotropic. *Beta*$_2$ selective agents become non-selective at higher doses. Additive with other sympatholytic drugs (e.g., methyldopa, reserpine). **SIDE EFFECTS: Common** (early; usually disappear/decrease with continued treatment): Nausea, diarrhea, wheezing, muscle aches, rash. CNS effects (esp. lipid soluble agents): tiredness, depression, nightmares, paresthesias. Transient falsely high elevations in LFT's and BUN. **Uncommon:** Sinus bradycardia (may be assoc'd with hypotension, syncope, shock, or angina); may precipitate CHF in cardiac patients; AV block. Increased hypoglycemic response to insulin/oral hypoglycemics. Claudication; Raynaud's syndrome; rare blood dyscrasias. **CAUTIONS:** MI, angina, HTN rebound, tachycardia can occur with sudden discontinuance. Avoid if possible in diabetics (may mask hypoglycemia). May mask signs of early hyperthyroidism. May be inadvisable in myasthenia gravis or within 2 wk of MAO inhibitor use. Cimetadine can decrease clearance. May require lower dose in hepatic disease. Discontinue if patient develops: bradycardia; CHF; high degree AV block; bronchospasm. **CONTRAINDICATIONS:** Manifest or impending CHF; non-arrhythmogenic hypotension; cardiogenic shock; complete heart block; asthma/obstructive lung diease; Raynaud's syndrome; malignant hypertension; allergic rhinitis (during pollen season). **RECOMMEND:** Base choice on *beta*-selectivity, dosing interval, S.E.s, and excretion route. Always discontinue over 2 wk. If on quinidine, reduce dose of both. Manufacturer suggests discontinue 48 h before surgery. **NOTE:** Full *beta*-blockade: heart rate = 55- 60/min with mild exertion.

DRUG	INDICATIONS & DOSAGE	SIDE EFFECTS & REMARKS
NON-SELECTIVE *beta*-BLOCKERS		
PROPRANOLOL (Inderal)	**Hypertension**: **PO:** 40 mg bid initially; 80-640 mg/d maintenance in 2-4 doses. **Angina**: **PO:** 10-20 mg tid initially; 30-320 mg/d maintenance in 3-4 doses. **Arrhythmias**: **PO:** 10 mg tid initially; 30-120 mg/d maintenance in 3-4 doses. **Migraine**: **PO:** 40 mg bid initially; 160-240 mg/d maintenance in 2-4 doses. **IHSS**: **PO:** 20 mg tid initially; 60-160 mg/d maintenance in 3-4 doses. **Post-MI**: **PO:** 60 mg tid initially; 180-240 mg/d maintenance in 3-4 doses. **Pheochromocytoma**: **Operable**: **PO:** 60 mg/d + alpha blocker 3d prior to surgery. **Inoperable**: **PO:** 10 mg tid + alpha blocker. **Emergency**: **IV:** 0.5-3 mg (rate < 1 mg/min); may repeat (once) in 2 min. **Pediatric HTN**: **PO:** 0.5-1 mg/kg/d initially; 0.5-4 mg/kg/d maintenance in 2-3 doses. **Pediatric Arrhythmias**: **PO:** 0.2-4 mg/kg/d in 3-4 doses.	Therapeutic response occurs over a wide range of oral doses, treatment must be individualized. Longer acting forms available, but usually yield lower plasma concentrations (may need to incease dose). Treatment failure if no response to migraine therapy within 4-6 weeks. Post-MI therapy may continue for up to 3 years. **NOTE:** Emergency IV administration should NOT be repeated for 4 hours after first two doses. **Hypertension Maintenance Changes**: **Early:** 3-5 d **Late:** 7-28 d **DOSE FORMS**: PO (Tab's): 20, 40,60, 80 mg Extended release (Cap's): 80, 120, 160 mg

beta-BLOCKERS: NON-SELECTIVE *Continued*

DRUG	INDICATIONS & DOSAGE	SIDE EFFECTS & REMARKS
TIMOLOL (Blokadren) (Timoptic)	**Hypertension:** **PO:** 10 mg bid initially; 20-60mg/d maintenance in 1-2 doses. **Post-MI:** **PO:** 10 mg bid. **Angina:** **PO:** 15 mg tid initially; 15-45 mg/d maintenance in 3-4 doses. **Increased Intraocular Pressure:** 1 drop of 0.25-0.5% solution, bid.	Group Remarks EXCEPT: No membrane-stabilizing action. **Hypertension Maintenance Changes:** **Early:** 7 d **Late:** 7 d **DOSE FORMS:** PO (Tab's): 5, 10, 20 mg
NADOLOL (Corgard)	**Hypertension:** **PO:** 40 mg/d initially; 40-320 mg/d maintenance as 1 dose. **Angina:** **PO:** 40 mg/d initially; 40-240 mg/d maintenance as 1 dose. **DOSE FORMS:** PO (Tab's): 40, 80, 120, 160 mg	Group Remarks EXCEPT: No hepatic metabolism. Normal excretion: renal, fecal. Prolonged action relative to propranolol. Can be cleared by hemolysis. **Hypertension Maintenance Changes:** **Early:** 2 d **Late:** 6-14 d
PINDOLOL (Visken)	**Hypertension:** **PO:** 5 mg bid initially; 10-60 mg/d maintenance in 2-3 doses. Dosage can be increased in 10 mg/d increments at 3-4 week intervals (if needed). **DOSE FORMS:** PO (Tab's): 5, 10 mg	Group Remarks EXCEPT: Only minimal first pass hepatic metabolism. No quinidine-like effect in therapeutic range. Doesn't suppress plasma renin activity. Less hypotensive action than others ("intrinsic sympathometic activity"). NOT indicated for resting angina (only for exertional). **SIDE EFFECTS:** Edema, dyspnea, GI, visual and CNS effects prominent. Rarely insomnia. **RECOMMEND:** Reduce dose in renal failure. Preferred *beta*-blocker in patients prone to bradycardia. **CAUTIONS:** AVOID when decreased cardiac contractility desired (IHSS, dissecting aortic aneursm). **NOTE:** Abrupt discontinuance may be better tolerated than with other *beta*-blockers. **Hypertension Maintenance Changes: Early:** 7-14 d; **Late:** 21-28 d
***beta*$_1$-SELECTIVE**		
METOPROLOL (Lopressor)	**Hypertension:** **PO:** 100 mg/d initially; 100-450 mg/d maint. in 1-3 doses. **Angina:** **PO:** 50 mg bid initially; 100-450 mg/d maintenance in 2-3 doses. Increase at weekly intervals (if needed). **DOSE FORMS:** PO (Tab's): 50, 100 mg	Group Remarks EXCEPT: Lacks quinidine-like effect. Crosses placenta. Doses > 100 mg/d NOT cardioselective. **Hypertension Maintenance Changes:** **Early:** 7 d **Late:** 7 d

beta-BLOCKERS: *beta*$_1$-SELECTIVE *Continued*

DRUG	INDICATIONS & DOSAGE		SIDE EFFECTS & REMARKS
ATENOLOL (Tenormin)	**Hypertension & Angina:** **PO:** 50 mg/d initially; 50-100 mg/d maintenance as 1 dose.	**DOSE FORMS:** PO (Tab's): 50, 100 mg	Group Remarks EXCEPT: Little hepatic metabolism. Reduce dose in renal failure: maximum dose = 50 mg/d (GFR = 15-33 cc/min); 50 mg qod (GFR < 15 cc/min). Doses > 100 mg/d NOT cardioselective. **Hypertension Maintenance Changes:** **Early:** 7 d **Late:** 14 d
ACEBUTALOL (Sectral)	**Hypertension:** **PO:** 400 mg/d initially; 200-1200 mg/d maintenance in 1-2 doses. **Premature Ventricular Contractions:** **PO:** 200 mg bid initially; 400-1200 mg/d maintenance in 2 doses.	**DOSE FORMS:** PO (Tab's): 200, 400 mg	Group Remarks EXCEPT: No membrane-stabilizing effect. Some sympathomimetic action. Decrease dose in geriatrics (increased bioavailability); maintain < 800 mg/d. **CAUTIONS:** Hepatic dysfunction. Impaired creatinine clearance (decrease dose: by 50% when creatinine clearance < 50 cc/ml; by 75% when creatinine clearance < 25 cc/ml).
	***alpha/beta*-BLOCKER**		
LABETALOL (Normodyne) (Trandate)	**Hypertension:** **PO:** 100 mg bid initially; 200-1200 mg/d maintenance in 2-3 doses (maximum 2400 mg/d). Increase doses in 100 mg bid increments at 2-3 day intervals (as needed). **IV:** 20 mg initially, add 40-80 mg q10min (maximum: 300 mg). Each injection must be given over a 2 min period.	**DOSE FORMS:** PO (Tab's): 100, 200, 300 mg IV: 5 mg/ml (20 ml ampules)	Group Remarks. Dual *alpha*$_1$- and *beta*- blockade actions. Asthmatic exacerbation. Fatigue. Nausea. Headache. Scalp parasthesias (initially). **CAUTION:** In diabetes. **CONTRAINDICATIONS:** Chronic pulmonary disease. Sick sinus syndrome. CHF. Heart block greater than first degree.

ADRENERGIC INHIBITORS

DRUG	INDICATIONS & DOSAGE	DOSE FORMS	SIDE EFFECTS & REMARKS
CENTRALLY-ACTING			
CLONIDINE (Catapres)	**Hypertension:** **PO:** 0.1 mg bid or tid initialiy; 0.2-1.2 mg/d maintenance in 2-4 doses (maximum 2.4 mg/d). **Hypertensive Urgency:** **PO:** 0.2 mg, then 0.1 mg qh until BP normal; (maximum 0.8 mg). **Opiate Withdrawal** (not an approved indication): **PO:** 0.3-1.2 mg/d (in 3-4 doses) for 10 d, then decrease 50% each d for 3 d. **Dysmenorrhea** (not an approved indication): **PO:** 0.025 mg bid for 2 wk before & during menses. **Migraine:** **PO:** 0.025 mg bid up to 0.15 mg/d.	PO (Tab's): 0.1, 0.2, 0.3 mg Transdermal Patches: See Remarks	**SIDE EFFECTS:** Dry mouth, sedation, constipation, depression, restlessness, rash. Rare retinal degeneration. Transient elevation of LFTs. Rebound hypertensive syndrome upon abrupt cessation: headache (2-3 h) & increased BP (8-24 h). **RECOMMEND:** Adminst. bid or tid. Reduce dose 50-70% if creatinine clearance < 50 cc/min. Taper discontinuence for 2-4 d. **Transdermal Patches**: Suitable only for mild to moderate HTN. Deliver 0.1, 0.2 or 0.3 mg/d for 7 d; peak plasma levels at 48-72 h. Side effects similar, but may be less severe or frequent; rash may occur at patch site with hyperpigmentation from chronic use. **Hypertension Maintenance Changes:** **Early:** 2 d **Late:** 6-7 d
GUANABENZ ACETATE (Wytensin)	**Hypertension:** **PO:** 4 mg bid initially; 4-64 mg/d maintenance.	PO (Tab's): 4, 8 mg	**SIDE EFFECTS:** Dry mouth (30% patients), sedation (40%), dizziness, headache. May worsen vascular insufficiency Rare palpitations, chest pain, ataxia. **RECOMMEND:** CAUTION in situations requiring alertness. **Hypertension Maintenance Changes:** **Early:** 7 d **Late:** 14 d
METHYLDOPA (Aldomet)	**Hypertension:** **PO:** 250 mg bid or tid initially; 500-3000 mg/d maintenance in 2-4 doses. **IV:** 250-1000 mg q6h.	PO (Tab's): 125, 250, 500 mg	**SIDE EFFECTS:** Drowsiness, rash, decreased libido, orthostatic hypotension, nightmares. Hemolysis: rare, but occurs in some G-6-PD-deficient patients. Positive direct Coombs' test after 6 months treatment (10-20%). **RECOMMEND:** Baseline CBC, Coombs' test. Periodic CBC, LFTs. Discontinue treatment if: decreased mental concentration, jaundice, fever or evidence of hemolytic anemia (evaluate if positive Coombs' test). Reduce dose 30-50% if creatinine clearance < 50 cc/min. Discontinue treatment upon development of bradycardia, edema or drug fever (occurs within 21 d & assoc'd with preexisting liver abnormality). **Hypertension Maintenance Changes:** **Early:** 2 d **Late:** 7 d

ADRENERGIC INHIBITORS *Continued*

DRUG	INDICATIONS & DOSAGE	DOSE FORMS	SIDE EFFECTS & REMARKS
PERIPHERALLY-ACTING			
GUANETHIDINE (Esimel) (Ismelin)	<u>**Hypertension**</u>: **PO:** 10 mg/d initially (or load 10 mg tid over 3d); 10-50 mg/d maintenance. <u>**Hypertension Maintenance Changes**</u>: **Early:** 5-7 d **Late:** 21 d	PO (Tab's): 10, 25 mg	**SIDE EFFECTS:** Postural & post-exercise hypotension with occasional syncope (increased by alcohol). Dizziness, weakness, lassitide. Nasal congestion. Diarrhea. Bradycardia, Na^+ retention (add diuretic). Inhibition of ejaculation (NOT impotence). Rare increased BUN, heart block, urine retention asthma. **NOTE:** Therapeutic action blocked by tricyclic antidepressants. **RECOMMEND:** Warn patient of orthostatic hypotension. Reduce dose or discontinue if increased BUN. Discontinue treatment 2-3 wk prior to surgery. **CONTRAINDICATIONS:** CHF not due to HTN, pheochromocytoma.
GUANADREL (Hylorel)	<u>**Hypertension**</u>: **PO (outpatient)**: 10 mg/d initially; 20-75 mg/d maintenance as 2-4 doses/d. **PO (inpatient)**: 25-50 mg/d initially, increase by 25-50 mg/d q24-48h. **Pediatric PO**: 0.2 mg/kg/d initially, increase by 0.2 mg/kg/d q1wk; maximum 3 mg/kg/d. <u>**Hypertension Maintenance Changes**</u>: **Early**: 5-7 d **Late**: 7-10 d	PO (Tab's): 10, 25 mg	**SIDE EFFECTS**: Similar to guanethidine; paresthesias and drowsiness possibly more common. Causes less drowsiness than methyldopa. NOTE: Effects may be potentiated by *alpha-* or *beta-* blocking agents; may be antagonized by tricyclic antidepressants or phenothiazines. **RECOMMENDATIONS**: Monitor orthostatic changes and ask about any related symptoms at each blood pressure (bp) check. Reduce dose at any of the following: severe diarrhea, excessive orthostatic hypotension, normal supine bp. Advise patients to rise SLOWLY from supine position. **CONTRAINDICATIONS**: CHF, MAO inhibitor use within previous 1 wk, pheochromocytoma.
RESERPINE (Serpasil) (Sandril)	<u>**Hypertension**</u>: **PO:** 0.5 mg/d initially; 0.1-0.25 mg/d maintenance. <u>**Hypertension Maintenance Changes**</u>: **Early:** 7 d **Late:** 7 d	PO (Tab's): 0.1, 0.25, 1.0 mg	**SIDE EFFECTS:** Lethargy; depression (at 2-8 months), esp. if history of depression. Bradycardia (reversible by atropine). Flush, warmth. Cramps, nausea, vomiting, diarrhea, increased secretion of gastric acid. Na^+ retention & edema. **NOTES:** No orthostatic hypotension at usual doses (unless IM adminst.). Main effect is to increase action of concurrent diuretic. Other reserpine preparations: Rauwolfia serpentina (whole root, contains 0.15-0.2% reserpine), Deserpidine (Harmonyl), Alseroxylon (Rauwiloid, contains 7.5-10% reserpine) and Rescinnamine (Moderil, a related alkaloid). **CAUTIONS:** Increased cardiac depression with concurrent quinidine, procainamide. Concurrent cardiac glycosides may predispose to arrhythmias. **RECOMMEND:** Discontinue treatment if signs of depression develop.

ADRENERGIC INHIBITORS *Continued*

DRUG	INDICATIONS & DOSAGE	DOSE FORMS	SIDE EFFECTS & REMARKS
MISCELLANEOUS			
PRAZOSIN (Minipress) *alpha-Blocker*	**Hypertension:** **PO:** 1 mg bid or tid initially; 3-20 mg/d maintenance in 2-3 doses. **Hypertension Maintenance Changes:** **Early:** 3-4 d **Late:** 3-4 d	PO (Cap's): 1, 2, 5 mg	Prazosin is an *alpha*-blocker. Maximum BP drop at 2-4 h. 3 mg/d prazosin equivalent to: 750-2000 mg/d methyldopa, 120 mg/d propranolol. **SIDE EFFECTS:** Dizziness (10%), drowsiness, weakness, syncope (usually at 30-120 min.), vertigo, nausea, depression. Tachycardia, palpitations, angina. Orthostatic hypotension at first dose (1%). Slower excretion in CHF. **RECOMMEND:** Warn patient: postural dizziness, drowsiness. Administer first dose at bedtime, but do NOT administer qhs to avoid dizziness. Decrease dose in renal failure.
PARGYLINE (Eutonyl) *MAO Inhibitor*	**Hypertension:** **PO:** 25 mg/d initially, increase 10 mg/d q1wk; maintenance 25-50 mg/d (maximum 200 mg/d).	PO (Tab's): 10, 25 mg	Pargyline is a monoamine oxidase inhibitor; see Group Remarks for MAO Inhibitor Antidepressants. Hypotensive effect is mainly postural, similar to ganglionic blockade. Therapeutic effect develops slowly; tolerance develops rapidly. **SIDE EFFECTS:** GI disturbances, insomnia, urinary frequency, dry mouth, nightmares, impotence, edema. Congestive failure may occur in patients with reduced cardiac reserve. **CAUTIONS:** Adverse drug reactions with OTC cold preparations, antihistamines, alcohol, some cheeses, and foods with high tyramine content. Eutonyl 25 mg contains tartrazine dye (potential for allergic reactions, esp. in patients hypersensitive to aspirin).

ANGIOTENSIN CONVERTING ENZYME INHIBITORS

GROUP REMARKS: ACE Inhibitors (ACEI) decrease blood pressure by decreasing peripheral resistance; they increase or have no effect on cardiac output. They should be used in hypertension refractory to step 1 & 2 drugs (add a diuretic before adding a *beta*-blocker in combination). **NOTES**: Transient hypotension upon first dose is common (esp. in CHF pts); NOT a contraindication. Maximal therapeutic effect may be delayed for several weeks. Antihypertensive effects are additive with diuretics and LESS than additive with *beta*-blockers. Antihypertensive effect diminished by concurrent NSAIDs (e.g. indomethacin) or aspirin. **SIDE EFFECTS**: **Common**: headache, hypotension (esp. in dehydrated patients), rash, dizziness and fatigue. **Less common**: dyspepsia and elevated BUN/creatinine (usually transient, except for patients with renal disease or CHF). **Rare**: elevated LFTs, syncope, muscle cramps, angioedema (potentially FATAL). Proteinuria reported in 1-2% patients, esp. those with pre-existing renal failure; may progress to nephrotic syndrome. Neutropenia is rare, but more common in pre-existing renal failure; reversible upon discontinuence. **RECOMMENDATIONS**: For initial dose hypotension: place patient in supine position and infuse (IV) saline. Perform baseline urinalysis, BUN, creatinine. Monitor urine protein monthly during first 9 months; if 24 h urine protein > 1 gm consider discontinuing treatment. Perform CBC q2wk (first 3 months); discontinue if: WBC decreases > 50%, WBC < 4,000 or poly's < 1,000. AVOID concurrent sympathomimetic medications. Have patients report any swelling (esp. of mouth or face), mouth sores or persistent rash. **CAUTIONS**: ACE Inhibitors may elevate serum potassium; use potassium-sparing diuretics and salt substitutes carefully, or avoid. ACE Inhibitors may be teratogenic or embryotoxic; they are probably secreted in breast milk. ACE Inhibitors cause false positive urine albumin results. 20% of patients with renal artery stenosis develop azotemia; discontinue ACEI therapy.

DRUG	INDICATIONS & DOSAGE	DOSE FORMS	REMARKS
CAPTOPRIL (Capoten)	<u>**Hypertension**</u>: **PO:** 25 mg bid or tid initially; 50-150 mg/d maintenance in 3-4 doses (maximum 450 mg/d). <u>**Congestive Heart Failure**</u>: **PO:** 6.25-12.5 mg tid initially; 150-450 mg/d maintenance in 3 doses (maximum 450 mg/d).	PO (Tab's): 25, 50, 100 mg	**SIDE EFFECTS**: Rash occurs in 5-10% of patients, altered taste occurs during initial therapy in 5-10%; reversible at 2-3 months. <u>**Hypertension Maintenance Changes**</u>: **Early:** 7 d **Late:** 14 d (Can increase dose q24h if necessary)
ENALAPRIL (Vasotec)	<u>**Hypertension**</u>: **PO**: 5 mg once/d initially; 10-40 mg/d maintenance in 2-4 doses. **PO (diuretic patient)**: 2.5 mg test dose. <u>**Above in Renal Impairment**</u>: **PO**: 2.5 mg/d initially if creat. clearance ≤ 30 cc/min or serum creat. > 3 mg/l (maximum 40 mg/d). Administer following dialysis.	PO (Tab's): 5, 10, 20 mg	**SIDE EFFECTS**: Headache and dizziness (and possibly angioedema) are more common than with captopril; rash is less common. <u>**Hypertension Maintenance Changes**</u>: **Early**: 1-3 d **Late**: 7-14 d
LISINOPRIL (Prinivil) (Zestril)	<u>**Hypertension**</u>: **PO**: 10 mg/d initially; 20-40 mg/d maintenance (single dose). **PO (diuretic patient)**: 5 mg test dose (monitor for hypotension; discontinue diuretic for 2-3d prior to start of ACEI therapy). <u>**Above in Renal Insufficiency**</u>: **PO**: 5 mg/d initially if creat. clearance = 10-30 cc/min; 2.5 mg/d initially if < 10 cc/min. Increase incrementally to maintenance dose (maximum 40 mg/d).	PO (Tab's): 10, 20 mg	**SIDE EFFECTS**: Common: hyperkalemia (2.2% pts.; more marked with CHF), diarrhea. Less common: cough, nausea, vomiting, hypotension, orthostatic hypotension, rash, chest pain, dyspnea. Rare: impotence, muscle cramps, back pain, nasal congestion, vertigo, myalgias, angina pectoris, arrhythmias, palpatations, syncope. Small decreases in hemoglobin and HCT. **CAUTIONS**: Dangerous hypotension can occur in salt/volume-depleted patients. **RECOMMENDATIONS**: Measure blood pressure prior to daily dose to determine if adequate control exists. Periodically monitor WBC count in patients with collagen vascular disease or renal disease. Discontinue/alter therapy if light-headedness occurs often. **CONTRAINDICATIONS**: Hypersensitivity.

VASODILATORS

DRUG	INDICATIONS & DOSAGE	SIDE EFFECTS & REMARKS
HYDRALAZINE (Apresoline)	**Hypertension:** **PO:** 10 mg qid initially; 40-300 mg/d maintenance in 4 doses. **Hypertensive Crisis:** **IM, IV:** 20-40 mg PRN (Onset 10-30 min). Change to PO therapy w/in 1-2d. **Congestive Heart Failure** (not approved use): **PO:** 50-800 mg tid.	Reflex tachycardia prominent, may precipitate angina or palpitations. Na^+ & fluid retention; may need diuretic. SLE syndrome (esp. in slow acetylators): fever, arthralgia, splenomegaly, lymphadenopathy, malaise, rash. Positive ANA titer, LE preparation, Coomb`s test. Rare blood dyscrasias, neuropathy (treat with pyridoxine). May increase cerebral ischemia if increased ICP. **CAUTIONS:** Patients with CVA, renal disease, coronary artery disease & valvular disease. **RECOMMEND:** Increase dosing interval to bid/qd if GFR <10 cc/min. Discontinue if SLE syndrome (many recommend discontinue if positive LE prep or ANA develops). Baseline CBC, LE prep., ANA titer. **NOTE:** IV dose = 3-4 x PO dose. Contains tartrazine dye. **DOSE FORMS:** PO (Tab's): 10, 25, 50, 100 mg **Hypertension Maintenance Changes:** **Early:** 3 d **Late:** 3-4 d
MINOXIDIL (Loniten)	**Hypertension:** **PO:** 5 mg/d initially; 5-40 mg/d maintenance in 1-2 doses (maximum 100 mg/d). **DOSE FORMS:** PO (Tab's): 2.5, 5 mg **Hypertension Maintenance Changes:** **Early:** 2 d **Late:** 2-4 d	Most potent oral vasodilator. Reflex tachycardia may precipitate angina. Na^+ & water retention (secondary edema prominent, CHF, pulmonary edema) may offset therapeutic effect. Pericardial effusion (esp. with renal failure, autoimmune disease, CHF). Myocardial hypertrophy/damage noted in animal studies. Frequent hypertrichosis (reverts 1-6 months after discontinuance). T-wave depression early in therapy (NOT assoc'd with damage). Hemodilution (HCT decreases 7%). Rare rash, gynecomastia, nausea, headache. Removed by dialysis. **CAUTION:** Overly rapid decrease in BP may precipitate MI or CVA. **RECOMMEND:** Use only in hypertension refractory to other drugs. Add diuretic (Lasix) to counter fluid retention (except in dialysis patients). Add beta-blocker/central antagonist to counter tachycardia. Discontinue if refractory fluid retention, CHF, pericardial effusion. Dialysis patients may require smaller doses (decrease by 33%). **NOTE:** Can adjust dosage q6h for rapid hypertension treatment.

PERIPHERAL VASODILATORS

GROUP REMARKS: Efficacy unproven (in general) for peripheral vascular disease or cerebral ischemia. None of these drugs are substitutes for appropriate therapy. **SIDE EFFECTS:** Tachycardia, flush, sweating, nausea, dizziness, headache, vasomotor and blood pressure instability. **CAUTIONS:** Parenteral dosing may exaggerate vasomotor and CVS effects so extreme care needed where tachycardia, or hypotension can be a problem (coronary artery disease, cerebrovascular renal insufficiency).

DRUG	INDICATIONS & DOSAGE	SIDE EFFECTS & REMARKS
DIRECT SMOOTH MUSCLE RELAXANTS		
PAPAVERINE	<u>**Vasodilation**</u>: **PO:** 75 mg tid initially; 225-1500 mg/d maintenance as 3-5 doses. **Extended release:** 150 mg bid initially; 300-600 mg/d maintenace as 2-3 doses. **IV,IM:** 30 mg initially; 30-120 mg (inject slowly over 1-2 min, can repeat q3h PRN). <u>**Extrasystoles**</u>: Same as IV,IM above but 2 doses may be given 10 min apart.	Possible myocardial depression. IV injection may precipitate transient ectopic rhythms. Vasodilatation effect increased by concurrent reserpine. May interfere with antiparkinsonism action of L-dopa. **CONTRAINDICATIONS:** Glaucoma, complete AV block. <u>**DOSE FORMS**</u>: PO (Tab's): 30, 60, 75, 100, 150, 200, 300 mg Extended release (Cap's): 150, 200, 300 mg
CYCLANDELATE (Cyclospasmol)	<u>**Vasodilation**</u>: **PO:** 300 mg qid initially; 400-1600 mg/d maintenance as 2-4 doses.	Administer with food to minimize nausea. Maintenance: Decrease dose by 200 mg/d until lowest effective dose. **CAUTION:** Glaucoma; large doses may prolong bleeding time. <u>**DOSE FORMS**</u>: PO (Tab's): 100, 200, 400 mg; PO (Cap's): 200, 400 mg
DIPYRIDAMOLE (Persantine)	<u>**Antiplatelet Aggregation**</u>: **PO:** 50 mg tid initially; 150-400 mg/d maintenance as 2-4 doses (used with other agents). <u>**Chronic Angina**</u>: **PO:** 50 mg tid initially; 150-300 mg/d maintenance as 3 doses. (No proven efficacy.)	Antiplatelet aggregation action additive with aspirin. Prolongs platelet survival in hypertensive valve disease. May precipitate angina in coronary artery disease pts. IV use has precipitated acute MI. **CAUTION:** Bleeding disorders or concurrent anticoagulants. <u>**DOSE FORMS**</u>: PO (Tab's): 100, 200, 400 mg
SYMPATHOMIMETICS		
NYLIDRIN (Arlidin)	<u>**Vasodilation**</u>: **PO:** 3 mg tid initially; 9-48 mg/d maintenance as 3-4 doses. (No proven efficacy.)	Increased gastric acid secretion, caution with gastric ulcer. **CONTRAINDICATIONS**: Acute MI, paroxysmal tachycardia, thyrotoxicosis, progressive angina. <u>**DOSE FORMS**</u>: PO (Tab's): 6, 12 mg

PERIPHERAL VASODILATORS: SYMPATHOMIMETICS *Continued*

DRUG	INDICATIONS & DOSAGE	SIDE EFFECTS & REMARKS
ISOXSUPRINE (Vasodilan) (Vasoprine)	<u>**Vasodilation**</u>: **PO**: 10 mg tid initially; 30-80 mg/d maintenance as 3-4 doses. **IM**: 5 mg bid initially; 10-30 mg/d maintenance as 2-3 doses.	Discontinue if rash occurs. **CONTRAINDICATIONS**: Post-partum period, arterial bleeding. <u>**DOSE FORMS**</u>: PO (Tab's): 10, 20 mg
***alpha*-ADRENERGIC BLOCKERS**		
TOLAZOLINE (Priscoline)	<u>**Neonatal Hypoxemia**</u>: **IV**: 1-2 mg/kg over 10 min, then 1-2 mg/kg/h.	Less active than phentolamine. Histamine-like GI simulation effect (caution in gastric ulcer). **SIDE EFFECTS**: Blood dyscrasias, hematuria, hepatitis. Rare MI. **CAUTION**: Mitral stenosis. **CONTRAINDICATIONS**: Post-MI, post-CVA status. <u>**DOSE FORMS**</u>: Injection: 25 mg/ml.
PHENOXYBENZAMINE (Dibenzyline)	<u>**Catecholamine Excess States (Pheochromocytoma)**</u>: **PO**: 10 mg bid initially; 20-40 mg/d maintenance as 2-3 doses.	To reverse epinephrine pressor effect in pheochromocytoma, give PO: 10 mg/d for 4 days, then increase by 10 mg/d q4d (effect seen in 2 wk); taper to minimum effective dose. Longer duration (3-7 d) than phentolamine - used for preoperative or long-term control of symptoms. Propranolol adjunct for BP control in pheochromocytoma (start propranolol only after full *alpha*-blockade).
	Phentolamine preferred for HTN crisis 2° to sympathomimetics or MAO inhibitors (more rapid onset). **SIDE EFFECTS**: Profound postural hypotension, miosis. **CONTRAINDICATIONS**: Conditions where decreased BP dangerous (dehydration, shock).	
PHENTOLAMINE (Regitine)	<u>**Diagnosis of Pheochromocytoma**</u>: **IM,IV**: 5 mg (single dose). <u>**Pediatric Pheochromocytoma**</u>: **IM**: 3 mg. <u>**HTN Crisis**</u>: **IV**: 5-10 mg (secondary to adrenergics). <u>**Norepinephrine Extravasation**</u>: **Local infiltration**: 5-10 mg within 12h.	Additional activity = *beta*-blockade. Positively inotropic, chonotropic (may increase BP at low doses). Test for pheochromocytoma most effective in patients with sustained hypertension: monitor BP q10min, 3 times (baseline) and treat with phentolamine. Monitor BP q30sec for 3 min, then at 1 min intervals for 7 min. After IM dose, monitor q5min for 30-40 min. Patient should be supine. Positive test if BP decreases >35 mmHg systolic or > 25 mmHg diastolic. **SIDE EFFECTS:** Hypotension, tachycardia, arrhythmias, angina, exacerbation of peptic ulcer. <u>**DOSE FORMS**</u>: Injection: 5 mg/ml.

MISCELLANEOUS VASODILATORS

DRUG	INDICATIONS & DOSAGE	SIDE EFFECTS & REMARKS
NITROPRUSSIDE		
SODIUM NITROPRUSSIDE (Nipride) (Nitropress)	**Hypertensive Crisis:** **IV:** 0.5 µg/kg/min initially; 0.5-10 µg/kg/min range (discontinue if no response in 10 min). **Refractory CHF:** **IV:** 0.5 µg/kg/min initially; 0.5-6 µg/kg/min range. Maintain wedge pressure 14-18 mmHg, heart rate < 10% elevated; Monitor CO, TPR, BP.	Decreases peripheral resistance & preload. BP returns to pre-treatment levels within 10 min of discontinuance. **SIDE EFFECTS:** Nausea, vomiting, diarrhea. Headache, dizziness, profound orthostatic symptoms. Increased serum creatinine, slight reflex tachycardia (HR may slow in CHF patients). Thiocyanate accumulation may precipitate hypothyroidism. **Thiocyanate levels:** Toxic effects at 50-100 µg/ml, fatalities possible at 200 µg/ml. Thiocyanate metabolites excreted renally. Toxic effects: Weakness, confusion, lethargy, rash, tinnitus, blurred vision, seizures, cyanosis, decreased deep tendon reflexes, mydriasis, coma. Metabolic acidosis = most reliable sign of toxicity. **Overdose treatment:** Amyl nitrate inhaler & sodium nitrite. Thiocyanate removed by dialysis. **RECOMMENDATIONS:** In hypertensive crisis, adminst. oral anti-HTN's immediately. Follow daily thiocyanate levels after 48 h (start immediately if renal failure). Discontinue if thiocyanate >100 µg/ml or upon signs of toxicity. Do not exceed 10 µg/kg/min. Restrain patient (to avoid orthostatic syncope). Adminst. via infusion pump (arterial catheter preferable but q2min BP readings may suffice). Discontinue if no response to 10 µg/kg/min for 10 min. **CAUTIONS:** Renal impairment, hepatic insufficiency, hypothyroidism, hyponatremia, cerebral vascular insufficiency. General goal = lower diastolic BP to 100 mmHg, but over-vigorous lowering may precipitate cerebral, myocardial or renal ischemia. **CONTRAINDICATIONS:** Compensatory hypertension (aortic coarction, AV shunt), aortic stenosis.
NICOTINIC ACID DERIVATIVES		
Efficacy unproven (in general) for peripheral vascular disease or cerebral ischemia. **SIDE EFFECTS:** Tachycardia, flush, sweating, nausea, dizziness, headache, vasomotor and blood pressure instability. **CAUTIONS:** Parenteral dosing may exaggerate vasomotor and cardiovascular effects; use extreme care where tachycardia or hypotension may be a problem (coronary artery disease, cerebrovascular renal insufficiency).		
NICOTINIC ACID (Niacin)	**Vasodilation:** **PO:** 50 mg tid initially; 150-450 mg/d as 3 doses (maximum 6000 mg/d).	**DOSE FORMS:** PO (Tab's): 25, 50, 100, 500 mg
NICOTINYL ALCOHOL (Pyridl Carbinol)	**Vasodilation:** **PO:** 50 mg tid; 150-300 mg/d as 3 doses. **Extended release:** 150 mg bid; 300-600 mg/d as 2 doses.	Prominent flush, strong placebo effect. Converted to niacin. Increased gastric acid secretion. Large doses assoc'd with hepatocellular toxicity. **CONTRAINDICATIONS:** Active peptic ulcer, gastritis. **DOSE FORMS:** PO (Tab's): 50 mg Elixer: 50 mg/5 ml

ANTIARRHYTHMIC AGENTS

GROUP REMARKS:

Group I Agents:

These are local anesthetic and other agents with membrane-stabilizing action. All of these agents inhibit the return of excitability to recently depolarized tissue by blocking the fast sodium influx channel to slow initial (phase O) depolarization. Sub-groups within this class are often established on minor electrophysiological differences (e.g., flecainide and encainide cause QRS prolongation and may be more arrhythmogenic). The Group I drugs are essentially similar; dangerous combinations have been used. Note that the antipsychotics, tricyclic antidepressants and antihistamines are also quinidine-like.

PROCAINAMIDE	**LIDOCAINE**	**PHENYTOIN**
DISOPYRAMIDE	**TOCAINIDE**	**FLECAINIDE**
QUINIDINE	**MEXILETINE**	**ENCAINIDE**

Group II Agent:

This agent is a *beta*-blocker. The inherent *beta*-blocking activity has effects on the AV refractory period and conduction time comparable to digitalis and is useful in slowing ventricular rate in the presenCe of a rapid atrial rate. In addition, however, propranolol and related compounds are quinidine-like.

PROPRANOLOL (See Antihypertensive Agents:Adrenergic Inhibitors:*beta*-Blockers)

Group III Agents:

These agents prolong phase 3 repolarization to prolong action potential duration; they thus delay the return of excitability.

AMIODARONE **BRETYLIUM TOSYLATE**

GROUP I ANTIARRHYTHMIC AGENTS

GROUP NOTES: Useful in suppressing atrial and ventricular ectopy. Side effects potentiated by hypoxia, acid base and electrolyte imbalance (esp. K^+) and are much more likely with parenteral use. **SIDE EFFECTS:** May be additive with anticholinergic drugs. Increased QT and QRS intervals (predisposes to ventricular dysrhythmias). Asystole, sinus arrest, SA and AV nodal block, syncope. May dangerously increase ventricular response to atrial tachyarrhythmias - must control (with digoxin) AV nodal conduction before using agents. **RECOMMENDATIONS:** Two/more weeks of anticoagulation before conversion of chronic atrial fibrillation to decrease risk of embolization. Discontinue if increased AV block, increased PVC's, or ventricular tachycardia develops. EKG, CBC, before and regularly during therapy. All IV administration requires continuous EKG and BP monitoring. **CAUTIONS:** Toxic effects additive within group. Myocardial depression and vasodilatation may cause hypotension or aggravate CHF. May worsen myasthenia gravis or precipitate crisis. Can potentiate skeletal muscle relaxants (e.g., curare, succinylcholine - e.g., post-operative period). Drugs inducing hepatic enzymes may require increasing Group I agent dose. **CONTRAINDICATIONS:** Pre-existing 2° or 3° AV block (unless patient has pacemaker), intra-ventricular conduction delays, rhythms due to escape mechanisms, digitalis toxicity.

ANTIARRHYTHMIC AGENTS: GROUP I ANTIARRHYTHMIC AGENTS *Continued*

DRUG	INDICATIONS/DOSES	SIDE EFFECTS & REMARKS
PROCAINAMIDE (Procan) (Pronestyl) (Sub-Quin)	**Ventricular Tachycardia:** **IV:**100 mg q5min (rate not > 25-50 mg/min) until: 1. Arrhythmia suppressed. 2. 1 gm total administered. 3. BP decreases > 15 mmHg. 4. QRS widens > 50%. 5. PR interval increases. Follow by 0.02-0.08 mg/kg/min (IV maint. dose 200-1000 mg/d). **IM:** 0.5-1 gm loading dose, repeat q4-6h (convert to PO ASAP). **PO:** 1 gm load, followed by 6.25 mg/kg q3h. **Extended release**: usually 50 mg/kg/d in 4 doses. **PAT, Atrial Fibrillation Conversion:** **PO:** 1.25 gm, then 750 mg at 1h, followed by 500-1000 mg q2h until conversion or toxicity signs; maintenance 500-1000 mg q4-6h; usually 1 gm q6h.	Group Remarks, EXCEPT increased Q-T interval less common. **LEVELS:** Monitor regularly (esp. in renal failure).Therapeutic plasma levels= 4-8 µg/ml; toxicity > 12 µg/ml. NAPA is active metabolite, therapeutic levels = 15-25 µg/ml. **SIDE EFFECTS:** Hypersensitivity reactions - 50% develop positive ANA after 2-18 months of therapy; 30% will progress to develop SLE syndrome (arthralgias, pleural/pericardial effusions, pleuritis, pericarditis, rash, lupus nephritis, etc.) - usually reverses 2 weeks after discontinuence (but may persist). Also hypergammaglobulinemia, blood dyscrasias (including agranulocytosis), anorexia, nausea, vomiting, diarrhea. **CAUTION:** Possible increased plasma levels in CHF, renal or hepatic failure. **RECOMMEND:** Discontinue if QRS widens > 50% or QT increases > 35%, if positive ANA titer develops, or if signs of SLE develop. Do EKG, LE preparation, ANA titer, and CBC before and periodically during therapy. If GFR= 10-50 cc/min., increase dose interval to q6-12h; GFR < 10cc/min. increase to q8-24h. Extended release forms ONLY for maintenance. **DOSE FORMS:** PO (Tab's): 250, 375, 500 mg; PO (Cap's): 250, 375, 500 mg Extended release: 250, 500, 750 mg **Malignant Arrhythmia:** **IV:** 200-600 mg, not > 20-50 mg/min (IV maintenance: 200-1000 mg/d). **PVC Suppression:** **PO:** 6.25 mg/kg q3h. **Other Arrhythmia:** **IM:** 500-1000 mg q4-8h. **IV:** Load 20-80 mg/kg over 5-10 min, then 0.02-0.08 mg/kg/min maintenance infusion. **Pediatric Arrhythmias:** **PO:** 20-50 mg/kg/d in 4-6 doses (maximum 4000 mg/d). **IV:** 3-6 mg/kg over 5 min, then infusion 0.02-0.08 mg/kg/min (usual total < 1000mg/d; maximum 2000 mg/d).
DISOPYRAMIDE (Norpace)	**Paroxysmal Supraventricular Tachycardia, Premature Atrial/Ventricular Contraction:** **PO:** 150 mg q6h (extended release: 300 mg q12h). **Ventricular Arrhythmias:** **PO:** 300 mg initially; then 150 mg q 6h. If needed, increase to 200 mg q6h (if no response, discontinue or hospitalize & increase to 250-400 mg q6h).	Group remarks EXCEPT: QRS width rarely increased. Pronounced anticholinergic effects. **LEVELS:** Plasma levels: 2-4 µg/ml, occasionally up to 7 µg/ml needed for ventricular arrhythmia. Toxicity assoc'd with > 9 µg/ml. **CAUTION:** History of angle closure glaucoma or urinary retention. If primary AV block develops, decrease dose - if persistent, consider discontinuing therapy. May increase coumadin effect. **RECOMMEND:** Discontinue if > 25% increase in QRS width. Decrease dose in liver failure. In renal failure, increase dosing interval; if GFR = 10-50 cc/min adminst. q12-24h, if GFR < 10 cc/min, dose q24-40h. **CONTRAINDICATIONS:** As above. Bundle Branch Block NOT a contraindication. **DOSE FORMS:** PO (Cap's): 100, 150 mg Extended release: 100, 150 mg

ANTIARRHYTHMIC AGENTS: GROUP I ANTIARRHYTHMIC AGENTS *Continued*

DRUG	INDICATIONS & DOSAGES	SIDE EFFECTS & REMARKS
QUINIDINE (Quinaglute) (Cardioquin) (Duraquin) (Dura-Tabs) (Cin-Quin) (Quinora) (Quinadex Extentabs)	**Test Dose**: **PO, IM:** 200 mg several hours before full dosing (Pediatric: 2 mg/kg). **Atrial Fibrillation Conversion**: **PO (sulfate):** 300-400 mg q6h; maintenance: 200-300 mg q6-8h. **PO (polygalacturonate):** 275-825 mg q3-4h, for 3-4 doses. If necessary, increase to 400-1000 mg q3-4h. Maintenance: 275 mg q8-12h. **PO (extended release-maintenance):** 324-648 mg gluconate or 600 mg sulfate q8-12h. **Paroxysmal Supraventricular Tachycardia**: **PO (sulfate):** 400-600 mg q2-3h (maint. as for atrial fibrillation). **Premature Atrial/Ventricular Contraction Suppression**: **PO (sulfate):** 200-300 mg tid or qid. **Parenteral**: **IM (gluconate):** Load 600 mg, then 200-400 mg q2h or PRN. **IV (gluconate):** 16 mg/min infusion; usually > 300 mg required for ventricular arrhythmia. **Pediatric**: **PO (sulfate):** 15-60 mg/kg/d in 5 doses. **IM,IV (gluconate):** 2-100 mg/kg/d q3-6h.	QRS widening > 50% may precipitate ventricular tachycardia **NOTES:** 200 mg of sulfate = 267 mg gluconate = 267 mg polygalacturonate. **LEVELS:** Usually therapeutic plasma levels = 2-7 µg/ml. No benefit to levels > 9 µg/ml. In dosing, do NOT exceed 3-4 gm/d. **SIDE EFFECTS:** Nausea, vomiting, diarrhea, abdominal cramps (less common with polygalacturonate and extended release forms). Cinchonism (tinnitus, headache, dizziness, etc.), drug fever, bone marrow toxicity, hemolytic anemia (esp. in G-6-PD-deficient patients), hepatotoxicity, blurred vision. **CAUTION:** Curare-like muscle weakening (esp. post-operative patients). Interactions: decreased phenytoin and phenobarbital half-life, increased serum digoxin concentrations, increased coumadin effect. Antacids delay absorption. **RECOMMEND:** Discontinue if QRS width increases > 50% (or > 25% with preexisting conduction delays), blood dyscrasias, hepatic or renal dysfunction. Periodic EKG, CBC, LFT's, renal function evaluation. Dose unchanged in renal failure. **CONTRAINDICATIONS:** History of adverse reaction to cinchona derivatives and as in Group Remarks. **DOSE FORMS**: PO: (sulfate): 100, 200, 300 mg PO: (polygalacturonate): 275 mg Extended release (gluconate): 324, 330 mg
LIDOCAINE (Xylocaine) (Anestacon)	**Acute Ventricular Arrhythmias**: **IV**: 50-100 mg initially (rate: 20-50 mg/min), then 1-4 mg/min for 24-30 h. **IM**: 300 mg (10% solution). **DOSAGE FORMS**: Ampuls: 10 mg/ml Vials: 40, 100, 200 mg/ml Syringes: 10, 20 mg/ml	**SIDE EFFECTS**: CNS effects: drowsiness, dizziness, nausea, vomiting, paresthesias, tinnitus, visual disturbances, convulsions, loss of consciousness, respiratory depression, coma. CV effects: hypotension, bradycardia, ventricular arrhythmias. Malignant hyperthermia has occurred rarely. **LEVELS**: Effect of single bolus lasts 10-20 min, thereafter half-life about 2 h. Mild side effects at 1.4-5.0 µg/ml; serious toxicity > 9 µg/ml. **RECOMMENDATIONS**: Reduce dosage in patients with: low cardiac output, CHF, hepatic disease, concurrent *beta*-blockade, cimetidine or age > 60 y.o.
TOCAINIDE (Tonocard)	**Ventricular Arrhythmias**: **PO**: 400 mg initially, then 400-800 mg tid.	**SIDE EFFECTS**: CNS effects: dizziness, paresthesias, numbness, tremor. GI side-effects: nausea, vomiting. **LEVELS**: Therapeutic level: 4-10 µg/m. **DOSAGE FORMS**: PO (Tab's): 400, 600 mg

ANTIARRHYTHMIC AGENTS: GROUP I ANTIARRHYTHMIC AGENTS *Continued*

DRUG	INDICATIONS & DOSAGES	SIDE EFFECTS & REMARKS
MEXILETINE (Mexitil)	**Ventricular Arrhythmias**: **PO**: 200 mg q8h initially, then 200-400 mg q8-12h. **Rapid Onset**: **PO**: 400 mg initially, then 200 mg q8h.	**SIDE EFFECTS**: Upper GI distress common. CNS effects: dizziness common, tremor. **LEVELS**: Therapeutic level: 0.5-2 µg/ml. Concurrent cimetidine may increase levels. **DOSAGE FORMS**: PO (Cap's): 150, 200, 250 mg
PHENYTOIN (Dilantin)	**Ventricular Arrhythmias**: **PO**: 1 gm initially (divided in 3 doses at 0,2,4h), 500 mg/d for 2d, then 400-600 mg/d maintenance. **IV**: 100 mg q5min, up to 500 mg; repeat 2h PRN (maximum rate = 50 mg/min).	See Anticonvulsants for a more complete discussion, including drug interactions. **SIDE EFFECTS**: Hypotension, ataxia, dysarthria, nystagmus, lethargy, gingival hypertrophy, macrocytic anemia, lupus, pulmonary infiltrates. **LEVELS**: Therapeutic level 10-20 µg/ml; toxic level > 20 µg/ml. **RECOMMENDATIONS**: Maintain IV dosing ≤ 50 mg/min. Reduce dose in hepatic or renal disease. **DOSAGE FORMS**: PO (Cap's): 30, 50, 100 mg; (Liquid) : 6, 25 mg/ml Injection: 50 mg/ml
FLECAINIDE (Tambocor)	**Ventricular Arrhythmias**: **PO**: 100 mg q12h initially, increase by 50 mg q4d; maint. 100-200 mgq12h (maximum 600 mg/d). **DOSAGE FORMS**: PO (Tab's): 100 mg	**SIDE EFFECTS**: May precipitate or worsen CHF due to depression of LV function. CNS side effects most common: dizziness, visual disturbances and headache. Others: dyspnea and nausea. **LEVELS**: Therapeutic levels = 0.2-1 µg/ml; levels > 0.7-1 µg/ml associated with higher rate of conduction defects and bradycardia. **CAUTIONS**: Use cautiously in patients with CHF or previous MI. **RECOMMENDATIONS**: Increase dosage cautiously in patient with impaired renal function.
ENCAINIDE (Enkaid)	**Arrhythmias**: **PO**: 25 mg q8h; increase to 35 mg at 3-5 d, if needed; further increase to 50 mg after another 3-5 d, if needed. **Above with Renal Failure**: **PO**: 25 mg/d if creat. clearance < 20 cc/min; increase to 25 mg q12h at 7 d, if needed; further increase to 25 mg q8h after another 7 d, if needed (maximum 150 mg/d).	Metabolites share antiarrhythmic activity/toxicity. **SIDE EFFECTS**: Ventricular arrhythmias develop/worsen in 10% of patients. PR and QRS widening is dose-related. Dizziness and blurred vision are frequent. Sinus bradycardia, sinus pauses, sinus arrest, heart block (2° or 3°) and worsening of congestive heart failure (1% pts.). Asthenia, chest pain, headache, paresthesias, palpitations, PVCs, syncope, dyspnea, constipation, diarrhea, dry mouth, nausea, rash, tremor. Less common: ataxia, hypertension, confusion, dream abnormalities, photophobia, and periorbital edema. **RECOMMENDATIONS**: Side effects increase significantly at doses > 200 mg/d; manfacturer recommends hospitalization when instituting > 200 mg/d. **CAUTIONS**: Cimetidine increases encainide plasma levels; potential for toxicity. **DOSAGE FORMS**: PO (Cap's): 25, 35, 50 mg

ANTIARRHYTHMIC AGENTS: *Continued*

DRUG	INDICATIONS & DOSAGES	SIDE EFFECTS & REMARKS
GROUP II ANTIARRHYTHMIC AGENT		
PROPRANOLOL - See Antihypertensive Agents:Adrenergic Inhibitors:*beta*-Blockers. (Inderal)		
GROUP III ANTIARRHYTHMIC AGENTS		
AMIODARONE (Cordarone)	<u>**Life-Threatening Ventricular Arrhythmias**</u>: **PO**: 800-1600 mg/d for 1-3 wk, reduce to 600-800 mg/d for 3-4 wk, then maintenance of 200-400 mg/d. <u>**DOSAGE FORMS**</u>: PO (Tab's): 200 mg	ONLY for life-threatening ventricular arrhythmias refractory to other agents, NOT an agent of first choice. Side effects are common; develop in 75% patients on ≥ 400 mg/d. **SIDE EFFECTS**: Potentially fatal toxicity occurs in 10-15% patients receiving doses > 400 mg/d, mainly pulmonary (pneumonitis, alveolitis, fibrosis). Other potentially fatal side effects include liver injury and arrhythmias typical of this class of drugs. Elevated LFTs are common. Corneal deposits (microscopic) develop in ≤ 10% and may cause blurred or halo vision; usually reversable. Amiodarone alters circulating thyroid hormone levels and may precipitate hypothyroidism (rarely hyper-). Photosensitization occurs in ≤ 10% patients. Noncompetitive adrenergic inhibition may produce alpha/beta blockade. Others: nausea, vomiting, peripheral neuropathy, tiredness, tremor and lack of coordination. **LEVELS**: Therapeutic = 1.0-2.5 µg/ml. **CAUTIONS**: Pharmacokinetics vary widely between patients; careful dosage adjustment and monitoring is required. **RECOMMENDATIONS**: Hospitalize patient during initial therapy, usually 1-2 wk. Perform thorough pulmonary evaluation periodically and at the first sign of any respiratory symptom. Reduce dose or discontinue at first sign of toxicity. Perform baseline and periodic LFTs; reduce dose or discontinue if 3X normal or if increase 2X above elevated baseline. **CONTRAINDICATIONS**: Severe sinus-node dysfunction. <u>**DRUG INTERACTIONS**</u>: Potentiates action of ***warfarin-type anticoagulants*** and can produce serious or fatal bleeding. Increases serum ***digoxin, digitoxin*** levels and may precipitate toxicity. Also increases serum levels of other antiarrhythmics (***quinidine, procainamide, phenytoin***) and may precipitate toxicity. Potentiates cardiac effects of concurrent ***β-blockers*** and ***calcium antagonists***; may produce bradycardia, sinus arrest or AV block.
BRETYLIUM TOSYLATE (Bretylol)	<u>**Life-Threatening Ventricular Arrhythmias**</u>: **IV**: 5 mg/kg injection, repeat10 mg/kg. **IV Maintenance**: 1-2 mg/min continuous infusion or 5-10 mg/kg over 10-30 min q6h. <u>**Ventricular Arrhythmias**</u>: **IV**: 5-10 mg/kg over 10-30 min q1-2h until arrhythmia reverses, then IV Maintenance as above. **IM**: 5-10 mg/kg q6-8h at varying sites (< 5 ml/site).	Bretylium causes an initial release of norepinephrine (NE) from nerve terminals, then diminishes further NE release. **SIDE EFFECTS**: Sympathomimetic effects occur initially (transient tachycardia, hypertension). Hypotension (esp. postural) is common; may require treatment but tolerance usually develops. Local necrosis may occur if IM sites not varied. **LEVELS**: Therapeutic = 0.5-1.0 µg/ml. **RECOMMENDATIONS**: Decrease dose in renal failure. Switch to oral antiarrhythmic ASAP. AVOID, if possible, use in patients with fixed cardiac output. <u>**DRUG INTERACTIONS**</u>: Potentiates ***digoxin, digitoxin*** toxicity. <u>**DOSAGE FORMS**</u>: Injection: 50 mg/ml

CARDIAC GLYCOSIDES

GROUP REMARKS: Choice of agent based on onset/duration of action and mode of adminst. Higher doses needed for SVT than CHF therapy. Clinical response (rather than total dose) most important factor in determining acute and maintenance doses. Agents with more rapid onset have shorter duration of action). These drugs cause slowing of AV conduction (junctional escape rhythms and AV block can result). 10-20% patients develop increased PR interval of 20 to 40 millisec. (or more) - a therapeutic (not toxic) side effect. Prolongation of AV nodal refractory period occurs (decreases rapid ventricular response to atrial fibrillation). Ectopic impulses increased (PVC's, bigeminy, ventricular tachycardia, etc.). Long term efficacy assoc'd with pre-treatment third heart sound. **LEVELS**: Useful to evaluate drug interactions, renal failure, non-compliance & suspected toxicity. Plasma levels show variable relation to symptoms of toxicity - EKG & clinical evaluation more important. **SIDE EFFECTS**: EKG changes: sagging J-point, shorter QT interval (may obscure ischemic ST-T wave changes). Nausea, vomiting, anorexia, diarrhea (common early signs of toxicity). Yellow or green vision, halos around objects, scotomas. Drowsiness, confusion, headache, toxic psychosis, seizures, neuralgias. Estrogen-like effects (esp. in elderly). Rare hypersensitivity reactions (usually within 6-10d) with eosinophilia. **CAUTIONS**: Low therapeutic index. Cardiac toxicity manifested by HR < 50/min., 2º or 3º AV block, junctional arrhythmias, PVC's, PAC's, atrial or ventricular tachyarrhythmias. May potentiate AV block. Drugs increasing AV nodal block: verapamil, diltiazem, clonidine, propranolol (& other *beta*-blockers). Drugs adding to bradycardia: diltiazem, *beta*-blockers, reserpine, methyldopa. Drugs increasing digoxin blood levels: quinidine, amiodarone, verapamil. Drugs decreasing absorption: antacids, cholestyramine, sulfasalazine, neomycin, kaolin-pectin. Succinyl choline may increase myocardial irritability. Possible pressor effect with IV injection . Toxic effects exacerbated by hypokalemia, hypomagnesemia, hypercalcemia, older age, smaller body size, hypothyroidism, cor pulmonale, CHF (NYMA II or III). Higher risk of use in recent MI (arrythmogenic), pre-excitation syndromes (may worsen W-P-W), IHSS, constrictive pericarditis, renal/hepatic failure, AV block > 1º (may need prophylactic pacer), frequent PVC's, and acute rheumatic carditis. **RECOMMENDATIONS**: Monitor K^+ & Mg^{++} closely if concurrent diuretic use. Discontinue if: ventricular tachycardia ensues, complete heart block develops, toxic signs develop. Avoid quinidine & procainamide in treatment of dig-toxic arrhythmias (may increase AV block). Treat toxicity with K^+ adminst., phenytoin (also lidocaine, propranolol, overdrive pacing, atropine). Cardioversion as last resort (may worsen arrhythmia); start at lowest energy levels. K^+ infusion in normo-kalemic patients controversial (mix 40-100 mEq KCl in 500 cc D5W, give at 30-40 mEq/h with constant EKG monitoring). Discontinue digoxin 1-2 d before elective cardioversion. **CONTRAINDICATIONS**: Incomplete AV block. Impending need to DC countershock (use propranolol). Ventricular arrhythmias. **NOTES**: Dialysis NOT useful in treating toxicity.

DRUG	DOSES	KINETICS	SIDE EFFECTS & REMARKS
DIGOXIN (Lanoxin) (Lanoxicaps)	**PO**: 0.75-1.25 mg initially; 0.125-0.375 mg maintenance. **IV**: 0.6-1.0 mg initially; 0.1-0.375 maintenance.	**Onset**: 0.5-2 h (PO); 5-30 min (IV) **Peak**: 6-8 h (PO); 1-5 h (IV) **Duration**: 3-4 d after discontinue	Obtain plasma levels 6-8 h after dosing. Reduce dose 20-25% upon change from PO to parenteral adminst. If GFR = 10-50 cc/min, decrease maintenance dose by 25-75%. If GFR < 10 cc/min, decrease loading dose by 25% & maintenance dose by 75-90%. CHF therapy doses: 8-12 µg/kg. SVT doses: 10-15 µg/kg. Serum levels = 2-4 ng/ml used occasionally in SVT (must switch to another agent). **LEVELS**: **Therapeutic**: 0.5-2.0 ng/ml; **Toxic**: > 2.0 ng/ml
DESLANOSIDE (Cedilanid-D)	**IM,IV**: 0.8 mg intially; 0.4 mg q2-4h (maximum 2 mg/d).	**Onset**: 10-30 min **Peak**: 1-2 h **Duration**: 2-5 d after discontinue	IV = preferred route. IM inject: Adminst. < 0.8 mg at any one site. Rapid digitalization (IV, IM): 1.6 mg (1-2 doses) or 0.8 mg initial, then 0.2-0.4 mg q2-4h to total of 1.6-2 mg. Start PO maintenance (digoxin) 12-24 h post-digitalization.
OUABAIN	**IV**: 0.2-0.5 mg initially; 0.1 mg q1h PRN (maximum 1.0 mg/d).	**Onset**: 5-10 min **Peak**: 0.5-2 h	Parenteral use only. More rapid onset than digoxin, for use in emergency only.
DIGITOXIN (Crystodigin)	**PO,IM,IV**: 0.8 mg loading dose; then 0.2 mg q6-8h for 2-3 doses; maintenance 0.05-0.2 mg/d.	Concurrent hepatic enzyme inducers may decrease serum levels. Rapid digitalization (PO, IM, IV): 0.6 mg, then 0.4 mg in 4-6h, then 0.2 mg q4-6h (3 doses) or 0.6 mg q3h (2 doses). Slow digitalization (PO): 2 mg bid (4 doses) or 0.2 mg 1-3 doses/d until 1.2-1.8 mg total. Maintenance: 10% of digitalizing dose (if GFR < 10 cc/min, decrease maintenance dose by 25-50%). **LEVELS**: **Therapeutic**: 20-35 ng/ml; **Toxic**: > 40-45 ng/ml.	

CARDIAC INOTROPIC AGENT

DRUG	INDICATIONS & DOSAGE	DOSE FORMS	REMARKS
AMRINONE (Inocor)	<u>Congestive Heart Failure</u>: **IV**: 0.75 mg/kg bolus over 2-3 min initially, then 5-10 µg/kg/min (maximum 10 mg/kg/d).	Ampules: 5 mg/ml (20 ml)	Slightly enhances AV conduction and may increase ventricular response rate in atrial fibrillation or flutter. **SIDE EFFECTS**: Thrombocytopenia (in 2% of patients), nausea and vomiting (1-2%), anorexia, abdominal discomfort, hepatotoxicity (0.2%), arrhythmias (3%), hypotension (1-2%), fever, chest pain, rare hypersensitivity reactions including myositis, vasculitis, pleuritis, pericarditis, ascites. **CAUTIONS**: Vasodilator side effect may produce hypotension necessitating discontinuation or reduction in dose. **RECOMMENDATIONS**: Use only in patients who have NOT responded to vasodilators, diuretics or digitalis. Monitor patients closely. Discontinue if evidence of hypersensitivity reaction or hepatic toxicity. Lower dosage or discontinue if thrombocytopenia (< 150,000/cc). Baseline and periodic platelet counts with therapy. **CONTRAINDICATIONS**: Bisulfite hypersensitivity. Amrinone hypersensitivity.

NITRATE AND NITRITE VASODILATORS

GROUP REMARKS: All decrease preload and therefore decrease myocardial work. All increase subendocardial blood flow and shunt blood to ischemic myocardium. Subject to extensive first-pass hepatic metabolism. Prolonged use or oral long-acting forms may cause cross-tolerance to short-acting forms (controversial). **SIDE EFFECTS:** Headache (frequently disappears after days to weeks of therapy). Hypotension, syncope (esp. with decreased cardiac reserve). Flush, nausea, tachycardia, rash. May decrease splanchnic and renal blood flow. Transient increase in intraocular pressure. **RECOMMENDATIONS:** Use smallest effective dose and titrate upwards until side effects become limiting. Choice of preparation depends on desired onset and duration of action. **Patient Instructions:** See physician immediately if chest pain NOT relieved by short-acting preparation given q5min for 3 doses. Take prophylactic long-acting form before exertion known to evoke angina. **CONTRAINDICATIONS:** Increased intracranial pressure. Severe anemia. Hypotension. Hypovolemia. Cardiac constriction or tamponade.

DRUG	INDICATIONS & DOSAGE	SIDE EFFECTS & REMARKS
	NITRATES	
NITROGLYCERIN (Glyceryl Trinitrate) (Nitroglycerol) **Sublingual:** (Nitrostat) **Topical Ointment:** (Nitro-bid) (Nitrong) (Nitrol) **Patches:** (Nitrodisc) (Transderm) (Nitrodur) **IV:** (Nitro-bid IV) (Nitrol) (Tridil) **Oral Extended Release:** (Angiospan) (Cardabid) (Niong) (Nitrocels) (Nitro-bid plateau caps) (Diacels) (Klavikordal) (Nitrocot) (Nitroglyn) (Nitorlex-D) (Nitrolin) (Nitronet) (Nitrospan) (Nitrostat-SR)(N-G-C) (Nitrocaps)	**Angina Prophylaxis:** **Buccal:** 1 mg tid initially; 3-12 mg/d maintenance as 3-12 doses. **Extended release:** 1-2.5 mg tid-qid initially; 10-30 mg/d maintenance as 2,3 doses. **Topical ointment:** 0.5 inch q4h initially; 0.5-5 inch/d maintenance as 6-8 doses. **NTG Patches:** 1 patch/d initially; 1-2 patches/d maintenance (lowest effective strength). **Acute Angina:** **Sublingual:** 0.5 mg (range: 0.15-0.6 mg) q5min, (maximum 3 doses). **IV:** 5 µg/min; increase by 5 µg/min q3-5min to 20 µg/min, then increase by 10-20 µg/min. Maximum dose determined by tolerance & response. With PVC tubing, increase 1st dose to 25 µg/min. **CHF:** **Topical ointment:** 1.5 inch q4h; 6-24 inches/d as 4-6 doses (Investigational).	Slight burning sensation with sub-lingual therapy, absence may indicate lack of potency. PVC tubing absorbs 40-80% of IV NTG (pre-soak to saturate). **Anti-anginal kinetics:** Ointment onset =30 min, duration = 3 h; sublingual onset = 1-2 min, duration = 15-30 min. **DOSE FORMS:** Buccal: 1, 2, 3 mg Extended release: 2.5, 6.5, 9.0 mg Topical ointment: 2% ointment **Patches:** Order dose as # mg/d NTG delievered to patient (compare to proven ointment efficacy of 10 mg/d): 2.5 mg/d = Transderm-Nitro 2.5, Nitrodur-5 5.0 mg/d = Transderm-Nitro 5, Nitrodur-10, Nitrodisc-10 7.5 mg/d = Nitrodur-15 10.0 mg/d = Transderm-Nitro 10, Nitrodur-20, Nitrodisc-10 15.0 mg/d = Transderm-Nitro 15 Transderm-Nitro membrane can rupture with vigorous removal = "dose dumping" (produces hypotension). Remove patches before electric cardioversion (explosive). Patch application q12h may be necessary for sustained 24 h effect.
ERYTHRITYL TETRANITRATE (Cardilate) (Erythritol Tetranitrate) (Peritrate)	**Angina Prophylaxis:** **PO:** 10 mg PRN; 10-100 mg/d as 1-5 doses. (headache w/ higher doses) **Esophageal Spasm:** **PO:** 10 mg qid; 10-15 mg/d as 4 doses. (spasm without gastric reflux)	Maximum effects at 30-45 min, duration approximately 2 hours. Exfoliative dermatitis. **DOSE FORMS:** PO (Tab's): 5, 10 mg

NITRATE AND NITRITE VASODILATORS: NITRATES *Continued*

DRUG	INDICATIONS & DOSAGE	SIDE EFFECTS & REMARKS
ISOSORBIDE DINITRATE (Isordil) (Sorate) (Sorbitrate) (Onset) (Dilatrate) (Isobid) (Isotrate) (Sorbide-TD)	**Acute Angina:** **Sublingual:** 5-10 mg q2-3h PRN. **PO:** 5-10 mg q2-3h PRN. **Angina Prophylaxis:** **PO:** 20 mg initially; then 10-40 mg q6h. **Extended release:** 40 mg initially; then 40-80 mg q8-12h. (Give oral forms on empty stomach)	Limit chewable tabs to 5 mg for initial dose (to avoid hypotension). **Kinetics:** Sublingual: 2-3 min onset; 2 h duration Oral: 60 min onset; 4-6 h duration Extended release: 30 min onset; 6-8 h duration Chewable tabs: 2-3 min onset; 0.5-2 h duration **DOSE FORMS:** Sub-lingual: 2.5, 5, 10 mg PO (Tab's): 5, 10, 20, 30 mg Extended release: 40 mg Chewtabs: 5, 10 mg
NITRITES		
AMYL NITRITE (Isoamyl nitrite)	**Angina:** Inhale 0.18 ml or 0.3 ml q3-5min PRN. **Cyanide Poisoning:** Inhale 0.3 ml ampule q1min until IV nitrite available.	Group Remarks EXCEPT: NOT recommended for angina. **SIDE EFFECTS:** tachycardia, headache & orthostatic hypotension. Murmer diagnosis: Stenotic lesions & IHSS are louder; mitral regurgitation, atrial regurgitation are softer. **CAUTION:** Methemoglobin formation in children.
SODIUM NITRITE	**Cyanide Poisoning:** 300 mg in 10% sln. at 2.4-5 ml/min. Follow by 12.5 gm (IV as 25% sln., 10 min.) Na^+ Thiosulfate. In children: 6 mg/kg as 3% sln., max = 300 mg IV.	Group Remarks EXCEPT: NOT recommended for angina. Child dosage limited by methemoglobinemia. **RECOMMEND:** Repeat with 50% initial dose if signs of cyanide intoxication return.

CALCIUM CHANNEL BLOCKERS

GROUP REMARKS: Cardiac depression, CHF, arrhythmia, AV block (Verapamil > Diltiazem > Nifedipine), bradycardia, increased cardiac depression with *beta*-blockers. Nausea, flush, headache, symptomatic hypotension, edema (usually responds to a diuretic), dizziness. Rarely rash, confusion, nervousness. **CONTRAINDICATIONS**: Heart block > 2° or 3° degree. Hypotension (systolic BP < 90 mm Hg), cardiogenic shock, sick sinus syndrome (unless pacemaker), hypersensitivity. **CAUTIONS**: Patients with left ventricular dysfunction, moderate to severe chronic CHF, aortic stenosis. **RECOMMEND**: Evaluate development of edema to rule out exacerbation of CHF.

DRUG	INDICATIONS & DOSAGE	SIDE EFFECTS & REMARKS
VERAPAMIL (Iproveratril) (Calan) (Isoptin)	**Angina**: **PO**: 40-80 mg tid initially; 240-480 mg/d maintenance in 3 doses. **Supraventricular Tachycardia**: **Adult (IV):** 5-10 mg (75-150 μg/kg). **Pediatric (IV)**: 1-15 years old: 100-300 μg/kg. < 1 year old: 100-200 μg/kg. IV doses: Infuse over 2 min period; repeat (once) in 30 min.	AV nodal depressant effects prominent. Because of adverse effects: 6% patients must lower dose; 5% must discontinue (higher % in patients with IHSS, sick sinus syndrome, severe CHF, or on *beta*-blockers). CHF occurs in < 1% patients; in 5-10% BP drops briefly to < 90/60 when dosed IV (rarely serious). PO use: Constipation (7%), peripheral edema (2%), fatigue, transient LFT elevation. **RECOMMEND**: Continuous EKG monitoring-essential with IV treatment. Periodic LFTs. **CONTRAINDICATIONS**: As above or if pulmonary capillary wedge pressure > 20 mm Hg. **DOSE FORMS**: PO (Tab's): 80, 120 mg Injection: 5 mg/2 ml
NIFEDIPINE (Procardia)	**Angina**: **PO**: 10 mg tid initially; 30-120 mg/d maintenance in 3-4 doses (maximum 180 mg/d). **DOSE FORMS**: PO (Cap's): 10 mg	Least effects on cardiac conduction. Outpatient: can increase dose by 30 mg/d. Inpatient: can increase dose by 10 mg q4-6h. Weakness, dyspnea, wheezing. Possibly assoc'd with CHF, MI, and ventricular arrhythmias. Rare: Increased angina, GI complaints, nervousness, balance problems. May increase serum digoxin concentration. **RECOMMEND**: Cautious withdrawal of *beta*-blockers upon starting Nifedipine. Withold 36 h prior to surgery if fentanyl to be used. Monitor digoxin levels and toxic signs closely.
DILTIAZEM (Latiazem) (Cardizem)	**Angina**: **PO**: 30 mg qid initially (increased q1-2d); 120-360 mg/d maintenance as 4 doses. **DOSE FORMS**: PO (Tab's): 30, 60 mg	Extensive first-pass hepatic metabolism. 1% patients must discontinue because of bradycardia, rash or GI problems. Nausea and anorexia in 3% patients, 2° or 3° block in 0.5%. Digoxin increased in 14-19% patients. **RECOMMEND**: As above. Can increase dosage q1-2d until angina controlled.

VASOCONSTRICTORS AND OXYTOCICS

GROUP REMARKS: The ergot alkaloids and derivative listed in this section act to contract vascular and non-vascular smooth muscle. Their major uses are in the treatment of migraine and to control the post-partum uterus. Oxytocin (Pitocin) may be used to induce labor as well as to limit bleeding.

DRUG	INDICATIONS & DOSAGE	DOSE FORMS	REMARKS
ERGONOVINE (Ergotrate)	**Prevent Post-Partum Bleeding**: **PO**: 0.2-0.4 mg q6-12h until uterine atony resolves (average 2 days). **IM,IV**: 0.2 mg, after placenta delivered; may repeat q2-4h.	PO (Tab's): 0.2 mg Ampules: 0.2 mg/ml (1 ml)	Onset: within 1 min (IV) 5-10 min (IM), ≥ 10 min (PO). **SIDE EFFECTS**: Ergotism (arterial insufficiency). Hypertension, headache, nausea, vomiting, diarrhea and allergic reactions. **CAUTIONS**: Use during coronary angiography has provoked life-threatening arrhythmias and myocardial infarction. May decrease lactation. Avoid prolonged use. Caution in conditions where vasoconstriction may be dangerous (mitral valve stenosis, heart disease, renal impairment, vascular disease, shunts. **RECOMMENDATIONS**: Severe cramping may require reduction in dosage. Monitor blood pressure, pulse and uterine response. **CONTRAINDICATIONS**: History of allergic or idiosyncratic reactions to the drug, induction of labor, threatened spontaneous abortion.
METHYLERGONOVINE (Methergine)	**Prevent Post-Partum Bleeding**: **PO**: 0.2 mg q6-8h for a maximum of 1 week. **IM,IV**: 0.2 mg after placenta delivered; repeat q2-4h PRN. (Infuse IV dose over 1 min.)	PO (Tab's): 0.2 mg Ampules: 0.2 mg/ml (1 ml)	Onset: immediate (IV), < 5 min (IM), 5-10 min (PO). **SIDE EFFECTS**: Hypertension, headache, chest pain, dyspnea, tinnitus, vomiting, nausea and dizziness. **CAUTIONS**: Caution in conditions where vasoconstriction may be dangerous (mitral valve stenosis, heart disease, renal impairment, vascular disease, shunts. **RECOMMENDATIONS**: AVOID IV use except in emergencies because of complications of sudden marked rise in blood pressure. **CONTRAINDICATIONS**: Hypertension, eclampsia, pregnancy, drug hypersensitivity.
ERGOTAMINE (Gynergen) (Ergomat) (Ergostat)	**Migraine Headaches**: **PO**: 1-2 mg at onset; then 1-2 mg q30 min PRN (maximum 6 mg/d or 10 mg/week). **SL**: 2 mg at onset; then 2 mg q30 min PRN (maximum 6 mg/d or 10 mg/week). **Inhalation**: 1 puff at onset; then 1 puff q5min PRN (maximum 6 puffs/d or 15 puffs/week).	PO (Tab's): 1 mg SL (Tab's): 2 mg Aerosol: 9 mg/ml-0.36 mg/puff (2.5 ml vials=60 puffs)	Causes venoconstriction, which diminishes pulsations in meningeal vessels, and arteriolar constriction, which can cause gangrene. **SIDE EFFECTS**: Paresthesias, leg cramps, myalgia, muscle weakness, sinus tachycardia, bradycardia, pruritis, arterial insufficiency, coronary vasospasm, chest pain, uterine contraction. **CAUTIONS**: Prolonged use or excessive doses may produce gangrene and ergotism. With prolonged use, dependency may occur due to associated migraine pain relief. Dysphoric effect may follow withdrawal after prolonged use. **RECOMMENDATIONS**: Initiate therapy at first sign of attack. Warn patient NOT to exceed recommended dosage. **CONTRAINDICATIONS**: Pregnancy, hypersensitivity to ergot alkaloids, renal insufficiency, coronary artery disease, hypertension, sepsis, liver disease, conditions where vasoconstriction may be dangerous (mitral valve stenosis, heart disease, renal impairment, vascular disease, shunts).

VASOCONSTRICTORS AND OXYTOCICS *Continued*

DRUG	INDICATIONS & DOSAGE	DOSE FORMS	REMARKS
METHYSERGIDE (Sansert)	**Prevention of Migraine Attacks**: **PO**: 4-8 mg/d (discontinue after 3 wks if no benefit). Discontinue drug for 3-4 weeks q6months.	Tablets: 2 mg	Retroperitoneal, cardiac and pleuropulmonary fibroses (with ureteral occlusion) can result from extended therapy and manifest as flank pain, pleural effusion, pleural friction rubs, heart murmurs, lower extremity vascular insufficiency, dysuria. Note the availability of propranolol and clonidine as alternative prophylactic agents. **SIDE EFFECTS**: Side effects occur in 40% of patients. Vascular insufficiency, neutropenia, eosinophilia, nausea, vomiting, diarrhea, abdominal pain, constipation, insomnia, dizziness, drowsiness, hyperesthesia, vertigo, psychiatric symptoms of dissociation, flushing, rashes, edema, weakness, myalgia, arthralgia. **CAUTIONS**: Tablets contain tartrazine; some patients may experience allergic-type reactions including asthma. Oxytocic properties preclude its use during pregnancy. Excreted in breast milk; may cause ergotism in infants of nursing mothers. **RECOMMENDATIONS**: A drug-free interval of ≥ 3-4 wks MUST be instituted q6months. Discontinue if leg cramps, flank pain, chest pain, pale, cold, numb, or painful extremities. Taper dose during last 2-3 weeks of each treatment period; do NOT discontinue abruptly. **CONTRAINDICATIONS**: Pregnancy, severe hypertension, coronary artery insufficiency, lower extremity phlebitis, collagen vascular disease, peripheral vascular disease, renal insufficiency, liver disease, heart valvular disease, sepsis.
OXYTOCIN (Pitocin)	**Labor Induction**: **IV**: 0.001-0.002 units/min initial infusion rate; then gradually increase dose at a rate of an additional 0.001-0.002 units/min q15-30min (maximum 0.020 units/min). **Prevent Post-Partum Bleeding**: **IM**: 10 units after delivery of the placenta (single dose). **IV**: 0.1-0.4% sln PRN. **Incomplete/Inevitable Abortion**: **IV**: 0.01-0.02 units/min. **Initial Milk Let-Down**: **Nasal**: 1 spray into one or both nostrils 2-3 min prior to nursing.	Ampules: 10 units/ml (0.5, 1, 10 ml) Tubex: 10 units/ml (1 ml) Nasal Spray: 40 units/ml (2, 5 ml squeeze bottles)	10 units oxytocin + 500 ml physiologic saline solution (or 5% dextrose in saline solution) gives a solution containing 0.01 units/2 drops. **SIDE EFFECTS**: Cardiac arrhythmia, nausea, vomiting, postpartum hemorrhage, anaphylactic reaction, afibrinogenemia, fetal bradycardia, fetal jaundice, uterine rupture. **CAUTIONS**: Hypertensive episodes, subarachnoid hemorrhages, fetal death and distress must all be considered prior to initiating therapy. Oxytocin has anti-diuretic effect and will increase water retention; caution in volume overload or cardiac pathology. Pelvic adequacy for delivery and presentation must be evaluated prior to use. If fetal distress might occur, fetal monitoring should be considered. **CONTRAINDICATIONS**: Nasal oxytocin contraindicated in pregnancy. Hypersensitivity to oxytocin, cephalopelvic disproportion, uncorrected abnormal fetal presentations, fetal distress with delivery not imminent, hypertonic uterine pathology, induction of labor when vaginal delivery is contraindicated.

COMBINATION AGENTS

BUTALBITAL:ASPIRIN:CAFFEINE
50 mg butalbital
325 mg aspirin
40 mg caffeine
(Fiorgen)
(Fiorinol)
(Butal Compound)
(Lanorinol)

BUTALBITAL:ACETAMINOPHEN:CAFFEINE
50 mg butalbital
325 mg acetaminophen
40 mg caffeine
(Fioricet)
(Esgic)
(Endolor)
(Medigesic Plus)

BUTALBITAL:ACETAMINOPHEN
50 mg butalbital
650 mg acetaminophen
(Axotal)
(Phrenilin Forte)
(Sedipap-10)

BUTALBITAL:ACETAMINOPHEN
50 mg butalbital
325 mg acetaminophen
(Bancap)
(Phrenilin)
(Triaprin)

ERGOTAMINE:CAFFEINE
1 mg ergotamine
100 mg caffeine
(Caffergot)
(Cafatine)
(Cafetrate)
(Ercatab)
(Wigraine)

PO: 2 tab's with initial attack; then 1 tab q30min (maximum 6 tab's/attack or 10 tab's/weel.

ERGOTAMINE:CAFFEINE Suppositories
2 mg ergotamine
100 mg caffeine

ERGOTAMINE:CAFFEINE:BELLADONNA:PENTOBARBITAL Suppositories
2 mg ergotamine
100 mg caffeine
0.125 mg belladonna alkaloids
60 mg pentobarbital
(Cafergot P-B)
(Caetrate P-B)
(Migergot P-B)

Rectal: 1 suppository with initial attack; repeat one in 1h PRN (maximum 2/attack or 5/week).

PRESSORS AND INOTROPES USED FOR HEMODYNAMIC SUPPORT

GROUP REMARKS: These drugs are all cardiac stimulants but differ in that some (e.g., isoproterenol) dilate all vascular beds; some (e.g., norepinephrine) constrict all vascular beds; some (e.g., epinephrine) dilate vessels in voluntary muscle but constrict in the skin and splanchnic areas; and some (e.g., dopamine) are vasodilators but become constrictors as the dose is increased. Some may therefore lower diastolic and mean blood pressure in normals, but elevate blood pressure depressed by shock or drugs. Concomitant use of halogenated anesthetic gases or cyclopropane may cause sensitization of the myocardium to the effects of these agents and may precipitate LETHAL cardiac arrhythmias. Simultaneous use with monamine oxidase inhibitors, tricyclic antidepressants or oxytocic drugs may precipitate disastrous rise in blood pressure. NOT to be used until any hypovolemia corrected.

DRUG	INDICATIONS & DOSAGE	DOSE FORMS	REMARKS
	PRESSORS WITH INOTROPIC ACTION		
DOPAMINE (Intropin)	**IV**: 2-5 µg/kg/min initially, then increase gradually in 5-10 µg/kg/min increments until satisfactory perfusion is obtained (maximum: 20-50 µg/kg/min).	Vials: 5 ml (200 mg)	*Beta*-adrenergic blocking drug effects are reversible with dopamine. Dilates renal and mesenteric blood levels at 1-2 µg/kg/min. Increases cardiac output with *beta*-receptor stimulating action at 2-10 µg/kg/min. At > 10-12 µg/kg/min, vasoconstrictive alpha-adrenergic effects predominate and > 20 µg/kg/min renal and mesenteric perfusion may be compromised.
	Onset of action is within 2-4 min of infusion. Duration of action < 10 min. For IV infusion in shock, mix 200-400 mg in 250 or 500 ml in NS or D5W (400-1,600 µg/ml). **SIDE EFFECTS**: Tachycardia, ectopic beats, angina, vomiting, nausea, peripheral vasoconstriction, hypertension, hypotension. **CAUTIONS**: If diastolic pressure rises markedly, decrease infusion rate. Patients with peripheral vascular disease may experience hypoperfusion and tissue damage. Extravasation may cause tissue necrosis. **RECOMMENDATIONS**: If extravasation occurs, immediately infiltrate affected tissues with 30 cc of a 2:1 mixture of saline and phentolamine. Invasive hemodynamic monitoring essential during use. When possible, increase central venous pressure to 10-15 cm of water or increase pulmonary wedge pressure to 14-18 mm Hg. Avoid simultaneous use with diphenylhydantoin, if possible. **CONTRAINDICATIONS**: Cardiac tachyarrythmias, pheochromocytoma.		
DOBUTAMINE (Dobutrex)	**IV**: 0.5 µg/kg/min initially, then increase gradually until desired tissue perfusion is obtained. The usual range of doses is 2.5-10 µg/kg/min (maximum 40 µg/kg/min).	Ampules: 20 ml (250 mg)	Improves cardiac output especially well in patients with cardiomyopathy. Onset within 1-2 min; peak effect may require 5-10 min. Increase in cardiac output NOT accompanied by marked increase in heart rate. Systemic vascular resistance is usually decreased. For IV infusion in shock, mix 250 mg in 250 or 500 ml in NS or D5W (500-1,000 µg/ml). **SIDE EFFECTS**: Tachycardia, hypertension, precipitation of rapid ventricular response in patients with atriofibrillation, ectopic beats, nausea, angina, headache, shortness of breath. **LEVELS**: Therapeutic plasma levels: 40-190 ng/ml. **CAUTIONS**: No cardiac output improvement if aortic outflow is obstructed. Do NOT administer monamine-oxidase inhibitors, oxytocic agents or tricyclic depressants simultaneously due to possible marked pressor response. **RECOMMENDATIONS**: May be used with nitroprusside to enhance cardiac output. **CONTRAINDICATIONS**: Idiopathic hypertrophic subaortic stenosis.

PRESSORS AND INOTROPES USED FOR HEMODYNAMIC SUPPORT *Continued*

DRUG	INDICATIONS & DOSAGE	DOSE FORMS	REMARKS
ISOPROTERENOL (Isuprel)	**Bradycardia, Heart Block**: **IV**: 0.5-20 µg/min until desired heart rate is obtained. Bolus of 0.02-0.06 mg IV can be given; if less urgent, give 0.2 mg IM or SQ. **SL**: 10 mg initially, then 5-50 mg PRN to maintain heart rate; chronic maintenance, 10-30 mg SL q4-6h. **RECTAL**: 5 mg initially, then 5-15 mg q2-6h PRN to maintain heart rate.	Ampules: 1:5,000 solution 0.2 mg/ml (5,10 mg) Glossets: 10, 15 mg (SL)	For IV infusion in shock, mix 2 mg (10 ml) in 500 ml NS or D5W (4 µg/ml) and infuse at 125 cc/min (5 µg/min). **SIDE EFFECTS**: Arrhythmias, hypotension (may precipitate Adams-Stokes attacks in patients with A-V nodal disease), tachycardia, sweating, headache, flushing, tremors, anxiety, dizziness, weakness, nausea, vomiting. **CAUTIONS**: Use caution and monitor EKG when administering simultaneously with digitalis. Pressor effect may be potentiated when given simultaneously with monoamine-oxidase inhibitor, oxytocic drugs and with tricyclic antidepressants. Doses which increase heart rate > 130 beats/min may precipitate ventricular arrhythmia or angina. **RECOMMENDATIONS**: Do NOT administer simultaneously with epinephrine. If heart rate > 110 beats/min, decrease infusion rate or temporarily discontinue. **CONTRAINDICATIONS**: Digitalis-induced tachyarrhythmias and other tachyarrhythmias which will not benefit from increased inotropic and chronotropic cardiac activity.
EPINEPHRINE (Adrenaline)	**Cardiac Arrest**: **IV**: 0.5-1 mg (5-10 ml of 1:10,000 solution) initially, then 0.5 mg q5min.	Ampules,1:1,000 (1 mg/ml): 1 ml Tubex,1:1,000 (1 mg/ml): 1, 2 ml Tubex,1:10,000 (0.1 mg/ml): 5, 10 ml Vials,1:1,000 (1 mg/ml): 30 ml	Also used SC during acute asthmatic attacks for bronchodilation. **SIDE EFFECTS**: Tachycardia, arrhythmias, angina pectoris, pulmonary edema, tremors, dry mouth, cold extremities, reduced renal blood flow. **CAUTIONS**: Propranolol administered simultaneously may block *beta*-adrenergic effects of epinephrine and allow unopposed *alpha*-stimulation, leading to severe hypertension. In patients with prefibrillatory cardiac arrhythmia, epinephrine may worsen arrhythmias. **RECOMMENDATIONS**: Toxic effects can be counteracted by injecting an *alpha*-adrenergic and a *beta*-adrenergic blocker. **CONTRAINDICATIONS**: Non-anaphylactic shock, narrow-angle glaucoma, in labor, cardiac dilation, coronary insufficiency, thyrotoxicosis, diabetes, hypertension, aortic aneurysm and pregnancy when maternal blood pressure > 130/80.
PRESSORS WITH VASOCONSTRICTIVE ACTION			
NOREPINEPHRINE (Levarteranol) (Levophed)	**IV**: 8-12 µg/ml solution: 1-3 ml/min initially; adjust rate to establish blood pressure > 90 mm Hg systolic.	Ampules: 1 mg/ml (4 ml)	Hypoxia, acidosis and hypercapnea MUST be corrected prior to or with infusion. Prolonged use may diminish plasma volume and worsen shock. *Alpha*-adrenergic blocking drug (e.g., phentolamine) will antagonize pressor effects. Atropine blocks reflex bradycardia caused by norepinephrine. MAO inhibitors, guanethidine, methyldopa, antihistamines, and ergot alkaloids may potentiate hypertension. **SIDE EFFECTS**: Reflex bradycardia, headache, palpitations, anxiety, hypertension, angina, diaphoresis, vomiting, cardiac arrhythmias, uterine contractions, and sloughing at infusion site. Rare thyroid enlargement and swelling. **RECOMMENDATIONS**: Treatment of extravasation: infiltrate area with 5-10 mg phentolamine in 15 cc saline. Use long IV line for administration. AVOID dilution in saline alone, use 5% dextrose or dextrose and saline. In previously hypertensive pts, adjust bp to ≤ 40 mm Hg below pre-existing systolic pressure. **CONTRAINDICATION**: Pregnancy.

PRESSORS AND INOTROPES USED FOR HEMODYNAMIC SUPPORT *Continued*

DRUG	INDICATIONS & DOSAGE	DOSE FORMS	REMARKS
METARAMINOL (Aramine)	<u>**Hypotension**</u>: **IV**: 0.5-5 mg initially; then mix a 0.025-0.2 mg/ml sln and adjust rate to establish blood pressure at desired level. **IM, SC**: 2-10 mg initially; reassess blood pressure in 10 min and readminister PRN. <u>**Severe Shock**</u>: **IV**: 0.5-5 mg initially; then mix a 0.025-0.2 mg/ml sln and adjust rate to establish blood pressure > 90 mm Hg systolic.	Vials: 10 mg/ml (10 ml)	Pressor response starts 1-2 min after IV infusion and 5-10 min after IM administration. **SIDE EFFECTS**: Tachycardia, arrhythmia, respiratory distress, reduced renal blood flow, angina, sweating, nausea, tremor, headache, metabolic acidosis, increased myocardial oxygen consumption. Extravasation may cause tissue necrosis. **CAUTIONS**: Fetal anoxia may result. **RECOMMENDATIONS**: Use with caution in patients with occlusive vascular diseases, diabetes mellitus, Buerger's disease, cirrhosis, and in patients on digitalis.
EPHEDRINE	**PO, IM, SC**: 25-50 mg q3-4h. **IV**: 5-25 mg slow PUSH; may be repeated after 10-15 min. <u>**Acute Asthma**</u>: **IM, IV, SC**: smallest effective dose (0.25-0.5 ml).	Ampules: 25, 50 mg/ml (1 ml) PO (Cap's): 25, 50 mg Cap's extended-release: 15, 30, 60 mg Syrup: 1 mg/5 ml, 25 mg/5 ml Nasal sln: 0.5, 1, 3%	Bronchodilation occurs within 1/4-1 h after PO dose. **SIDE EFFECTS**: Tachycardia or reflex bradycardia, tremor, reduced renal blood flow, CNS depression, somnolence, hypertension, cardiac arrhythmias, decreased splanchnic blood flow, urinary retention in patients with prostatic hypertrophy. May precipitate narrow-angle glaucoma. **CAUTIONS**: May exacerbate side effects of theophylline. Nasal application may cause rebound sinus congestion. **RECOMMENDATIONS**: Correct hypoxia, acidosis and hypercapnia prior to use. **CONTRAINDICATIONS**: Severe coronary insufficiency, hyperthyroidism, hypertension, diabetes mellitus, cardiac asthma.
MEPHENTERAMINE (Wyamine)	<u>**Shock**</u> (not recommended): **IV**: 20-60 mg bolus; then 1.2 mg/ml infusion at 1-5 mg/min. **IM**: 10-30 mg initially (maximum 80 mg); repeat PRN.	Ampules: 15 mg/ml (2 ml) Vials: 15, 30 mg/ml (10 ml) Tubex: 30 mg/ml (1 ml)	**SIDE EFFECTS**: Hypertension, arrhythmia, anxiety, seizures, incoherence, paresthesias. **CAUTIONS**: Digitalis may increase arrythmogenic effect on heart. **RECOMMENDATIONS**: Arrhythmias during anesthesia can be treated by *beta*-blocking agents.

PRESSORS AND INOTROPES USED FOR HEMODYNAMIC SUPPORT *Continued*

DRUG	INDICATIONS & DOSAGE	DOSE FORMS	REMARKS
METHOXAMINE (Vasoxyl)	**Shock Emergencies**: **IV**: 3-5 mg SLOWLY. **Transient Hypotension**: **IM**: 5-15 mg, depending on degree of decrease; repeat PRN. **IV**: 3-5 mg if systolic pressure < 60 mm; may be given with 10-15 mg IM for prolonged effect. **Paroxysmal Supraventricular Tachycardia**: **IV**: 10 mg SLOWLY (over 3-5 min).	Ampules: 20 mg/ml (1 ml)	*Beta*-adrenergic blocking drugs may potentiate vasoconstrictive effects. **SIDE EFFECTS**: Hypertension, headache, bradycardia, anxiety, nervousness, angina, respiratory distress, tremor, projectile vomiting, pilomotor activation, micturition, seizures, cerebral hemorrhage. **CAUTIONS**: Severe bradycardia and decreased cardiac output common; especially of concern with poor cerebral or coronary circulation. May cause increased uterine contractility and fetal anoxia. Use with extreme caution. **RECOMMENDATIONS**: Bradycardia may be treated with atropine.
PHENYLEPHRINE (Neo-Synephrine)	**Mild or Moderate Hypotension**: **IV**: 0.1-0.5 mg; repeat q10-15 min PRN. **IM, SC**: 2-5 mg (maximum: 10 mg); repeat q1-2h PRN. **Severe Hypotension/Shock (including drug-related hypotension)**: **IV**: 100-180 μg/min to raise blood pressure rapidly; then 40-60 μg/min when blood pressure is stabilized. **Paroxysmal Supraventricular Tachycardia**: **IV**: 0.5 mg over 20-30 sec initially (maximum: 1 mg); then 0.6-0.7 mg PRN.	Ampules: 10 mg/ml (1 ml)	**SIDE EFFECTS**: Palpitations, hypertension with headache, vomiting, tachycardia or reflex bradycardia, tingling, pallor, arrhythmias (rare). **CAUTIONS**: Exercise extreme caution in hyperthyroidism, bradycardia, partial heart block, atherosclerosis and in elderly patients. **RECOMMENDATIONS**: EKG monitoring when using in patients receiving digitalis, *beta*-blocking drugs, guanethidine and reserpine. **CONTRAINDICATIONS**: Ventricular tachycardia, hypersensitivity, severe hypertension.

Section 2: ANTIBIOTIC AGENTS
Table of Contents and Spectra of Activity

Lactam Antibiotics-Penicillins & Cephalosporins

Benzyl Penicillins and Related Agents

Benzyl Penicillins

Spirochetes: T. pallidum.
Gram positive rods: Clostridium species (including anaerobes), B. anthracis, Listeria monocytogenes.
Gram positive cocci: Streptococci, S. pneumoniae, non-beta-lactamase-producing staphylococci.
Gram negative cocci: N. gonorrhoeae, N. meningotidis.
Gram negative rods: Effectiveness variable against: E. coli, Salmonella species, Shigella species, Fusobacterium species, H. influenzae, Streptobacilus moniliformis, Enterobacter species.
Other organisms: Actinomyces bovis.
***Note*:** All are excreted (and concentrated) in the urine.

Cephalosporins Equivalent to Benzyl Penicillins

Spectrum of activity equivalent to benzyl penicillins with the addition of increased coverage of staphylococcal organisms. All are excreted (and concentrated) in the urine.

Effective for streptococcus faecalis (urinary tract infections only).

Useful vs. B-Lactamase Staphylococci

Penicillins

Spectrum of activity equivalent to benzyl penicillins, but less active. Reserve for use against "resistant" (lactamase-producing) staphylococci.

Cephalosporins

Spectrum of activity equivalent to benzyl penicillins with the addition of increased coverage of staphylococcal organisms. All are excreted (and concentrated) in the urine.

Gram Positive & Some Gram Negative Coverage

Useful Against Hemophilus Influenzae

"1st Generation" Cephalosporins

Gram positive rods: Clostridium species.
Gram positive cocci: Streptococci, Staphylococci, S. pneumoniae
Gram negative cocci: N. gonorrhoeae, N. meningitidis.
Gram negative rods: Effectiveness variable against: E. coli, H. influenzae, Klebsiella species, Proteus mirabilis, Enterobacter species, Bacteroides fragilis, Salmonella, Shigella .
***Note*:** Generally similar to the benzyl penicillins, but with greater activity (lower inhibitory concentration) against Gram negative rods and H. influenzae.

Penicillins (Semi-Synthetic)

Gram positive rods: Clostridium species.
Gram positive cocci: S. pneumoniae, non-penicillinase-producing staphylococci, Streptococci, Streptococcus faecalis (except cyclacillin), N. meningitidis.
Gram negative cocci: N. gonorrhoeae (except cyclacillin).
Gram negative rods: E. coli, H. influenzae, Proteus mirabilis,

Salmonella, Shigella.
Note: Generally similar to the benzyl penicillins, but with greater activity (lower inhibitory concentration) against Gram negative rods and H. influenzae.

AMOXICILLIN........52
Amoxil, Larotid, Polymox, Trimox

AMPICILLIN........53
Omnipen, Penbritin, Polycillin, Polycillin-N, Principen
Also: Bacillus anthracis, Listeria monocytogenes species.

BACAMPICILLIN........53
Spectrobid
Also: Streptococci

CYCLACILLIN........53
Cyclapen
ONLY effective against E. coli and Proteus mirabilis in urinary tract.

HETACILLIN........54
Versapen, Versapen K
Also: Bacillus anthracis, Listeria monocytogenes.

Useful vs. ß-Lactamase-Producing N. gonorrhoeae

Generally similar to the benzyl penicillins, but with greater activity (lower inhibitory concentration) against Gram negative rods and H. influenzae. Also active against lactamase-producing N. gonorrhoeae.

CEFOXITIN........54
Mefoxin

CEFONICID........55
Monocid

CEFOTAXIME
Claforan
(See section: Lactams; Gram Positive & Some Gram Negative Coverage; Useful vs. H. influenzae; "1st Generation Cephalosporins)

CEFUROXIME
Zinacef
(See section: Lactams; Gram Positive & Some Gram Negative Coverage; Useful vs. H. influenzae; "1st Generation Cephalosporins)

Ineffective vs. ß-Lactamase Producing N. Gonorrhoeae

Generally similar to the benzyl penicillins, including minimal activity against beta-lactamase-producing N. gonorrhoeae.

CEFACLOR........56
Ceclor

CEFOPERAZONE........56
Cefobid

CEFORANIDE........56
Precef

CEFAMANDOLE
Mandol
(See section: Lactams; Gram Positive & Some Gram Negative Coverage; Useful vs. H. influenzae; "1st Generation Cephalosporins)

MOXALACTAM
Moxam
(See section: Lactams; Extended Gram Negative & Other Coverage; Effective in Meningitis; Some Activity vs. P. aeruginosa)

Extended Gram Negative & Other Coverage

The semi-synthetic penicillins and cephalosporins listed below are used against serious Gram negative and mixed infections, often in combination with aminoglycosides. Based on clinical effectiveness and penetration into the CNS, they are divided into those effective and those ineffective in meningitis. They are further subdivided according to their relative activity against pseudomonas. Differences in uses are summarized in the following chart:

	Effective in Meningitis	Active vs. P. aeruginosa
MOXALACTAM (Moxam)	+	+
CEFOPERAZONE (Cefobid)	+	+
CEFOTAXIME (Claforan)	+	+
CEFTRIAXONE (Rocephin)	+	+/-, -
CEFUROXIME (Zinacef)	+	-
CEFTAZIDIME (Fortaz)	-	+
CEFSULODIN (Cefomonil)	-	+
PIPERACILLIN (Pipracil)	-	+
AZLOCILLIN (Azlin)	-	+
CEFTIZOXIME (Cefizox)	-	+
CARBENICILLIN (Pyopen, Geocillin)	-	+/- , -
MEZLOCILLIN (Mezlin)	-	+/- , -
TICARCILLIN (Ticar)	-	+/- , -

Effective in Meningitis

Effective in Meningitis and Some Activity vs. P. aeruginosa

MOXALACTAM........57
Moxam

CEFOPERAZONE
Cefobid
(See section: Lactams; Gram Negative & Some Gram Positive Coverage; Ineffective vs. ß-Lactamase Producing N. gonorrhoeae)

Sulfonamides and Urinary Tract Agents

Spectrum of action includes Gram positive and Gram negative bacteria, Nocardia, Chlamydia trachomatis and some protozoa. NOT Pseudomonas, Serratia or most Proteus. Used with other agents for: T. gondii, P. falciparum and H. influenza. Used in first urinary tract infections, nocardiosis, and toxoplasmosis. Often effective in urinary tract infections due to E. coli, P. mirabilis, P. vulgaris, S. aureus and Klebsiella-Enterobacter.

Related Agents

Gram positive: most cocci.
Gram negative: ampicillin-resistant H. influenzae, chloramphenicol-resistant S. typhi, Ps. pseudomallei; variable against Shigella dysenteriae.
Other: Mycobacterium marinum, Nocardia asteroides, Pneumocystis carinii.

Indications in Addition to Urinary Tract Infections

Gram positive: Most Streptococcus pneumoniae, Staphylococcus aureus, Streptococcus pyogenes, Nocardia.
Gram negative: Most Enterobacteriaceae (including Acinetobacter, Enterobacter, E. coli, Klebsiella pneumoniae, P. mirabilis, Salmonella, Shigella), H. influenzae, H. ducreyi, N. gonorrhoeae, 70% of indole-positive proteus, 50% providencia and Serratia.
Anaerobes: Most Bacteroides.
Protozoa: Pneumocystis carinii.

Non-Sulfonamide Urinary Tract Agents

Gram negative: E. coli, Proteus vulgaris and P. mirabilis, Klebsiella species, Enterobacter, Serratia species.

Gram negative: E. coli, Proteus species (mirabilis, vulgaris, rettgeri-including indole-positive forms), Morganella morganii, Pseudomonas species, Enterobacter and enterococci.

Gram positive: Strptococcus faecalis, Staphylococcus aureus, S. epidermidis.
Gram negative: E. coli, Klebsiella, Proteus, Pseudomonas aeruginosa.

Gram negative: E. coli, Proteus species (mirabilis and indole-positive forms), Klebsiella, some strains of Salmonella and Shigella, Enterobacter and the majority of Enterobacteriaceae species.

Gram positive: Staphylococcus aureus, S. epidermidis, Streptococcus faecalis.
Gram negative: Citrobacter, Corynebacterium, Enterobacter, E. coli, Klebsiella, Neisseria, Salmonella and Shigella.

Miscellaneous Antibacterial Agents

Gram positive: Staphylococci, Streptococci, Bacillus anthracis, Corynebacterium species, Clostridium species, Erysipelothrix species, and Listeria monocytogenes.
Gram negative: Neisseria species, some strains of H. influenzae, Legionella pneumophila, Pasteurella, Brucella and Bordetella pertussis.
Others: Chlamydiae and Actinomyces species, Mycoplasma pneumoniae, rickettsiae, treponema, trachoma, and lymphogranuloma inguinale.

Infrequently Used Miscellaneous Agents

CLINDAMYCIN 75

Cleocin

Gram positive: Staphylococci, Streptococci, Corynebacterium diphtheriae, Nocardia asteroides, some N. gonorrheae.
Gram negative: Some H. influenzae.

LINCOMYCIN 75

Lincocin

Same as Clindamycin.

VANCOMYCIN 75

Vancocin

Gram positive: Staphylococci, Group A ß-hemolytic Streptococci, Pneumococci, Enterococci, Corynebacteria, and Clostridia.

METRONIDAZOLE 76

Flagyl

Gram positive: Clostridium, peptococcus, and peptostreptococcus.
Gram negative: Bacteroides, Fusobacterium, Veillonella, Gardnerella vaginalis and Campylobacter fetus.
Others: Entamoeba histolytica, Trichomonas vaginalis, Giardia lamblia, and Balantidium coli.

CHLORAMPHENICOL 77

Chloromycetin

Gram positive: Streptococcus pneumoniae and many others.
Gram negative: Salmonella, H. influenzae and Neisseria species.
Others: Rickettsia, Vibrio cholera, Chlamydia and Mycoplasma.

Polymyxins

Gram negative: Acinetobacter, Citrobacter, E. coli, Enterobacter, H. influenzae, Klebsiella pneumoniae, P. aeruginosa, Salmonella, Shigella, and some strains of Bordetella and Vibrio.

COLISTIMETHATE 78

Coly-Mycin M

COLISTIN 78

Coly-Mycin S

POLYMYXIN B 78

Aerosporin

Antituberculous and Related Agents

Agents of First Choice

ISONIAZID 79

Laniazid, Niconyl, Nydrazid, Teebaconin

Mycobacterium: M. tuberculosis, M. bovis, some strains of M. kansasii.

ETHAMBUTOL 79

Myambutol

Myobacterium: M. tuberculosis, M. bovis, M. marinum, some M. kansasii, M. acium, M. fortuitum, M. intracellulare.

RIFAMPIN 80

Rifadin, Rifocin, Rimactane

Mycobacterium: M. tuberculosis, M. bovis, M. marinum, M. kansasii, some strains of M. fortuitum, M. avium, M. intracellulare, M. leprae.
Gram positive: Staphylococcus aureus.
Gram negative: Neisseria, H. influenzae, Legionella pneumophila.

STREPTOMYCIN

Strycin

See section: Aminoglycosides and Related Agents.

Second Line Agents

PYRAZINAMIDE (PZA) 80

Aldinamide

Mycobacterium: Mycobacterium tuberculosis.

CAPREOMYCIN 81

Capastat sulfate

Mycobacterium: M. tuberculosis, M. bovis, M. kansasii, some M. avium and M. intracellulare.

ETHIONAMIDE 81

Trecator SC

Mycobacterium: M. tuberculosis, M. bovis, M. kansasii some strains of M. avium and M. intracellulare

AMINOSALICYLIC ACID 82

p-aminosalicylic acid, PAS, Pamisyl, Parasal, Teebacin

Mycobacterium: M. tuberculosis.

CYCLOSERINE 82

Seromycin

Gram positive: Staphylococcus aureus.
Gram negative: Enterobacter, Escherichia coli.
Mycobacterium: M. tuberculosis, M. bovis, some M. kansasii, M. marinum, M. ulcerans, M. avium, M. smegmatis, and M. intracellulare.

Antifungal Agents

AMPHOTERICIN B 83

Fungizone, Mysteclin-F

Fungi: Aspergillus fumigatus, Paracoccidioides brasiliensis, Coccidioides immitis, Cryptococcus neoformans, Histoplasma capsulatum, Mucor mucedo, Rhodotorula species, Sporothrix schenckii,

Antiviral Agents

Effective against: HSV-1 and HSV-2, varicella-zostervirus, Epstein-Barr virus, herpesvirus simiae, cytomegalovirus.

Effective against: several strains of influenza A.

Effective against: HSV-1 and HSV-2, varicella-zoster, cytomegalovirus, vaccinia, hepatitis B virus, Epstein-Barr virus, various animal DNA viruses, rhabdoviruses, oncornaviruses.

LACTAM ANTIBIOTICS: PENICILLINS AND CEPHALOSPORINS

PENICILLIN GROUP REMARKS:
Penicillins are bacteriocidal antibiotics active against many Gram positive and some Gram negative bacteria. Most penicillins contain the ß-lactam ring which is responsible for many of their unique properties. Cleavage of this ring causes complete loss of antibacterial activity. For this presentation, cephalosporins and penicillins are organized in three ways: by overall spectrum of activity, by effectiveness against specific important pathogens and by effectiveness in specific disease states. The term "penicillin" refers to natural penicillins and semi-synthetics.

HYPERSENSITIVITY REACTIONS: Between 1% and 10% of patients are allergic to penicillins; following injection, anaphylaxis occurs in 0.01-0.05%, with fatal shock in 0.002% of all patients. Fever and eosinophilia may be the only manifestations of hypersensitivity; other common reactions include: utricaria, pruritus, rash (maculopapular, erythematous, or morbilliform), chills, serum sickness-like reactions, bronchospasm, joint pain, Arthus reactions, edema, erythema, angioedema, and exfoliative dermatitis. Very rarely: Stevens-Johnson syndrome, erythema nodosum, and purpuric or vesiculobullous eruptions.

SIDE EFFECTS: **GI effects** most common: nausea, vomiting, diarrhea; also black hairy tongue and colitis **Hematologic effects**: Neutropenia, eosinophilia, leukopenia, thrombocytopenia, thrombocytopenic purpura, agranulocytosis, granulocytopenia and hemolytic anemia. Penicillins prolong bleeding/prothrombin times and interfere with hemostasis via hypokalemia and platelet dysfunction. Coagulation abnormalities and clinical bleeding are more common with: ticarcillin, carbenicillin, mezlocillin, piperacillin, azlocillin and nafcillin. **Renal effects**: Acute interstitial nephritis (characterized by hematuria, albuminuria and oliguria) has occurred with all penicillins. These reactions are allergic and are usually associated with fever, skin rash and eosinophilia. Acute glomerulonephritis, encarteritis, acute tubular necrosis, and elevations of creatinine or BUN have rarely been reported. **CNS effects**: Most common: headache, dizziness, giddiness, fatigue, and prolonged muscle relaxation. Neurotoxicity (lethargy, neuromuscular irritability, hallucinations, convulsions, hyperreflexia, myoclonus, asterixis, and seizures) may occur with transient high serum levels following large IV doses (especially in patients with renal failure). **Miscellaneous**: Hyperkalemia (possibly fatal) may occur during continuous high dose IV therapy (10-100 million units/d) with potassium Pen G, especially in pre-existing renal impairment; signs include hyperreflexia, convulsion, coma, and cardiac arrhythmias. High doses of sodium salts of penicillins may produce/worsen CHF.

Continued, next page

CEPHALOSPORIN GROUP REMARKS:
Cephalosporins are bacteriocidal antibiotics active against many Gram positive and some Gram negative bacteria. Cephalosporins contain a ß-lactam or equivalent ring. Cleavage of this ring causes complete loss of antibacterial activity. For this presentation, cephalosporins and penicillins are organized in three ways: by overall spectrum of activity, by effectiveness against specific important pathogens and by effectiveness in specific disease states. The term "cephalosporin" is used to refer to cephalosporins, cephamycins and 1-oxa-ß-lactams. Cephalosporins are only stable for a short time in solution.

HYPERSENSITIVITY REACTIONS: Approximately 5% of patients are allergic to cephalosporins; of these, 5-15% are cross-reactive to penicillins. Most common hypersensitivity reactions: utricaria, pruritus, rash (maculopapular, erythematous, or morbilliform), fever and chills, serum sickness-like reactions, bronchospasm, eosinophilia, joint pain, edema, erythema, angioedema, and exfoliative dermatitis. Hypersensitivity reactions occur most frequently in patients with a history of allergy, particularly to penicillins. Anaphylaxis has occurred rarely.

SIDE EFFECTS: **GI effects**: Most common (33% patients following PO, 23% following parenteral dosing): nausea, vomiting, diarrhea; also anorexia, abdominal pain/upset, altered taste and colitis. **Hematologic effects**: Non-immunologic positive direct and indirect Coomb's tests occur in 3% patients, most commonly with high doses in the presence of hypoalbuminemia/renal failure. Other hematologic effects include: neutropenia, leukopenia, thrombocytopenia, agranulocytosis, granulocytopenia and hemolytic anemia. Neutropenia is more common with prolonged high doses and may require discontinuance. Cephalosporins prolong bleeding/prothrombin times and interfere with hemostasis via hypoprothrombinemia, platelet dysfunction or immune thrombocytopenia (rarely). Coagulation abnormalities and clinical bleeding are more common with: moxalactam, cefaperazone, cefalothin, cefamandole. **Renal effects**: Transient increases in BUN and serum creatinine occur; pyuria, dysuria and hematuria occur less frequently. Renal toxicity is more likely in elderly patients or those with pre-existing renal impairment or receiving other nephrotoxic agents. Acute renal failure is rare. **CNS effects**: Most common: dizziness, headache, malaise, fatigue and vertigo. Rare: paranoid reactions (especially in patients with renal impairment receiving cephalexin or cephalothin). Large intrathecal doses have produced hallucinations, nystagmus and seizures. **Local effects**: IM administration (especially cephalothin and cefoxitin) causes pain, induration, tenderness, and tissue sloughing. Accidental SC administration may produce a sterile abcess. **Miscellaneous**: hypotension, fever, dyspnea and interstitial pneumonitis.

Continued, next page

LACTAM ANTIBIOTICS: PENICILLINS AND CEPHALOSPORINS *Continued*

PENICILLIN GROUP REMARKS Continued

PREGNANCY: Penicillins are Category B agents; they cross the placenta and are excreted in breast milk in small quantities.

RECOMMENDATIONS: In streptococcal infections, continue treatment for at least 10d to avoid late sequelae. Periodically monitor LFTs, BUN, creatinine and CBC during extended therapy with penicillinase-resistent penicillins.

CAUTIONS: Use with caution in patients with history of any allergies (especially to drugs); avoid if allergy is to cephalosporins. Use cautiously when renal impairment is present or suspected; perform periodic observation and monitoring prior to and during therapy. Reduce daily dose in patients with transient or persistent reduction of urinary output due to renal insufficiency; elevated serum levels can occur from usual doses. Bacterial or fungal superinfections can occur with prolonged or repeated courses of therapy. Jarisch-Herxheimer reactions (fever/chills, muscle aches, leukocytosis, skin lesions) have been reported during the treatment of syphilis. Some preparations contain tartrazine dye (potential for allergic reactions, esp. in patients hypersensitive to aspirin).

CONTRAINDICATIONS: Penicillins are contraindicated in any patient with a history of severe hypersensitivity reactions to any penicillin.

DRUG INTERACTIONS:

Probenecid increases serum levels of penicillins via interference with tubular secretion. ***Salicylates*** and ***indomethacin*** increase the half-life of the penicillins.

CEPHALOSPORIN GROUP REMARKS Continued

PREGNANCY: Usage in pregnancy: Cephalosporins are Category B agents (Moxalactam is Category C). They cross the placenta are excreted in breast milk in small quantities. Cephalosporin pharmacokinetics change in the pregnant woman: half-lives shorten and serum levels decrease.

RECOMMENDATIONS: Most manufacturers recommend periodic assessment of renal, hepatic and hematopoietic systems during extended or high dose therapy. IM injections should be administered deep within the muscle to avoid local inflammatory reactions. In streptococcal infections, continue treatment for at least 10d to avoid late sequelae.

CAUTIONS: Use with caution in patients with histories of any allergies (especially to drugs); avoid, if possible, if allergy is to penicillins. Use cautiously when renal function impaired or in the elderly and other patients with suspected renal impairment; periodic observation and monitoring prior to and during therapy. Reduce daily dose in patients with transient or persistent reduction of urinary output due to renal insufficiency; elevated serum levels can occur from usual doses. Bacterial or fungal superinfections can occur with prolonged or repeated courses of therapy.

CONTRAINDICATIONS: Cephalosporins are contraindicated in any patient with a history of severe hypersensitivity reactions to any cephalosporin.

DRUG INTERACTIONS:

Probenecid increases serum levels of cephalosporins via interference with tubular secretion. Additive nephrotoxicity may occur with ***colistin, vancomycin, polymyxin B*** and ***aminoglycosides***.

LAB INTERACTIONS:

False-positives for urine glucose may occur with all procedures, EXCEPT enzyme-based (Clinistix, Tes-Tape) tests; moxalactam does NOT interfere with Clinitest. False-positives for proteinuria with acid precipitation tests. Cephalosporins may falsely elevate urinary 17-ketosteroid values.

BENZYL PENICILLINS

SPECTRUM OF ACTIVITY - BENZYL PENICILLINS:
Spirochetes: T. pallidum and organisms of yaws and pinta.
Gram positive rods: Clostridium species (including anaerobes), B. anthracis, Listeria monocytogenes.
Gram positive cocci: Streptococci, S. pneumoniae, non-ß-lactamase-producing staphylococci.
Gram negative cocci: N. gonorrhoeae, N. meningococci.
Gram negative rods: Effectiveness variable (often minimal) against: E. coli, Salmonella species, Shigella species, Fusobacterium species, H. influenzae, Streptobacilus moniliformis, Enterobacter species.
Other organisms: Actinomyces bovis.
Note: All are excreted (and concentrated) in the urine and are therefore especially effective in urinary tract infections.

BENZYL PENICILLINS *Continued*

DRUG	INDICATIONS & DOSAGE	DOSE FORMS	REMARKS
PENICILLIN G (Penicillin G Sodium) (Penicillin G Potassium)	**Mild Infections**: **PO**: 250 mg (400,000 units) qid. **Pediatric PO**: 25,000 -100,000 units/kg/d in 4-6 doses. **Serious Infections** : **IM, IV**: 6-24 million units/d. **Pediatric IV**: 100,000-500,000 units/kg/d in 6-12 doses. **Rheumatic Fever-Prophylaxis**: **PO**: 200,000-250,000 units bid. **Bacterial Endocarditis Prophylaxis**: **(dental procedures)**: **IM**: 1 million units Pcn G (pediatric-30,000 units/kg) plus 600,000 units Pcn G Procaine (pediatric-600,000 units) 30-60min prior to procedure, then PO: 500 mg Pcn V (pediatric-250mg), q6h for 8 doses.	PO (Tab's): 100,000; 200,000 (125 mg); 250,000; 400,000 (250 mg); 500,000; 800,000 units. **(genitourinary procedures)**: **IM, IV**: 2 million units Pcn G (pediatric-30,000 units/kg); plus gentamycin, 1.5 mg/kg (pediatric-2mg/kg) or IM streptomycin, 1 gm (pediatric-20mg/kg) 30-60min prior to procedure; repeat q8h for gentamycin or q12h for strptomycin.	NOTES: Contains approximately 1.7 mEq Na^+ or K^+ per 1 million units.
PENICILLIN V (Phenoxymethyl penicillin) **Acid**: (Pen-Vee) (V-Cillin) **K+ salt**: (Penicillin VK) (Pen-Vee K) (V-Cillin-K) Various others	**Mild Infections**: **PO**: 125- 500 mg q6h. **Rheumatic Fever (prophylaxis)**: **PO**: 125 mg bid. **Pediatric PO**: 15-60 mg/kg/d as 3-6 doses. **Bacterial Endocarditis Prophylaxis (GU or dental procedures)**: Same as Pcn G Na^+ or K^+ (250 mg = 400,000 units).	PO (Tab's): 125, 250, 500 mg. PO (Liquid): 125 mg/0.6 ml, 125 mg/5 ml, 250 mg/5 ml	Penicillin Group Remarks. More resistant to gastric acid inactivation than Pcn G; absorption more reliable, serum levels higher and may be given with meals. Pcn VK absorbed mainly from the stomach; Pcn V absorbed mainly from the small intestine. Enterococci, Haemophilus influenzae, and N. meningitidis require relatively high concentrations of Pcn V for inhibition. 250 mg is equivalent to 400,000 units of the antibiotic. **CAUTIONS**: Potassium content: 0.7 mEq K^+/250 mg of Pcn VK (caution with renal failure).
PENICILLIN G PROCAINE (Crysticillin) (Wycillin)	**General Infections**: **IM**: 600,000-1.2 million units/d as1-2 doses. **Pediatric IM**: 100,000-600,000 units/d as1-2 doses. **Uncomplicated Gonorrhea**: **IM** (women): 4.8 million units (split at 2 sites); 1 gm of probenecid PO 30 min prior to injection. **Bacterial Endocarditis Prophylaxis (GU or dental procedures)**: Same as Pcn G Na^+ or K^+.		ONLY for IM use. Slow release form of Pcn providing sustained levels for 2-4d. Clinical use should be limited to mild infections caused by organisms very susceptible to Pcn G procaine. **SIDE EFFECTS**: Penicillin Group Remarks. Also, sterile abscesses at injection site and CNS stimulation, seizures, myocardial depression, conduction disturbances, systemic vasodilation. **CONTRA-INDICATIONS**: History of procaine or penicillin hypersensitivity.

BENZYL PENICILLINS *Continued*

DRUG	INDICATIONS & DOSAGE	DOSE FORMS	REMARKS
BENZATHINE PENICILLIN G (Bicillin) (Permapen)	**Minor Infections**: **PO**: 400,000-600,000 units q4-6h. **Pediatric PO**: 25,000-90,000 units/kg/d in 3-6 doses. **Group A Streptococcal Infections**: **IM**: 1.2 million units (single dose). **Pediatric IM**: 900,000 units (BW > 27 kg) as a single dose; 300,000-600,000 units (BW < 27 kg) as a single dose. **ß-hemolytic Steptococcal Prophylaxis**: **PO**: 200,000 units bid **IM**: 1.2 million units/month or 600,000 units q2wk. **Syphilis (acute)**: **IM**: 2.4 million units (single dose). **Neurosyphilis/Syphilis (latent)**: **IM**: 2.4-3 million units/wk for 3 wks.	PO (Tab's): 200,000 units Deep IM Injection: 300,000; 600,000 units **Yaws, Pinta or Bejel**: **IM**: 1.2 million units (single dose). **C. Diptheriae Prophylaxis**: **IM**: 600,000 units (single dose). **IM (< 6 y.o.)**: 600,000 units (single dose).	Slowly released form providing sustained levels for 2-4 weeks; dosage increase prolongs action but does not yield higher peak levels. Use only for organisms highly susceptible to Pcn G. For IM use, use tissue depot form-single 600,000 unit dose maintains therapeutic levels for 4-5 d. **CAUTION**: Benzathine Pcn G crystals can precipitate and cause vascular occlusion.

CEPHALOSPORINS EQUIVALENT TO BENZYL PENICILLINS

SPECTRUM OF ACTIVITY - CEPHALOSPORINS EQUIVALENT TO BENZYL PENICILLINS:
Gram positive rods: Clostridium species (including anaerobes).
Gram positive cocci: Peptococci, Peptostreptococci, Streptococci, S. pneumoniae, non-ß-lactamase-producing staphylococci.
Gram negative cocci: N. gonorrhoeae, N. meningitidis.
Gram negative rods: Effectiveness variable against: E. coli, Salmonella species, Shigella species, H. influenzae, Klebsiella species, Proteus mirabilis.
Note: Spectrum of activity equivalent to the benzyl penicillins with the addition of increased coverage of staphylococcal oraganisms. All are excreted (and concentrated) in the urine and are therefore especially effective in urinary tract infections.

DRUG	INDICATIONS & DOSAGE	DOSE FORMS	REMARKS
CEFACLOR (Ceclor)	**General Infections**: **PO**: 250-500 mg q8h; maximum 4 gm/d. **Pediatric Infections**: **Minor**: 20 mg/kg/d in 3 doses. **Severe**: 40 mg/kg/d in 3 doses; maximum 1 gm/d.	PO (Cap's): 250, 500 mg PO (Liquid): 25, 50 mg/ml	Cephalosporin Group Remarks. Mainly excreted in the urine. Food in stomach delays absorption. More active than cephalexin against H. influenzae. **SIDE EFFECTS**: Nausea is prominent.
CEPHALEXIN (Keflex)	**General Infections**: **PO**: 250-500 mg in 2-4 doses; maximum 4 gm/d. **Pediatric PO**: 25-100 mg/kg/d in 4 doses.	PO (Tab's): 1 gm PO (Cap's): 250, 500 mg PO (Liquid): 25, 50 mg/ml Pediatric Drops: 100 mg/ml	Cephalosporin Group Remarks. Excreted via the kidneys. False-positive test for urinary reducing substances. **RECOMMEND**: Reduce dose or increase dosage interval if creatinine clearance < 40 cc/min.

CEPHALOSPORINS EQUIVALENT TO BENZYL PENICILLINS *Continued*

DRUG	INDICATIONS & DOSAGE	DOSE FORMS	REMARKS
CEPHRADINE (Velosef) (Anspor)	<u>**Infections**</u>: **PO**: 250 mg q6h or 500 mg q12h (Minor); 500 mg-1 gm q12h (Severe). **IM, IV**: 2-4 gm qid; maximum 8 gm/d. **Pediatric PO**: 25-50 mg/kg/d in 2-4 doses (maximum 4 gm/d). **Pediatric IV, IM**: 50-100 mg/kg/d as 4 doses. <u>**Surgical Prophylaxis**</u>: **IM, IV**: 1 gm 30-90 min before surgery; repeat q4-6h for 2 doses.	PO (Cap's): 250, 500 mg PO (Tab's): 1.0 gm PO (Liquid): 25, 50 mg/ml	Cephalosporin Group Remarks. 6 mEq of Na+/gm cephradine; may cause fluid overload. Use for S. fecalis ONLY in urinary tract infections. **SIDE EFFECTS**: Occasional tightness of the chest and paresthesias. - - - - - - - - - - ***Note***: In addition to Group Spectrum of Activity: Effective for streptococcus faecalis (urinary tract infections only).
CEFADROXIL (Duricef) (Ultracef)	<u>**Urinary Tract Infections**</u>: **PO**: 1-2 gm/d in 1-2 doses. <u>**Skin**</u>: **PO**: 1 gm/d in 1-2 doses. <u>**Pharyngitis, Tonsillitis (ß-hemolytic streptococci)**</u>: **PO**: 0.5 gm bid for 10d. <u>**Pediatric Infections**</u>: **PO**: 15 mg/kg bid.	PO (Cap's): 500 mg PO (Tab's): 1000 mg PO (Liquid): 25, 50, 100 mg/ml	Cephalosporin Group Remarks. Dosage in renal impairment: PO: 1 gm initially; 500 mg maintenance (q12h if creat. clearance = 25-50 cc/min, q24h if 10-25 cc/ min, q36h if ≤ 10 cc/min). **RECOMMEND**: Administer with meals to minimize GI effects. Monitor renal patients closely.

AGENTS USEFUL vs. ß-LACTAMASE-PRODUCING STAPHYLOCOCCI

SPECTRUM OF ACTIVITY- AGENTS USEFUL vs. ß-LACTAMASE PRODUCING STAPHYLOCOCCI:
Gram positive cocci: S. pneumoniae, ß-lactamase-producing staphylococci, S. aureus, Beta-hemolytic streptococci (except Oxacillin).
Note: Methicillin-resistant staphylococci and 5-10% of staph epidermidis are resistant.

PENICILLINS

DRUG	INDICATIONS & DOSAGE	DOSE FORMS	REMARKS
CLOXACILLIN (Tegopen)	<u>**Infections**</u>: **PO**: 250-500 mg q6h. **Pediatric PO**: 50-100 mg/kg/d in 4 doses.	PO (Cap's): 250, 500 mg PO (Liquid): 25 mg/ml	Penicillin Group Remarks. Na+: capsules = 0.6 mEq/250 mg; oral sln =1.4 mEq/5 ml. **SIDE EFFECTS**: Penicillin Group Remarks.

AGENTS USEFUL vs. ß-LACTAMASE-PRODUCING STAPHYLOCOCCI: PENICILLINS *Continued*

DRUG	INDICATIONS & DOSAGE	DOSE FORMS	REMARKS
METHICILLIN (Azapen) (Celbenin) (Staphcillin)	<u>**Infections**</u>: **IM**: 1000 mg q4-6h. **IV**:1000 mg q6h. <u>**Pediatric (< 20 kg) Infections**</u>: **IM**: 25 mg/kg/d in 4 doses. **IV**: 200-300 mg/kg/d in 4 doses.	Injection: 1, 2, 4, 6, 10 gm (powder)	Penicillin Group Remarks. Na+: 2.9 mEq/gm. Some S. aureus and S. epidermidis are resistant to methicillin (usually when MIC > 12.5 µg/ml). **SIDE EFFECTS**: Interstitial nephritis with hematuria sometimes occurs 1-4 wk after starting therapy (≤ 17% patients with doses > 200 mg/kg/d or long term therapy); usually reversible with discontinuation. **RECOMMEND**: Manufacturer recommends periodic urinalysis, for interstitial nephritis, and frequent CBC, for marrow suppression; discontinue immediately if either occur. ***Note***: In addition to Group Spectrum of Activity: Effective for streptococci.
NAFCILLIN (Unipen)	<u>**Infections**</u>: **PO**: 250 mg-1 gm q4-6h. **IM**: 500 mg q4-6h. **IV**:3000-6000 mg/d in 6 doses. <u>**Pediatric Infections**</u>: **PO**: 50 mg/kg/d in 4 doses. **IM**: 50 mg/kg/d in 2 doses. **IV**: 150-200 mg/kg/d in 4-6 doses.	PO (Cap's): 250 mg PO (Tab's): 500 mg PO (Liquid): 50 mg/ml Injection: 500 mg, 1, 1.5, 2, 4, 10 gm (powder)	Penicillin Group Remarks. Na+: capsules = 0.6 mEq/250 mg; oral sln = 0.7 mEq/5 ml; IV sln = 2.9 mEq/gm. More resistant to acid inactivation than Pcn G, but irregular absorption. Serum levels of 0.06-1.9 µg/ml inhibit most strains of S. aureus. **SIDE EFFECTS**: Rare interstitial nephritis. **RECOMMEND**: Administer 1 h before or 2 h after meals. Periodic renal function tests during long-term therapy. ***Note***: In addition to Group Spectrum of Activity: Effective for streptococcus viridans.
DICLOXACILLIN (Dycil) (Dynapen) (Pathocil) (Veracillin)	<u>**Mild Infections**</u>: **PO**: 125-250 mg q6h. <u>**Pediatric (< 40 kg) Infections**</u>: **PO**: 12.5 mg/kg/d in 4 doses.	PO (Cap's): 125, 250, 500 mg PO (Liquid): 12.5 mg/ml	Penicillin Group Remarks. PO administration ONLY. Na+: capsules = 0.6 mEq/250 mg; oral sln = 1.1-3 mEq/5 ml. At 1 h: serum level = 5-9 µg/ml after 250 mg dose, 10-20 µg/ml after 500 mg dose. In vitro concentrations of 0.05-0.8 µg/ml inhibit most strains of S. aureus. **CAUTIONS**: Crosses placenta, safety in pregnancy and neonates NOT established. **CONTRAINDICATIONS**: NOT for use in neonates. NOT for severe, life-threatening infections.

AGENTS USEFUL vs. β-LACTAMASE PRODUCING STAPHYLOCOCCI: PENICILLINS *Continued*

DRUG	INDICATIONS & DOSAGE	DOSE FORMS	REMARKS
OXACILLIN (Bactocil) (Prostaphlin) (Resistopen)	**Infections**: **PO**: 500-1000 mg q4-6h for ≥ 5d. **IM, IV**: 250-500 mg q4-6h. **Pediatric (< 40 kg) Infections**: **PO**: 50-100 mg/kg/d in 4 doses. **IM, IV**: 50-100 mg/kg/d in 4-6 doses.	PO (Cap's): 250, 500 mg PO (Liquid): 50 mg/ml Injection: 0.25, 0.5, 1, 2, 4, 10 gm	Penicillin Group Remarks. Na+: capsules = 0.6 mEq/250 mg; oral sln = 0.9 mEq/5 ml; IV sln = 2.8-3.1 mEq/gm. In vitro, oxacillin = 0.4-6.3 µg/ml inhibits most S. aureus (including penicillinase-producing strains); however, some are resistant. S. pneumoniae and group A streptococci often inhibited at 0.06-0.25 µg/ml in vitro. **SIDE EFFECTS**: With IV use: hepatic dysfunction and transient renal dysfunction in neonates. **CAUTIONS**: Safe use in pregnancy NOT established. **RECOMMEND**: Administer 1 h before or 2 h after meals. Closely monitor renal function in neonates and infants. ***Note***: In addition to Group Spectrum of Activity: Effective for streptococci.

CEPHALOSPORINS

SPECTRUM OF ACTIVITY - CEPHALOSPORINS USEFUL vs. β-LACTAMASE-PRODUCING STAPHYLOCOCCI:
Gram positive rods: Clostridium species.
Gram positive cocci: Streptococci, S. pneumoniae, Staphylococci, Peptococci, Peptostreptococci.
Gram negative cocci: N. gonorrhoeae, N. meningitidis.
Gram negative rods: Effectiveness variable against: E. coli, Salmonella species, Shigella species, H. influenzae, Klebsiella species, Proteus mirabilis.
Note: Spectrum of activity equivalent to benzyl penicillins with the addition of increased coverage of staphylococcal organisms. All are excreted (and concentrated) in the urine and are therefore especially effective in urinary tract infections.

DRUG	INDICATIONS & DOSAGE	DOSE FORMS	REMARKS
CEFAZOLIN (Ancef) (Kefzol)	**Minor Infections**: **IM, IV**: 750-4000 mg/d in 3-4 doses. **Severe Infections**: **IM, IV**: 4000-6000 mg/d in 3-4 doses (maximum 12 gm/d). **Pediatric (> 1 mo) Infections**: **IM, IV**: 25-100 mg/kg/d in 3-4 doses. **Surgical Prophylaxis**: **IM, IV**: 1 gm 30-90 min before surgery; 500-1000 mg repeated q6-8h for 24h after surgery.	Injection: 250, 500 mg; 1, 5, 10 gm	Cephalosporin Group Remarks. **SIDE EFFECTS**: False positive tests for urine reducing substances. Na+ salt has 2 mEq Na+/gm. **CAUTIONS**: Protect from light. **Renal Impairment**: **IM, IV**: Full dose if creat. clearance ≥ 55 cc/min or if serum creat. ≤ 1.5 mg/dl. Full dose ≥ q8h if creat. clearance = 35-54 cc/min or if serum creat. = 1.6-3.0 mg/dl. Half dose ≥ q12h if creat. clearance = 11-34 cc/min or if serum creat. = 3.1-4.5 mgdl. Half dose q18-24h if creat. clearance ≤ 10 cc/min or if serum creat. ≥ 4.6 mg/dl.(Many other schemes proposed.)

AGENTS USEFUL vs. ß-LACTAMASE-PRODUCING STAPHYLOCOCCI: CEPHALOSPORINS *Continued*

DRUG	INDICATIONS & DOSAGE	DOSE FORMS	REMARKS
CEPHALOTHIN (Keflin) (Seffin)	**Infections**: **IM, IV**: 4-12 gm/d in 4-6 doses. **Pediatric Infections**: **IM, IV**: 80-160 mg/kg/d in 4-6 doses. **Surgical Prophylaxis**: **IV**: 1-2 gm 30-60 min before surgery; 1-2 gm q6hs for 24 h after surgery. **Renal Impairment**: **IV**: 1-2 gm initially; then 2 gm q6h if creat. clearance = 50-80 cc/min; 1.5 gm q6h if 25-50 cc/min; 1 gm q6h if 10-25 cc/min; 500 mg q6h if 2-10 cc/min; 500 mg q8h if < 2 cc/min.	Injection: 1, 2, 4, 20 gm (powder)	Cephalosporin Group Remarks. **SIDE EFFECTS**: Rare increase in prothrombin time (especially in elderly, debilitated or vitamin K-deficient patients). Cephalothin produces severe local reactions (especially phlebitis) more frequently than other cephalosporins. **RECOMMEND**: Administer via small needles in large veins to reduce the risk of phlebitis (and add 10-25 mg hydrocortisone to IV sln's containing 4-6 gm of cephalothin).
CEPHAPIRIN (Cefadyl)	**Infections**: **IM, IV**: 500 mg-1 gm q4-6 h; maximum 12 gm/d. **Pediatric Infections**: **IM, IV**: 40-80 mg/kg/d in 3-4 doses. **Surgical Prophylaxis**: **IM, IV**: 1-2 gm 30-60 min before surgery, 1-2 gm during surgery; then q6h for 24h after surgery. **Renal Impairment**: **IM, IV**: 7.5-15 mg/kg q12h if creat. clearance = 5-10 cc/min or serum creat. > 5 mg/dl; same for dialysis patients (administer immediately before dialysis and q12h thereafter).	Injection: 5, 1, 2, 4, 20 gm	Cephalosporin Group Remarks. Contains 2.36 mEq Na^+/gm. Usual doses sometimes acceptable if creat. clearance ≥ 10 cc/min; caution recommemded with oliguria. **CAUTIONS**: Should not be mixed with other antibiotics.

LACTAM ANTIBIOTICS: GRAM POSITIVE & SOME GRAM NEGATIVE COVERAGE

AGENTS USEFUL vs. H. INFLUENZAE

"1st GENERATION" CEPHALOSPORINS

SPECTRA OF ACTIVITY - "1st GENERATION" CEPHALOSPORINS USEFUL vs. H. INFLUENZAE:
Gram positive rods: Clostridium species.
Gram positive cocci: S. pneumoniae, Peptococci, Peptostreptococci, staphylococci
Gram negative cocci: N. gonorrhoeae, N. meningitidis.
Gram negative rods: Effectiveness variable against: E. coli, H. influenzae, Klebsiella species, Proteus mirabilis, Enterobacter species, Providencia rettgeri.
Note: Generally similar to the benzyl penicillins, but with greater activity (lower inhibitory concentration) against Gram negative rods and H. influenzae.

DRUG	INDICATIONS & DOSAGE	DOSE FORMS	REMARKS
CEFOTAXIME (Claforan)	**General Infections**: **IM, IV**: 1 gm q6-8h; maximum 12 gm/d. **Severe Infections**: **IV**: 2 gm q4-8h; maximum 12 gm/d. **Simple Gonococcal Infections**: **IM**: 1 gm (single dose). **Surgical Prophylaxis**: **IM, IV**: 1 gm 30-90min before surgery, repeat at 30-120min (additional intraoperative doses may be given); 1 gm within 2 h after surgery. **Cesarean Section**: **IV**: 1 gm as umbilical cord is clamped, repeat q6h for 2 doses. **Renal Impairment**: Reduce dosage by one-half if creat. clearances < 20 cc/min.	Injection: 0.5, 1, 2 gm **Pediatric (< 50 kg) Infections**: **IM, IV**: 50-180 mg/kg/d in 4-6 doses. **Neonate Infections**: **IV (age 0-1 wk)**: 50 mg/kg q12h. **IV (age 1-4 wk)**: 50 mg/kg q8h.	Use > 2h after surgery does not reduce the incidence of infections. Na+: 2.2-2.6 mEq/gm. **CAUTIONS**: Safe use in infants and children NOT established. **RECOMMEND**: Protect from light. ***Note***: In addition to Group Spectrum of Activity: Effective for Bacteroides fragilis, Serratia species and Proteus vulgaris.
CEFUROXIME (Zinacef) *Continued, next page*	**General Infections**: **IM, IV**: 750-1500 mg q8h for 5-10 d. **Pediatric IM, IV**: 50-100 mg/kg/d in 3-4 doses. **Simple Gonococcal Infections**: **IM**: 1.5 gm (single dose). *Continued, next page*	Injection: 0.75, 1.5 gm	Cephalosporin Group Remarks. Hypersensitivity reactions occur in 2% of patients. Na+: 2.4 mEq/gm. M. morgani, Citrobacter species sometimes resistant. **SIDE EFFECTS**: Positive direct Coomb's test. **RECOMMEND**: In children with renal impairment, decrease frequency of dosage per the adult recommendations. *Continued, next page*

LACTAM ANTIBIOTICS: "1st GENERATION" CEPHALOSPORINS USEFUL vs. H. INFLUENZAE *Continued*

DRUG	INDICATIONS & DOSAGE	DOSE FORMS	REMARKS
CEFUROXIME *Continued*	<u>**Surgical Prophylaxis**</u>: **IV**: 1500 mg 30-60 min before surgery, then 750 mg q8h intra-operatively. <u>**Open Heart Surgery**</u>: **IV**: 1500 mg during anesthesia, then q12h (maximum 6000 mg). <u>**Renal Impairment**</u>: **IM, IV**: 750 mg-1.5 gm q8h if creat. clearance > 20cc/min; 750 mg q12h if 10-20 cc/min; 750 mg q24h if < 10cc/min.	See previous page. <u>**Bacterial Meningitis**</u>: **IV**: 200-240 mg/kg/d initially in 3-4 doses; 100 mg/kg/d upon clinical improvement.	See previous page. - - - - - ***Note***: In addition to Group Spectrum of Activity: Effective for Fusobacterium species, Salmonella species, Shigella species, Providencia species and some Citrobacter species.
CEFAMANDOLE (Mandol)	<u>**General Infections**</u>: **IM, IV**: 500-1000 mg q4-8h. **Pediatric IM, IV**: 50-150 mg/kg/d in 3-6 doses. <u>**Severe Infections**</u>: **IM, IV**: 4-12 gm/d in 4-6 doses (maximum 2 gm/dose, 12 gm/d).	Injection: 0.5, 1, 2,10 gm	Cephalosporin Group Remarks. Na+: 3.3 mEq/gm. **SIDE EFFECTS**: Transient neutropenia, positive urine tests for reducing substances. - - - - - ***Note***: In addition to Group Spectrum of Activity: Effective for Fusobacterium species, Salmonella species, Shigella species, Providencia species and some Proteus vulgaris.

PENICILLINS

SPECTRA OF ACTIVITY - PENICILLINS USEFUL vs. H. INFLUENZAE:
Gram positive cocci: S. pneumoniae, non-penicillinase-producing staphylococci, beta-hemolytic streptococci, Streptococcus faecalis (except cyclacillin).
Gram negative cocci: N. gonorrhoeae (except cyclacillin).
Gram negative rods: E. coli, H. influenzae, Proteus mirabilis.
Note: Generally similar to the benzyl penicillins, but with greater activity (lower inhibitory concentration) against Gram negative rods and H. influenzae.

DRUG	INDICATIONS & DOSAGE	DOSE FORMS	REMARKS
AMOXICILLIN (Amoxil) (Larotid) (Polymox) (Trimox)	<u>**General Infections**</u>: **PO**: 250-500 mg q8h. **Pediatric PO**: 20-40 mg/kg/d in 3 doses.	PO (Cap's): 250, 500 mg PO (Tab's): 125, 250 mg PO (Liquid): 10, 25, 50 mg/ml Pediatric Drops: 50 mg/ml	Penicillin Group Remarks. Complete cross-resistance occurs between amoxicillin and ampicillin. In vitro, 0.01-1.0 µg/ml amoxicillin inhibits Gram positive cocci and Gram negative organisms including N. gonorrhoeae, N. meningitidis, and H. influenzae. - - - - - ***Note***: In addition to Group Spectrum of Activity: Effective for Streptococcus viridans.

LACTAM ANTIBIOTICS: PENICILLINS USEFUL vs. H. INFLUENZAE *Continued*

DRUG	INDICATIONS & DOSAGE	DOSE FORMS	REMARKS
AMPICILLIN (Omnipen) (Penbritin) (Polycillin) (Principen)	**General Infections**: **PO**: 250-500 mg q6h. **IM, IV**: 500 mg q6h. **Pediatric (< 40 kg) Infections**: **PO**: 50 mg/kg/d in 4 doses (maximum 250 mg/dose). **IM, IV**: 50 mg/kg/d in 4-6 doses. **Meningitis**: **IV**: 150-200 mg/kg/d in 6-8 doses. **Gonorrhea**: **PO**: 3500 mg, with 1 gm probenicid. **IM**: 500 mg q8-12h for 2 doses.	PO (Tab's): 125 mg PO (Cap's): 125, 250, 500 mg PO (Liquid): 20, 25, 50 mg/ml Injection: 125, 250, 500, 1000, 2000, 4000 mg (powder)	Penicillin Group Remarks. Resistant to acid; only 30-60% of PO dose absorbed. No advantage over Pcn G or V for infections by Gram positive organisms. Some strains of E. coli, Salmonella, and P. mirabilis are highly resistant. Contains approximately 3 mEq Na+/gm. **SIDE EFFECTS**: Non-allergic Rubella-like rash (especially common in patients receiving allopurinol or with infectious mononucleosis), pruritis, urticaria, abdominal discomfort, nausea, vomiting, eosinophilia, superinfection, overgrowth of bowel flora, diarrhea (usually mild). Very rarely: interstitial nephritis, crystalluria. **CAUTIONS**: Unlike other penicillins, causes dose-related rash. ***Note***: In addition to Group Spectrum of Action: Effective in Streptococci, Bacillus anthracis, Listeria monocytogenes, Salmonella species, Shigella species, Clostridium species, N. meningitidis.
BACAMPICILLIN (Spectrobid)	**General Infections**: **PO**: 400-800 mg q12h. **Pediatric PO**: 25-50 mg/kg/d in 2 doses.	PO (Tab's): 400 mg PO (Liquid): 25 mg/ml	Penicillin Group Remarks. Hydrolyzed to ampicillin in intestine; can be given q12h. ***Note***: In addition to Group Spectrum of Action: Effective in Streptococci.
CYCLACILLIN (Cyclapen)	**General Infections**: **PO**: 250-500 mg q6h. **Pediatric PO (> 20 kg)**: 250 mg q8h. **Pediatric PO (< 20 kg)**: 125 mg q8h. **Tonsillitis/Pharyngitis**: **PO**: 250 mg q6h. **Pediatric PO**: same as above. **Bronchitis/Pneumonia**: **PO**: 250 mg q6h (mild-moderate cases), 500 mg q6h (severe cases). **Pediatric PO**: 50 mg/kg/d (mild-moderate cases), 100 mg/kg/d q6h (severe cases). **Otitis Media/Skin Infections**: **PO**: 250-500 mg q6h. **Pediatric PO**: 50-100 mg/kg/d in 3-4 doses. **Genitourinary**: **PO**: 250-500 mg q6h. **Pediatric PO**: 100 mg/kg/d in 3-4 doses.	PO (Tab's): 250, 500 mg	Penicillin Group Remarks. Essentially identical to ampicillin but more completely absorbed and produces less diarrhea. **SIDE EFFECTS**: Elevated SGOT. ***Note***: In addition to Group Spectrum of Action: Effective only in E. coli and Proteus mirabilis urinary tract infections.

LACTAM ANTIBIOTICS: PENICILLINS USEFUL vs. H. INFLUENZAE *Continued*

DRUG	INDICATIONS & DOSAGE	DOSE FORMS	REMARKS
HETACILLIN (Veraspen) (Veraspen K)	<u>**General Infections**</u>: **PO**: 225-450 mg q6h. **Pediatric PO (< 40 kg)**: 22.5-45 mg/kg/d in 4 doses.	PO (Cap's): 225 mg PO (Liquid): 112.5 , 225 mg/5 ml Powder equivalent to: 112.5, 225 mg/5 ml PO (Cap's) [K+ salt]: equivalent to: 225 mg	Penicillin Group Remarks. Hetacillin is hydrolyzed to ampicillin in vivo; it is inactive until hydrolyzed. **SIDE EFFECTS**: Fewer GI problems than ampicillin. **CAUTIONS**: Possibility of superinfections with mycotic or bacterial pathogens. **RECOMMEND**: In very severe infections, initiate treatment with parenteral ampicillin. Periodically assess hepatic, hematopoietic and renal function when used long-term, especially in prematures, neonates, infants.
		Note: In addition to Group Spectrum of Action: Effective in Streptococci, Bacillus anthracis, Listeria monocytogenes, Salmonella species, Shigella species, Clostridium species, N. meningitidis.	

AGENTS USEFUL vs. ß-LACTAMASE PRODUCING N. GONORRHOEAE

SPECTRUM OF ACTIVITY - AGENTS USEFUL vs. ß-LACTAMASE-PRODUCING N. GONORRHOEAE:
Gram positive rods: Clostridium species (except cefonicid).
Gram positive cocci: S. pneumoniae, beta-hemolytic streptococci, Peptococci (except cefonicid), Peptostreptococci (except cefonicid), non-ß-lactamase-producing staphylococci.
Gram negative cocci: N. gonorrhoeae (except cefonicid), N. meningitidis (except cefonicid).
Gram negative rods: E. coli, H. influenzae, Klebsiella species, Proteus mirabilis, Providencia rettgeri (except cefonicid).
Other organisms: Morganella morganii (except cefonicid).
Note: Generally similar to the benzyl penicillins, but with greater activity (lower inhibitory concentration) against Gram negative rods and H. influenzae.

DRUG	INDICATIONS & DOSAGE	DOSE FORMS	REMARKS
CEFOXITIN (Mefoxin) *Continued, next page*	<u>**General Infections**</u>: **IM, IV**: 1 gm q6-8h. <u>**Moderate-Severe Infections**</u>: **IM, IV**: 1 gm q4-6h or 2-3 gm q6-8h (maximum 12 gm/d). **Pediatric IM, IV**: 80-160 mg/kg/d in 4-6 doses. <u>**Renal Impairment**</u>: **IM, IV**: 1-2 gm initially, then: 1-2 gm q8-12h if creat. clearance = 30-50 cc/min; 1-2 gm q12-24h if 10-29 cc/min; 0.5-1 gm q12-24h if 5-9 cc/min; 0.5-1 gm q24-48h if < 5 cc/min. <u>**Gonorrhea**</u>: **IM**: 2 gm with 1 gm PO probenecid given 30 min before injection.	Injection: 1, 2, 10 gm (powder) *Continued, next page*	Cephalosporin Group Remarks. Patients > 50 y.o. may be more susceptible to renal toxicity. Contains 2.3 mEq Na+/gm. Unlike most other cephalosporins, cefoxitin is active against many strains of B. fragilis. **SIDE EFFECTS**: Pain at the site of IM injections (reduced by reconstitution with 0.5-1% lidocaine solution). **CAUTIONS**: Benzyl alcohol used in IV solutions may cause toxicity in neonates. ***Note***: In addition to Group Spectrum of Action: Effective in Salmonella species, Shigella species, Proteus vulgaris and Providencia species.

LACTAM ANTIBIOTICS: AGENTS USEFUL vs. ß-LACTAMASE PRODUCING N. GONORRHOEAE *Continued*

DRUG	INDICATIONS & DOSAGE	DOSE FORMS	REMARKS
CEFOXITIN *Continued*	**Acute Pelvic Inflammatory Disease**: **IM**: 2 gm with 1 gm PO probenecid given 30 min before injection, plus doxycycline100 mg bid for 10-14 d. **Surgical Prophylaxis**: **IM, IV**: 2 gm 30-60min before surgery; then 2 gm q6h for 4 doses (12 doses after prosthetic joint implantation).	See previous page.	See previous page.
CEFONICID (Monocid)	**General Infections**: **IM, IV**: 1-2 gm/d. **Surgical Prophylaxis**: **IM, IV**: 1 gm 60min before surgery, then 1 gm/d for 2 d. **Renal Impairment**: **IM, IV**: 7.5 mg/kg initially; then 10-25 mg/kg q24h if creat. clearance = 60-79 cc/min; 8-20 mg/kg q24h if 40-59 cc/min; 4-15 mg/kg q24h if 20-39 cc/min; 4-15 q48h if 10-19cc/min; 4-15 mg/kg q3-5d if 5-9 cc/min; 3-4 mg/kg q3-5d if < 5 cc/min.	Injection: 1, 2, 10 gm (powder)	Cephalosporin Group Remarks. Contains 3.7 mEq Na+/gm. **RECOMMEND**: For IM injection use large muscle and < 1 gm per injection.
CEFOTAXIME (Claforan)	See section: Lactams; Gram Positive & Some Gram Negative Coverage; Useful vs. Hemophilus influenzae; "1st Generation" Cepahalosporins		
CEFUROXIME (Zinacef)	See section: Lactams; Gram Positive & Some Gram Negative Coverage; Useful vs. Hemophilus influenzae; "1st Generation" Cepahalosporins		

AGENTS INEFFECTIVE vs. ß-LACTAMASE-PRODUCING N. GONORRHOEAE

SPECTRUM OF ACTIVITY - AGENTS INEFFECTIVE vs. ß-LACTAMASE-PRODUCING N. GONORRHOEAE:
Gram positive rods: Clostridium species.
Gram positive cocci: S. pneumoniae, beta-hemolytic streptococci (except ceforanide), Peptococci, Peptostreptococci, non-beta-lactamase-producing staphylococci.
Gram negative cocci: Non-beta-lactamase-producing N. gonorrhoeae.
Gram negative rods: E. coli, H. influenzae, Klebsiella species, Proteus mirabilis (except moxalactam), Enterobacter species (except cefaclor), Providencia rettgeri (except cefaclor).
Note: Generally similar to the benzyl penicillins, but with minimal activity against ß-lactamase-producing N. gonorrhoeae.

LACTAM ANTIBIOTICS: AGENTS INEFFECTIVE vs. ß-LACTAMASE-PRODUCING N. GONORRHOEAE *Continued*

DRUG	INDICATIONS & DOSAGE	DOSE FORMS	REMARKS
CEFACLOR (Ceclor)	**General Infections**: **PO**: 250-500 mg q8h (maximum 4 gm/d). **Pediatric PO**: 20 mg/kg/d in 3 doses. **Severe Infections (Pneumonia, Otitis media)**: **Pediatric PO**: 40 mg/kg/d in 3 doses (maximum 1 gm/d).	PO (Cap's): 250, 500 mg PO (Liquid): 25, 50 mg/ml	Cephalosporin Group Remarks. Similar to cephalexin. ***Note***: In addition to Group Spectrum of Action: Effective in N. meningitidis, Salmonella species, Shigella species.
CEFOPERAZONE (Cefobid)	**General Infections**: **IM, IV**: 2-4 gm/d in 2 doses.	Injection: 1, 2 gm	Cephalosporin Group Remarks. Half-life is reduced slightly during hemodialysis. Contains 1.5 mEq Na+/gm. Resistance sometimes encountered in H. influenza, N. gonorrhoeae, P. aeruginosa, Acinetobacter species. **RECOMMEND**: In pre-existing hepatic dysfunction or renal impairment, dosage should NOT exceed 1-2 gm/d without monitoring serum concentration. ***Note***: In addition to Group Spectrum of Action: Effective in Morganella morganii, Proteus vulgaris, Citrobacter species, Serratia species, Bacteroides fragilis, Fusobacter species, Eubacterium species, some Pseudomonas aeruginosa.
CEFORANIDE (Precef)	**General Infections**: **IM, IV**: 500-1000 mg q12h. **Pediatric IM, IV**: 20-40 mg/kg/d in 2 doses. **Surgical Prophylaxis**: **IM, IV**:500-1000 mg 60 min prior to surgery, one time only (for prosthetic device implantation, follow with 500-1000 mg bid for 2 d after surgery). **Renal Impairment**: **IM, IV**: Vary dosage intervals: q12h if creat. clearance ≥ 60 cc/min; q24h if 20-59 cc/min; q48h if 5-19 cc/min; q48-72h if < 5cc/min.	Injection: 0.5, 1 gm	Cephalosporin Group Remarks. Similar to cephamandole, but less active vs. Staph. aureus. ***Note***: In addition to Group Spectrum of Action: Effective in Citrobacter species, Fusobacterium species.
CEFAMANDOLE (Mandol)	See section: Lactams; Gram Positive & Some Gram Negative Coverage; Useful vs. Hemophilus influenzae; "1st Generation" Cephalosporins		
MOXALACTAM (Moxam)	See section: Lactams; Extended Gram Negative & Other Coverage; Effective in Meningitis; Some Activity vs. P. aeruginosa		

LACTAM ANTIBIOTICS WITH EXTENDED GRAM NEGATIVE & OTHER COVERAGE

GROUP REMARKS ON SPECTRUM OF ACTIVITY:
The spectra of activities listed in this section detail the organisms that an individual agent is SIGNIFICANTLY active against. This section, Extended Gram Negative Agents, is divided into the clinical categories of Effective and Ineffective in meningitis (based on clinical effectiveness and penetration into the CNS). These clinical categories are subdivided into Active and Inactive against pseudomonas. When an agent is described as being "inactive against pseudomonas" what is meant is a RELATIVE inactivity when compared with agents considered to be "effective against pseudomonas". For example, any given strain of pseudomonas has unpredictable sensitivity against both carbenicillin and moxalactam; however, moxalactam is much more likely (statistically) to be active against that strain than is carbenicillin.

Differences of USES (not exact differences in sensitivities) can be summarized by the chart in the adjacent column:

	Effective in Meningitis	Active vs. P. aeruginosa
MOXALACTAM (Moxam)	+	+
CEFOPERAZONE (Cefobid)	+	+
CEFOTAXIME (Claforan)	+	+
CEFTRIAXONE (Rocephin)	+	+/-, -
CEFUROXIME (Zinacef)	+	-
CEFTAZIDIME (Fortaz)	-	+
CEFSULODIN (Cefomonil)	-	+
PIPERACILLIN (Pipracil)	-	+
AZLOCILLIN (Azlin)	-	+
CEFTIZOXIME (Cefizox)	-	+
CARBENICILLIN (Pyopen, Geocillin)	-	+/- , -
MEZLOCILLIN (Mezlin)	-	+/- , -
TICARCILLIN (Ticar)	-	+/- , -

DRUG	INDICATIONS & DOSAGE	DOSE FORMS	REMARKS

AGENTS EFFECTIVE IN MENINGITIS

SPECTRUM OF ACTIVITY-LACTAMS WITH EXTENDED GRAM NEGATIVE COVERAGE AND EFFECTIVE IN MENINGITIS:
Generally similar to the benzyl penicillins, but with greater activity in meningitis and variable activity against P. aeruginosa. Specific activities common to all agents in the "Effective in Meningitis" include:
Gram negative rods: E. coli, H. influenza, Klebsiella species, M. morgani, P. vulgaris, Enterobacter species, Serratia species.

AGENTS WITH SOME ACITIVITY vs. P. AERUGINOSA

DRUG	INDICATIONS & DOSAGE	DOSE FORMS	REMARKS
MOXALACTAM (Moxam) *Continued, next page.*	<u>General Infections</u>: **IM, IV**: 2-6 gm/d in 3 doses, for 5-14 d (maximum 4 gm q8h). **Pediatric IM, IV**: 50 mg/kg q6-8h (maximum 200 mg/kg/d); 100 mg/kg loading dose in Gram negative meningitis. **Neonate IM, IV**: 50 mg/kg q12h. <u>Renal Impairment</u>: **IM, IV**: 3 gm q8h if creat. clearance = 50-80 cc/min, q12h if 25-49 cc/min; 1.25 gm q12h if 2-24 cc/min; 1 gm q24h if < 2 cc/min.	Injection: 1, 2 gm	Restrict use to severe infections caused by bacteria resistant to other, safer agents. 3.8 mEq Na+/gm. **SIDE EFFECTS**: Cephalosporin Group Remarks. Disulfuram-like reactions can occur if alcohol ingested within 48 h of last dose. Life-threatening bleeding diatheses (2.5% of patients treated > 4 d). May interfere with platelet aggregation/coagulation and prolong prothrombin time. **RECOMMEND**: Administer < 4 gm/d to avoid platelet dysfunction. Add prophylactic vitamin K (10 mg/wk, parenterally), unless contraindicated. Monitor bleeding and prothrombin times q2d. If bleeding occurs: discontinue use; treat with fresh frozen plasma, prothrombin complex and/or platelet concentrate and rule out disseminated intravascular coagulation. *Continued, next page.*

LACTAM ANTIBIOTICS WITH EXTENDED GRAM NEGATIVE & OTHER COVERAGE *Continued*

DRUG	INDICATIONS & DOSAGE	DOSE FORMS	REMARKS
MOXALACTAM *Continued*	See previous page.	See previous page.	***Note***: In addition to Group Spectrum of Activity: Effective in P. rettgeri, Citrobacter species, Peptococcus species, Peptostreptococcus species, B. fragilis, Fusobacterium species, Eubacterium species; P. aeruginosa sometimes resistant.
CEFOPERAZONE (Cefobid)	See section: Lactams; Gram Negative & Some Gram Positive Coverage; Ineffective vs. ß-Lactamase-Producing N. gonorrhoeae.		
CEFOTAXIME (Claforan)	See section: Lactams; Gram Negative & Some Gram Positive Coverage; Useful vs. Heamophilus influenzae; "1st Generation" Cephalosporins.		
AGENTS WITH NO/MARGINAL ACTIVITY vs. P. AERUGINOSA			
CEFTRIAXONE (Rocephin)	<u>**General Infections**</u>: **IM, IV**: 500-1000 mg q12-24h for 4-14 d (maximum 4 gm/d). **Pediatric IM, IV**: 50-75 mg/kg/d in 2 dose (maximum 2 gm/d). <u>**Meningitis**</u>: **IM, IV**: 75 mg/kg initially; then 50 mg/kg q12h (maximum 4 gm/d). <u>**Uncomplicated Gonococcal Infections**</u>: **IM**: 250 mg (single dose). <u>**Surgical Prophylaxis**</u>: **IM**: 1 gm 30-120 min prior to surgery.		Cephalosporin Group Remarks. 3.6 mEq Na+/gm. Activity against: N. gonorrhoeae, P. mirabilis. Anti-pseudomonal effect is marginal; enterococci and C difficile are resistant. Occasional urinary casts. **SIDE EFFECTS**: Allergic side effects may be more common than with other cephalosporins. Bleeding may occur. **CAUTIONS**: Prescribe with caution in patients with GI disease, especially colitis. **RECOMMEND**: Continue therapy for at least 2 days after resolution of symptoms (10 days in S. pyogenes infections). Monitor blood levels and reduce dose with severe renal or hepatic disease. - - - - - - - - - - ***Note***: In addition to Group Spectrum of Activity: Effective in N. gonorrhoeae, P. mirabilis. Anti-pseudomonal effect is marginal; enterococci and C difficile are resistant.
CEFUROXIME (Zinacef)	See section: Lactams; Gram Negative & Some Gram Positive Coverage; Useful vs. Heamophilus influenzae; "1st Generation" Cephalosporins.		

AGENTS WITH NO/MARGINAL EFFECTIVENESS IN MENINGITIS

SPECTRUM OF ACTIVITY - LACTAMS WITH EXTENDED GRAM NEGATIVE COVERAGE AND NO/MARGINAL EFFECTIVENESS IN MENINGITIS: Generally similar to the benzyl penicillins, but with minimal activity in meningitis and variable activity against P. aeruginosa. In actual practice the spectrums and efficacy of these agents are augmented by the combined use with an aminoglycoside; when this is done, any differences among the sensitivites of the drugs in this class are reduced significantly. Specific activities common to all agents in the "No/Marginal Effectiveness in Meningitis" include:

Continued, next page.

LACTAM ANTIBIOTICS: AGENTS WITH EXTENDED GRAM NEGATIVE & OTHER COVERAGE *Continued*

DRUG	INDICATIONS & DOSAGE	DOSE FORMS	REMARKS
SPECTRUM OF ACTIVITY - LACTAMS WITH EXTENDED GRAM NEGATIVE COVERAGE AND NO/MARGINAL EFFECTIVE IN MENINGITIS *Continued* **Gram positive rods**: Clostridium species, Bacteroides species. **Gram positive cocci**: Staphylococci, S. pneumoniae (except ceftazidime), Peptococci (except ceftazidime and cefsulodin), Peptostreptococci (except ceftazidime and cefsulodin). **Gram negative cocci**: N. gonorrhoeae (except ceftazidime). **Gram negative rods**: Pseudomonas aeruginosa, Fusobacterium species (except ceftazidime, cefsulodin and carbenicillin).			
AGENTS WITH SOME ACITIVITY vs. P. AERUGINOSA			
CEFTAZIDIME (Fortaz)	<u>**General Infections**</u>: **IM, IV**:1000 mg q8-12h; maximum 6 gm/d. **Pediatric IV**: 30-50 mg/kg/d in 3 doses (maximum 6 gm/d). **Neonate IV**: 30 mg/kg q12h. <u>**Renal Impairment**</u>: **IM, IV**: 1000 mg q12h if creat. clearance = 31-50 cc/min, q24h if 16-30 cc/min; half dose q24h if 6-15 c/min, q48h if < 5 cc/min.	Injection: 0.5, 1. 2 gm	Cephalosporin Group Remarks. 2.3 mEq Na+/gm. Alcohol intolerance, bleeding disorders not seen in clinical trials. Half-life = 2-5 h with dialysis. **RECOMMEND**: Repeat maintenance dose after each dialysis treatment. - ***Note***: In addition to Group Spectrum of Activity: Anti-staphylococcal activity marginal, especially good against pseudomonas. (Greater activity against P. aeruginosa than cefoperazone, cefsulodin, or piperacillin.) Proteus vulgaris, Acinetobacter species, S. marcescens. Enterobacter cloacae, P. vulgaris, NO activity against B. fragilis.
PIPERACILLIN (Pipracil) (Pipril) (Pentcillyn) (Avocin)	<u>**General Infections**</u>: **IM, IV**: 3-4 gm q4-6h (maximum 24 gm/d). <u>**Severe Infections**</u>: **IV**: 6-18 gm (200-300 mg/kg) q4-6h. <u>**Uncomplicated Gonorrhea**</u>: **IM**: 2 gm (single dose) with 1000 mg PO probenecid 30 min prior injection. <u>**Hemodialysis**</u>: **IM, IV**: 2 gm q8h (maximum 6 gm/d); add 1 gm after each dialysis. <u>**Intra-abdominal Surgery**</u>: **IV**: 2 gm immediately prior; 2 gm during surgery; then 2 gm q6h for 24 h after surgery.	Injection: 2, 3, 4 gm	Penicillin Group Remarks. Most active broad-spectrum penicillin to date. Can inactivate aminoglycosides. 1.85 mEq (42.5 mg) Na+/gm. **SIDE EFFECTS**: Local reactions prominent: thrombophlebitis in 4% of patients; pain, erythema, induration and GI symptoms in 2%. **RECOMMEND**: Limit IM injections to 2 gm/site. Administer IM into large muscle. Give in combination with an aminoglycoside or a cephalosporin for initial treatment of life-threatening infections. - ***Note***: In addition to Group Spectrum of Activity: Active against ß-lactamase-producing gonococci but NOT against other Gram negative or staphylococcal ß-lactamase producers. Active against: S. fecalis, S. viridans, E. coli, H. influenzae, Klebsiella species, N. meningitidis, P. mirabilis, Salmonella, Enterobacter, P. vulgaris, P. rettgeri, Citrobacter, Serratia, Acinetobacter, Peptococci, Peptostreptococci, Bacteroides, Fusobacterium species, Eubacterium species, Veillonella species.

LACTAM ANTIBIOTICS: AGENTS WITH EXTENDED GRAM NEGATIVE & OTHER COVERAGE *Continued*

DRUG	INDICATIONS & DOSAGE	DOSE FORMS	REMARKS
AZLOCILLIN (Azlin)	<u>**General Infections**</u>: **IV**: 3 gm q4h or 4 gm q6h (maximum 24 gm/d). <u>**Complicated UTIs**</u>: **IV**: 3 gm q6h. <u>**Renal Failure**</u>: **IV**: 2 gm q8h if creat. clearance = 10-30 cc/min; 3 gm q12h if < 10 cc/min.	Injection: 2, 3, 4 gm	Penicillin Group Remarks. Skin rashes less common than with ampicillin. 2.17 mEq (49.8 mg) Na^+/gm. False-positive tests for urinary sugar and urobilinogen may occur. **SIDE EFFECTS**: Rapid IV use has been associated with chest discomfort (infuse over > 5 min). **CAUTIONS**: Excreted in human milk. Will neutralize aminoglycosides in solution. **RECOMMEND**: Serum levels may aid dosage adjustment in patients with renal failure or hepatic insufficiency. - - - - - - - - - - ***Note***: In addition to Group Spectrum of Activity: Active against: S. fecalis, L. monocytogenes, E. coli, H. influenzae, Klebsiella species, P. mirabilis, Salmonella, Enterobacter, M. morgani, P. vulgaris, P. stuartii, Enterobacter, Citrobacter, Acinetobacter, Peptococci, Peptostreptococci, Bacteroides, Fusobacterium, Eubacterium, Veillonella and non-beta-lactamase-producing staphylococci only. ***Note***: All penicillinase-producing staphylococci and most enterobacters/serratias are resistant.
CEFTIZOXIME (Cefizox)	<u>**General Infections**</u>: **IM, IV**: 1-2 gm q8-12h (maximum 12 gm/d). **Pediatric IM, IV**: 50 mg/kg q6-8h (maximum 200 mg/kg/d). <u>**Renal Impairment**</u>: **IM, IV**: 500-1000 mg initially; then 750-1500 mg q8h if creat. clearance = 50-80 cc/min; 500-1000 mg q12h if 5-49 cc/min. <u>**Dialysis Patients**</u>: **IM, IV**: 500-1000 mg q48h or 500 mg q24h.	Injection: 1, 2 gm	Cephalosporin Group Remarks. 2.6 mEq Na^+/gm. **SIDE EFFECTS**: Disulfuram-like reaction prominent with concurrent alcohol ingestion. **CAUTIONS**: Cephalosporin group remarks; also, only slightly active against pseudomonas. **RECOMMEND**: Combine with an aminoglycoside or an acylamino penicillin in severe systemic infections. - - - - - - - - - - ***Note***: In addition to Group Spectrum of Activity: E. coli, H. influenza, Klebsiella species, P. mirabilis, M. morgani, P. vulgaris, P. rettgeri, Enterobacter, Serratia, Acinetobacter, Peptococci, Peptostreptococci, B. fragilis. NOT active against C. difficile-if suspected, also use metronidazole. Less active than cefotaxime or moxalactam for Gram positive infections.

LACTAM ANTIBIOTICS: AGENTS WITH EXTENDED GRAM NEGATIVE & OTHER COVERAGE *Continued*

DRUG	INDICATIONS & DOSAGE	DOSE FORMS	REMARKS
AGENTS WITH NO/MARGINAL ACITIVITY vs. MENINGITIS & P. AERUGINOSA			
CARBENICILLIN (Pyopen) (Geopen) (Geocillin)	**General Infections**: **PO**: 382-764 mg q6h. **IM, IV**: 1 -2 gm q6h. **Pediatric IM, IV**: 50 - 200mg/kg/d in 4-6 doses. **Serious Infections**: **IV**: 200-500 mg/kg/d as 6-12 doses (maximum 40 gm/d). **Pediatric IM, IV**: 250-500 mg/kg/d in 4-6 doses. **Renal Impairment**: **IV**: 2 gm q8h if creat. clearance < 5 cc/min. **Uncomplicated Gonorrhea**: **IM**: 4 gm (one dose split at two sites); 1 gm probenicid PO 30 min prior to injection.	Injection: 1, 2, 5, 10, 20, 30 gm PO (Tab's): 382 mg	Penicillin Group Remarks. Pipracillin, azlocillin, and ticarcillin have replaced carbenicillin as first-line therapy for serious pseudomonas infection. Especially useful in UTI due to high urinary tract levels. 4.7 or 5.3 mEq Na^+/gm. Aminoglycoside half-life decreased if given concurrently. **SIDE EFFECTS**: Inhibition of platelet aggregation, bleeding diathesis, hypernatremia. Sensation of bad taste, nausea, vomiting and diarrhea is relatively frequent. **RECOMMEND**: Do NOT exceed 2 gm/dose in IM injection. PO therapy reserved for urinary tract infections. - - - - - - - - - - ***Note***: In addition to Group Spectrum of Activity: beta-hemolytic streptococci, E. coli, H. influenzae, Proteus mirabilis, Enterobacter species, M. morganii, S. faecalis, Serratia species, Salmonella species, Citrobacter species, P. rettgeri. NOT effective against Klebsiella and affects Bacteroides only at high doses.
MEZLOCILLIN (Mezlin) *Continued, next page.*	**General Infections**: **IM, IV**: 4 gm q6h (maximum 16 gm/d). **Pediatric IM, IV**: 50 mg/kg q4h. **Severe Infections**: **IM, IV**: 200-350 mg/kg/d in 4-6 doses (maximum 24 gm/d). **Uncomplicated Gonorrhea**: **IM, IV**: 1-2 gm (single dose); 1 gm probenicid PO 30 min prior to injection. *Continued, next page.*	Injection: 1, 2, 3, 4 gm	Penicillin Group Remarks. Can produce false positives in non-enzymatic urinary tests for sugar and urobillinogen. 1.85 mEq Na+/gm. Local pain with IM injection. Inactivates aminoglycosides if mixed in solution. **RECOMMEND**: Administer IV doses SLOWLY (> 5 min). Dissolve in 1% lidocaine for IM use. Slow IM injection will minimize discomfort. Venous irritation minimized if drug concentrations < 10%. *Continued, next page.*

DRUG	INDICATIONS & DOSAGE	DOSE FORMS	REMARKS
MEZLOCILLIN *Continued*	**Renal Impairment**: **IM, IV**: 1.5-3 gm q8h if creat.clearance =10-30 cc/min; 1.5-2 gm q8h (maximum 3 gm q6h) if < 10 cc/min. **Hemodialysis**: **IM, IV**: 3-4 gm after each dialysis, then q12h (3 gm q12h during peritoneal dialysis).	See previous page.	***Note***: In addition to Group Spectrum of Activity: beta-hemolytic streptococci, E. coli, H. influenzae, Klebsiella species, Proteus mirabilis, Enterobacter species, M. morganii, Eubacterium species, Veillonella species, S. faecalis, Serratia species, Citrobacter species, Acinetobacter species, P. rettgeri, P. stuartii. NOT effective against any ampicillin-resistant H. influenzae; synergy against Klebsiella, Serratia, Pseudomonas, and Proteus occurs with concurrent aminoglycoside use.
TICARCILLIN (Ticar)	**General Infections**: **IM, IV**: 1000 mg q6h. **Pediatric IM, IV**: 50-100 mg/kg/d in 4-6 doses. **Severe Infections**: **IV**: 150-300 mg/kg/d in 4-8 doses. **Pediatric IV**: 150-200 mg/kg/d in 4-6 doses. **Renal Impairment**: **IV**: 3 gm initially; then 2 gm q4h if creat. clearance = 31-60 cc/min, q8h if 10-30 cc/min, q12h if < 10 cc/min; q24h if creat. clearance < 10 cc/mi <u>and</u> concurrent hepatic dysfunction.	Injection: 1, 2, 3, 6, 20 gm	Penicillin Group Remarks. 5.2 mEq Na+/gm. Inactivates aminoglycosides in solution. **CAUTIONS**: May increase bleeding time in patients on anticoagulants. **RECOMMEND**: Concurrent aminoglycoside for serious pseudomonas infections. **CONTRAINDICATIONS**: Concurrent use of anticoagulants may be a reason to avoid ticarcillin. - - - - - - - - - - ***Note***: In addition to Group Spectrum of Activity: beta-hemolytic streptococci, E. coli, H. influenzae, Proteus mirabilis, Enterobacter species, Morganelli morganii, Eubacterium species, Veillonella species, Streptococcus faecalis, Serratia species, Salmonella species, Citrobacter species, Proteus vulgaris, Proteus rettgeri. Less active than piperacillin or azlocillin in Pseudomonas infections.

AMINOGLYCOSIDES AND RELATED AGENTS

GROUP REMARKS: Aminoglycosides are used most widely against Gram negative enteric bacteria or when there is suspicion of sepsis. In treating bacterial endocarditis caused by fecal streptococci or some Gram negative bacteria, the aminoglycoside is given with a penicillin (enhances bacterial wall permeability to facilitate the entry of the aminoglycoside). Amikacin is likely to be more active than others against coliform bacteria resistant to other aminoglycosides. Kanamycin is not effective against Pseudomonas aeruginosa; other aminoglycosides are effective.

DOSAGE CALCULATION: This is one of many schemes for calculating dosage intervals. The optimum guide to individual dosing is monitoring of serum levels.

Dosing weight: Calculated using lean body weight (LBW):

Males: LBW = 50 kg +/- 3.2 kg for each inch above/below 5 feet.

Females: LBW = 45 kg +/- 2.3 kg for each inch above/below 5 feet.

Obese patients: dosing weight = LBW + [0.4 x (actual weight - LBW)].

Dosing interval with impaired renal function:

Gentamycin, tobramycin and netilmicin :

Dosing interval (hours) = 8 x [serum creatinine (mg/100ml)].

Amikacin and Kanamycin:

Dosing interval (hours) = 9 x [serum creatinine (mg/100ml)].

SIDE EFFECTS: All aminoglycosides can cause varying degrees of ototoxicity and nephrotoxicity. Ototoxicity can manifest as either hearing loss (cochlear damage; noted first with high-frequency tones) or as vestibular damage (vertigo, ataxia, and loss of balance). Nephrotoxicity may increase creatinine levels or reduce creatinine clearance. Very high doses produce curare-like effects, resulting in respiratory paralysis (treat with neostigmine). Gentamycin, tobramycin, and streptomycin are associated more with vestibular toxicity; amakacin, kanamycin, netilmicin, tobramycin and neomycin are associated more with auditory toxicity. Hypersensitivity occurs rarely. **CAUTIONS**: In renal function impairment, excretion is greatly reduced and drug accumulation and toxicity may occur. Therefore, either reduce dosage or increase the interval between doses. Earliest sign of renal damage is granular casts in urine (nonspecific). Low therapeutic index necessitates monitoring serum drug levels. Unexpectedly rising aminoglycoside serum levels despite stable BUN and creatinine may indicate altered renal function. **RECOMMENDATIONS**: Monitor serum levels to avoid severe toxicity if renal function changes rapidly. Measure peak levels 1 hour after infusion, trough levels just prior to the next infusion. Obtain peak and trough levels 48 hours after initiating therapy and then, if renal function is stable, every 3-4 days. Toxicity is more closely associated with elevated trough levels. Perform BUN, serum creatinine and urinalysis q2d. Monitor eighth cranial nerve function via audiometric testing. **CONTRAINDICATIONS**: Known hypersensitivity to aminoglycosides.

DRUG	INDICATIONS & DOSAGE	DOSE FORMS	REMARKS
AMIKACIN (Amikin)	**Bacterial Infections**: **IM, IV**: 15 mg/kg/d in 2-3 doses (maximum 1.5 gm/d). **Uncomplicated UTI**: **IM, IV**: 250 mg q12h.	Injection: 50, 250 mg/ml	**SPECTRUM OF ACTIVITY**: **Gram positive**: Staphylococcus aureus. **Gram negative**: Pseudomonas (EXCEPT P. cepacia and P. maltophilia), E. coli, Proteus species, Providencia, Klebsiella species, Enterobacter, Serratia species , Citrobacter freundii, Acinetobacter. **Other**: Nocardia asteroides, Mycobacterium avium-intracellulare. ***Note***: Synergistic against Pseudomonas aeruginosa and other Enterobacteriaceae when used in combination with ticarcillin or azlocillin. NOT effective against S. pneumoniae or other streptococci, H. influenza, neisseria, or anaerobes. - - - - - - - - - - Therapeutic serum level should be 8-16, and NOT > 35 µg/ml; trough serum level should be NOT > 5 µg/ml. Not affected by most bacterial aminoglycosidases; therefore often useful against tobramicin and gentamicin-resistant organisms. **RECOMMEND**: Only use in uncomplicated UTI if other, less toxic antibiotics are not effective.

AMINOGLYCOSIDES AND RELATED AGENTS *Continued*

DRUG	INDICATIONS & DOSAGE	DOSE FORMS	REMARKS
KANAMYCIN (Kantrex)	<u>Bacterial Infections</u>: **IM, IV**: 15 mg/kg/d in 2-4 doses for 7-10 d (maximum 1.5 gm/d). **Pediatric IM, IV**: 15 mg/kg/d in 3-4 doses (maximum 1.5 gm/d). <u>Hepatic Encephalopathy</u>: **PO**: 8-12 gm/d in 4 doses. <u>Perioperative Bowel Preparation</u>: **PO**: 1 gm q1h for 4 doses; then 1 gm q6h for 36-72 h.	PO (Cap's): 500 mg Injection: 37.5, 250, 330 mg	**SPECTRUM OF ACTIVITY**: **Gram positive**: Staphylococcus aureus. **Gram negative**: **Good activity**: Most Pseudomonas aeruginosa, E. coli, some Proteus and Serratia, Klebsiella pneumoniae, Enterobacter aerogenes. ***Note***: Cross-resistance with Neomycin is complete. NOT effective against: S. pneumoniae, group A streptococci, enterococci, bacteroides, clostridia or fungi. Therapeutic serum levesl should be 8-16 µg/ml and NOT > 30 µg/ml; trough level should NOT be > 5 µg/ml.
GENTAMICIN (Garamycin)	<u>Severe Infections</u>: **IM, IV**: 3-5 mg/kg/d in 3-4 doses. **Pediatric IM, IV**: 2-2.5 mg/kg q8h (180 mg/m^2/d in 3 doses). <u>Mild to Moderate Infections</u>: **IM, IV**: 2-3 mg/kg/d in 2-3 doses. **Pediatric IM, IV**: 2-2.5 mg/kg q8h (180 mg/m^2/d in 3 doses). <u>Intrathecal or Intraventricular</u>: **Adults**: 4-8 mg/d. **Infants & Children**: 1-2 mg/d.	Injection: 0.4, 0.6, 0.8, 1, 1.2, 1.6, 2, 2.4, 10, 40 mg/ml Intrathecal: 2 mg/ml	**SPECTRUM OF ACTIVITY**: **Gram positive**: Staphylococcus aureus. **Gram negative**: <u>Good activity</u>: most Pseudomonas aeruginosa, E. coli, Proteus vulgaris, Klebsiella pneumoniae, Enterobacter aerogenes, Serratia species, Yersinia species, Brucellae, Campylobacters, Pasturellae, Acinetobacter. <u>Moderate activity</u>: Proteus mirabilis, salmonellae, H. influenzae, Listeria, gonococci. ***Note***: Synergistic against P. aeruginosa when used in combination with piperacillin or azlocillin; against Klebsiella when used in combination with cephalosporins; and against enterococci when used in combination with ampicillin. NOT effective against: S. pneumoniae, group A streptococci, enterococci, meningococci, clostridia, Pseudomonas cepacia, Pseudomonas pseudomaelli, or Nocardia asteroides. Therpeutic serum concentrations should be 4-8l µg/ml and NOT > 12 µg/m; troughs should NOT be < 2 µg/ml (preferably < 1 µg/l). May elevate SGOT.
STREPTOMYCIN (Strycin)	<u>Severe Fulminating Infections</u>: **IM**: 2-4 gm/d in 2-4 doses. **Pediatric IM**: 20-40 mg/kg/d in 2-4 doses. <u>Tuberculosis</u>: **IM**: 1 gm/d initially, reduce to 1 gm 2-3 times/wk. <u>Tularemia</u>: **IM**: 1-2 gm/d in 2-4 doses for 7-10d or until patient afebrile for 5-7d. *Continued, next page.*	Injection: 400, 500 mg/ml Powder: 1, 5 gm	**SPECTRUM OF ACTIVITY**: **Gram positive**: Mycobacterium tuberculosis, Streptococci (including faecalis). **Gram negative**: Enterobacter species (including E. aerogenes), E. coli, H. influenzae, H. ducreyi, Neisseria species (including N. gonorrhoeae), Proteus species, Salmonella species, Shigella species, Yersina pestis. ***Note***: 2-30% of M. tuberculosis show primary resistance (more common in patients from developing countries). In general, do NOT exceed a maximum peak serum level of 25 mg/l; higher levels useful in meningitis. CSF penetration very poor (2-4% of serum concentrations present in breast milk). **SIDE EFFECTS**: Vestibular ototoxicity (25-30% of patients) occurs in a dose-dependent manner (especially if *Continued, next page.*

AMINOGLYCOSIDES AND RELATED AGENTS *Continued*

DRUG	INDICATIONS & DOSAGE	DOSE FORMS	REMARKS
STREPTOMYCIN *Continued*	**Plague**: **IM**: 2-4 gm/d in 3-4 doses until patient afebrile for 3d. **Bacterial Endocarditis (penicillin-sensitive alpha and non-hemolytic streptococci)**: **IM**: 1 gm q12h for 1 wk, then 0.5 gm q12h for 2nd wk (with penicillin). **Geriatric IM**: 0.5 gm q12h for 2 wks.	See previous page.	daily dose ≥ 1 gm or total dose > 60 gm); total deafness occurs in approximately 6% of cases. Others include: CNS and respiratory depression, marrow suppression and renal injury. Allergic reactions occur; eosinophilia and rashes more common, anaphylactic shock relatively rare. May cause cardiovascular collapse similar to the "gray-baby syndrome" in infants. **RECOMMEND**: Evaluate audiometric, vestibular and renal function q2wks. Discontinue at first sign of hearing/balance disorder. Use ONLY in combination with other agent(s) to avoid emergence of resistent strains. **CONTRAINDICATIONS**: AVOID use during pregnancy.
NEOMYCIN (Mycifradin) (Neobiotic)	**Preoperative Gut Sterilization**: **PO**:1000 mg in the afternoon, then 1000 mg in 1h, then 1000 mg at bedtime. Give 1000 mg erythromycin base with each 1000 mg neomycin. Give on 3rd day of bowel preparation. **Hepatic Coma**: **PO**: 4-12 gm/d (in 3-6 doses) for 5-6 d. **Pediatric PO**: 50-100 mg/kg/d (in 3-6 doses) for 5-6 d.	PO (Tab's): 500 mg PO (Liquid): 125 mg/5 ml (60 ml)	**SPECTRUM OF ACTIVITY**: **Gram positive**: Staphylococci. **Gram negative**: Enterobacter aerogenes, E. coli, Klebsiella species, Proteus species (including P. vulgaris), Pseudomonas aeruginosia. ***Note***: Cross-resistance is complete with kanamycin and partial with streptomycin and gentamicin. --- **SIDE EFFECTS**: With oral administration, candida overgrowth may occur and a malabsorption syndrome with steatorrhea and diarrhea can result, especially with prolonged therapy. Others: sensitization leading to allergic reactions; renal or eighth nerve injury.
TOBRAMYCIN (Nebcin)	**Bacterial Infections**: **IM, IV**: 3-5 mg/kg/d in 3-4 doses. **Pediatric IM, IV**: 6-7.5 mg/kg/d in 3-4 doses.	Injection: 10, 40 mg/ml	**SPECTRUM OF ACTIVITY**: **Gram positive**: Staphylococci (including S. aureus, S. epidermidis). **Gram negative**: Pseudomonas aerugonisa, E. coli, Proteus species (including indole-positive, indole-negative P. mirabilis, P. vulgaris), Providencia species (including P. rettgeri), Klebsiella species, Enterobacter species, Serratia species, Citrobacter freundii, Acinetobacter, Shigella species, Yersinia pestis. ***Note***: Synergistic against P. aeruginosa and other Enterobacteriaceae when used in combination with ticarcillin or azlocillin. NOT effective against: S. pneumoniae or other streptococci, H. influenza, neisseria or anaerobes. Pseudomonas resistant to gentamicin may be sensitive to tobramycin and amikacin. --- Some cross-resistance with gentamicin and amikacin. **SIDE EFFECTS**: Vestibular and renal injury.

TETRACYCLINES

SPECTRUM OF ACTIVITY: **Bacteriostatic**: Many Gram positive (though usually NOT drugs of first choice) and Gram negative (bacteroides species, H. ducreyi, P. tularensis, P. pestis, V. comma, V. fetus, B. bacilliformis) microorganisms, some other anaerobes, rickettsiae, mycoplasmas, L-forms, chlamydiae, some protozoans (e.g., amebae), trachoma, psittacosis and ornithosis agents. A 5 d course of tetracycline is effective in eliminating penicillinase-producing gonococci (however some forms resistant). Useful in respiratory tract infections and non-gonococcal urethritis. **Sensitivity testing usually needed to predict efficacy**: Streptococcus, Klebsiella, Acintobacter and Shigella species; H. influenzae, E. coli, E. aerogenes. **Often effective as an alternative to penicillin**: Niesseria (IV administration only for N. meningitidis-except PO minocycline in the treatment of asymptomatic nasopharyngeal carrier state), Treponema, Clostridium, and Actinomyces species; B. anthracis, F. fusiforme, L. monocytogenes.

GROUP REMARKS: Activity of the tetracyclines extends somewhat further into the Gram negative area than the penicillins (but are more likely to be ineffective against streptococci) and were the first antibiotics to be labeled "broad-spectrum". All tetracyclines are equivalent in their bacteriostatic effects. **NOTES**: GI absorption is irregular; fecal excretion is high. Agents which are more slowly excreted: demeclocycline, methacycline, minocycline (yields higher blood levels); doxycycline (does not accumulate in renal failure), minocycline (absorbed well). Complete tetracycline group cross resistance usually occurs (EXCEPT for minocycline; only partial cross-resistance occurs). Food, milk, antacids and other sources of divalent calcium reduce oral GI absorption of the tetracyclines by 50% or more. Demeclocycline, tetracycline, oxytetracycline, and methacycline are excreted unchanged in urine (glomerular filtration); doxycycline and minocycline are NOT excreted renally. **SIDE EFFECTS**: Deposited in growing bones and teeth causing tooth dysplasia. GI side effects: nausea, vomiting, and diarrhea (commonest reasons for discontinuance). Others: anal pruritis, vaginal or oral candidiasis, staphylococcal enterocolitis and esophageal ulcers. Rarely, doxycycline hyclate and tetracycline cause esophagitis. Rarely associated with impaired hepatic function, especially (1) during pregnancy, (2) with pre-existing hepatic insufficiency, and (3) with high doses given IV. May increase BUN and cause renal insufficiency (except doxycycline; can exacerbate pre-existing renal failure or produce it in cirrhotics). Can induce sensitivity to sunlight or U.V. light (esp. demeclocycline and particularly in blonds). Dizziness, vertigo, nausea, and vomiting (esp. minocycline; with 200 to 400 mg/day, 35-70% of patients affected). Outdated citrate preparations (no longer available) associated with Fanconi like syndrome. Rare blood dyscrasia seen (associated with long term treatment). IV use may cause venous thrombosis. IM injection produces painful local irritation. Hypersensitivity reactions are rare. **RECOMMENDATIONS**: Avoid sunlight or UV radiation. Pre-existing renal or hepatic impairment warrants baseline function studies. AVOID during the last half of pregnancy or in children < 12 y.o.. Do NOT administer with iron, aluminum, calcium, or magnesium-containing compounds such as milk, antacids, laxatives (markedly decreases absorption). May potentiate oral anticoagulants and thus may warrant more frequent coagulation monitoring.

DRUG	INDICATIONS & DOSAGE	DOSE FORMS	REMARKS
TETRACYCLINE (Achromycin) (Panmycin) (Cefracycline) (Muracin) (Neo-Tetrine) (Sumycin) (Tetrosol) *Continued, next page*	**Mild to Moderate Infections**: **PO**: 500 mg q12h or 250 mg q6h. **Severe Infections**: **PO**: 500 mg q6h. **IM**: 250 mg q24h or 300 mg in 1-2 doses. **IV**: 250-500 mg q12h (maximum 500 mg q6h). **Brucellosis**: **PO**: 500 mg q6h for 3 wk (add 1 gm IM streptomycin; bid for 1 wk; then q24h for 2nd wk). **Syphilis (primary, secondary or latency <1 year)**: **PO**: 50 mg q6h for 15d (maximum 4o gm/10d) [penicillin is first-choice drug]. *Continued, next page*	PO (Cap's): 100, 250, 500 mg PO (Tab's): 250, 500 mg IM Powder: 100, 250 mg IV Powder: 250, 500 mg PO (Liquid): 25 mg/ml Syrup: 25 mg/ml	Claims of enhanced absorption of tetracycline-phosphate complex are NOT established. Increasing oral dose > 250 mg usually does NOT increase absorption. Excretion predominantly via kidney. **SIDE EFFECTS**: May give rise to reversible increase in intracranial pressure. Esophageal ulceration has occurred following capsule administration.

TETRACYCLINES *Continued*

DRUG	INDICATIONS & DOSAGE	DOSE FORMS	REMARKS
TETRACYCLINE *Continued*	**Syphilis (Latency >1 year or complicated)**: **PO**: 500 mg q6h for 30 d (Penicillin is first-choice treatment). **Uncomplicated Gonorrhea**: **PO**: 500 mg q6h for 7 d. **Adjunct for Pelvic Inflammatory Disease**: **PO**: 500 mg q6h for 10-14 d. **Non-gonococcal Urethritis**: **PO**: 500 mg q6h for 7 d. **Chlamydia Trachomatis Infections (Urethral, Endocervical, Rectal)**: **PO**: 500 mg q6h for 7 d. **Severe Acne**: **PO**: 1 gm/d (divided) for 1-2 wk; then 125-500 mg/d maintenance. **Sexually Transmitted Epididymitis**: **PO**: 500 mg q6h for 10 d. **Lymphogranuloma Venereum**: **PO**: 500 mg q6h for 14 d.	See previous page.	See previous page.
OXYTETRACYCLINE (Terramycin)	**Bacterial Infections**: **PO**: 500 mg initially; then 250 mg q6h (maximum 4 gm/d). **IM**: 250 mg q24h or 300 mg/d in 1-3 doses. **IV**: 250-500 mg q12h (maximum 500 mg q6h). **Pediatric PO**: 25-50 mg/kg/d in 4 doses. **Pediatric IM**: 15-25 mg/kg/d in 2-3 doses (maximum single dose = 250 mg). **Pediatric IV**: 5-10mg/kg q12h.	PO (Cap's): 125, 250 mg PO (Tab's): 250 mg Injection: 50, 125 mg/ml Powder: 250, 500 mg PO (Liquid): 5 mg/ml	
DEMECLOCYCLINE (Declomycin)	**Bacterial Infections**: **PO**: 600 mg/d, divided q6-12h. **Pediatric PO**: 6-12 mg/kg/d in 2-4 doses. **Gonorrhea Patients Sensitive to Penicillin**: **PO**: 600 mg initially; then 300 mg q12h (for 4 d or to 3 gm total). **Chlamydia Trachomatis Infections (Urethral, Endocervical, Rectal)**: **PO**: 300 mg q6h for ≥ 7 d.	PO (Cap's): 150 mg PO (Tab's): 150, 300 mg **SIADH**: **PO**: 600 mg-1.2 gm/d (divided q6-8h)	Used for chronic SIADH; diuresis usually occurs ≤5d after start of therapy. Also available in capsules and tablets with Nystatin. **SIDE EFFECTS**: Photosensitivity reactions prominent. May increase BUN and depress plasma prothrombin activity. A vasopressin-resistant nephrogenic diabetes insipidus is occasionally caused by demeclocycline. **CAUTIONS**: Crosses placental barrrier and may be toxic to fetus; enters human milk. **RECOMMENDATIONS**: Must lower dose in renal failure.

TETRACYCLINES *Continued*

DRUG	INDICATIONS & DOSAGE	DOSE FORMS	REMARKS
DOXYCYCLINE (Vibramycin)	**Bacterial Infections**: **PO, IV**: 100 mg q12h for 1 d; then 100 mg/d in 1-2 doses. **Pediatric PO, IV**: 2.2 mg/kg q12h for 1 d; then 2.2 mg/kg/d in 1-2 doses (maximum 4.4 mg/kg/d). **Acute Gonococcal Infection**: **PO**: 100 mg bid for 7 d. **Adjunct in Pelvic Inflammatory Disease**: **PO**: 100 mg bid for 10-14 d. **Chlamydia Trachomatis Infections (Urethral, Endocervical, Rectal)**: **PO**: 100 mg bid for 7 d. **"Traveller's Diarrhea" Prophylaxis**: **PO**: 100 mg/d. **Sexually Transmitted Epididymitis**: **PO**: 100 mg bid for 10d. **Lymphogranuloma Venereum**: **PO**: 100 mg bid for 14d. **Primary/Secondary Syphilis**: **PO, IV**: 300 mg/d for 10 d.	PO (Cap's): 50, 100 mg PO (Tab's): 100 mg Powder: 100, 200 mg PO (Liquid): 5, 10 mg/ml	Long-acting tetracycline derivative. IV administration: infuse as 0.5 mg/ml sln over ≥ 1 h. Blood levels double when dose increased from 100-200 or from 200-400 mg. **SIDE EFFECTS**: Esophogeal mucosal ulceration sometimes seen after capsule ingestion (especially with hiatus-hernia patients).
MINOCYCLINE (Minocin) (Vectrin)	**Bacterial Infections**: **PO, IV**: 200 mg initially; then 100 mg bid (maximum 400 mg/d). **Pediatric PO, IV**: 4 mg/kg initially; then 2 mg/kg bid. **Syphilis**: **PO**: 200 mg initially; then 100 mg bid for 10-15 d. **Chlamydia Trachomatis or U. Urealyticum**: **PO**: 100 mg bid for 7 d. **Penicillin-Sensitive Gonorrhea Patients**: **PO**: 200 mg initially; then 100 mg bid for ≥ 4 d. **Meningococcal-Carrier State**: **PO**: 100 mg bid for 5 d. **Mycobacterium Marinum Infections**: **PO**: 100 mg bid for 6-8 wk.	PO (Cap's): 50, 100 mg PO (Tab's): 50 mg Powder: 100 mg PO (Liquid): 10 mg/ml	**SPECTRUM OF ACTIVITY**: Only tetracycline derivative which retains activity against strains of Staphylococci resistant to the other tetracyclines. **NOTES**: Long-acting tetracycline derivative. Blood levels double when dose increased from 100-200 or from 200-400 mg. Good penetration into CSF (20-40%). **SIDE EFFECTS**: CNS effects prominent; CDC recommends that Rifampin be used in the treatment of meningococcal carriers unless contraindicated. Transient common dizziness (especially females) at the beginning of treatment; may affect driving ability. **CAUTIONS**: Warn patient of initial dizziness and instruct NOT to drive or operate machinery when starting therapy.

SULFONAMIDES AND URINARY TRACT AGENTS

SPECTRUM OF ACTIVITY: Sulfonamides were originally active against a wide range of Gram positive and Gram negative bacteria; however, the increasing incidence of resistance in these bacteria has decreased the clinical usefulness of the group. Quantitative but not necessarily qualitative differences in activity exist between different sulfonamides. Spectrum of action includes: Gram positive and Gram negative bacteria, Nocardia, Chlamydia trachomatis and some protozoa. Sulfonamides inhibit some enteric bacteria but NOT Pseudomonas, Serratia or most Proteus. Used in conjunction with other agents for: T. gondii, P. falciparum and H. influenza. Sulfonamides (often with trimethoprim) are used in first urinary tract infections, nocardiosis, and toxoplasmosis. Often effective in urinary tract infections due to E. coli, P. mirabilis, P. vulgaris, S. aureus and Klebsiella-Enterobacter.

GROUP REMARKS: The sulfonamides are bacteriostatic by antagonizing bacterial folic acid synthesis. Some agents are more water soluble than others. Sulfonamides enter well into pleural, ocular, cerebrospinal and synovial fluids. **LEVELS**: Peak blood levels generally occur 2-3 h after oral intake. Therapeutic effect occurs at serum unbound sulfonamide levels = 5-15 mg/dl; increased toxicity at levels > 20 mg/dl. Silver sulfadiazine used on burn wounds develops only low systemic levels. Sulfonamides cross the placenta and are excreted in breast milk. **SIDE EFFECTS**: Side-effects occur in ≤ 5% of patients and must be considered wherever unexplained symptoms or signs develop. Incidence of side effects is higher with slowly excreted "long-acting" sulfonamides than with the rapidly excreted ones. **Common**: Fever, rashes, photosensitivity, urticaria, nausea, vomiting and diarrhea. **Urinary Tract**: Sulfonamides may cause nephrosis and/or allergic nephritis, proteinuria and hematuria. May precipitate crystalluria (especially at neutral or acid urine pH) with hematuria, proteinuria, or obstruction possible-may be prevented by using the more soluble sulfonamides (e.g., sulfisoxazole), alkalinizing urine (5-15 gm sodium bicarbonate daily), forcing fluids and performing urinalysis every 3-5 d. Deterioration of renal function can occur with cotrimoxazole. **Hematopoietic Disturbances**: Hemolytic anemia (associated with G-6-PD deficiency), aplastic anemia, granulocytopenia, thrombocytopenia, hypoprothrombinemia, methemoglobinemia and leukomoid reactions. Discontinue therapy before the reaction has advanced to a severe or life-threatening stage. **Other**: Pancreatitis, stomatitis, hepatic inflammation and necrosis. Depression neuropathy, headache, vertigo, transverse myelitis, seizures, hallucinations, psychosis, tinnitus, vertigo, hearing loss and ataxia. Conjunctivitis, arthritis, hepatitis, exfoliative dermatitis, polyarteritis nodosa, serum sickness, allergic myocarditis, eosinophillic pneumonia, fibrosing alveolitis and Stevens-Johnson syndrome. At the end of pregnancy sulfonamides increase the risk of kernicterus and hemolytic jaundice in newborns. Oligospermia, infertility, goiter, diuretic effect and low blood glucose have been reported. **RECOMMENDATIONS**: Perform CBC every 3-5 d and complete urinalysis every wk; hepatic and renal function evaluation during prolonged treatments. Avoid rapid IV administration. Maintain adequate fluid intake to prevent crystalluria. **CONTRAINDICATIONS**: Sulfonamide hypersensitivity, infants (< 2 months old), porphyria, term pregnancy, during lactation, hypersensitivity to sulfonureas, hypersensitivity to thiazide-type agents.

DRUG	INDICATIONS & DOSAGE	DOSE FORMS	REMARKS
FOR URINARY TRACT INFECTIONS ONLY			
SULFISOXAZOLE (Gantrisin) (SK-Soxazole) (Sulfizin)	<u>**Urinary Tract Infections**</u>: **PO**: 2-4 gm initially, then 4-8 gm/d in 4-6 doses. **Pediatric PO**: 75 mg/kg or 2 gm/m^2 initially, then 150 mg/kg/d or 4 gm/m^2/d in 4-6 doses (maximum 6 gm/d). **IM, IV**: 50 mg/kg initially, then 100 mg/kg/d. (Total daily dosage may be given IV in 4 doses or IM in 2-3 doses.)	PO (Tab's): 500 mg PO (Liquid): 100 mg/ml Syrup: 100 mg/ml Emulsion: 200 mg/ml Vaginal cream: 10% Injection: 400 mg/ml	For IM use: administer ≤ 10 ml, NOT > 5 ml in any one site. For children, the volume given IM in any one site should be correspondingly less than in adults. - - - - - - - - - - **Combinations with Phenazopyradine**: (Aqua-Ton-S) (Azo-Gantrisin) (Azo-Sulfisocon) (Suldiazo) (Uridium) **Vaginal preparations**: (Koro-Sulf) (Vagilia) (Cantri)

SULFONAMIDES AND URINARY TRACT AGENTS *Continued*

DRUG	INDICATIONS & DOSAGE	DOSE FORMS	REMARKS
SULFAMETHOXAZOLE (Gantanol)	<u>Urinary Tract Infections</u>: **PO**: 2 gm initially, then 1 gm bid; maximum 2 gm/d. **Pediatric PO**: 50-60 mg/kg initially, then 25-30 mg/kg bid; maximum 75 mg/kg/d.	PO (Tab's): 0.5, 1 gm PO (Liquid): 100 mg/ml	Alkalinization of the urine is not required.
RELATED URINARY TRACT AGENT			
SPECTRUM OF ACTIVITY: **Gram positive**: Most cocci (including penicillinase-producing gonococci). **Gram negative**: Ampicillin-resistant H. influenzae, chloramphenicol-resistant S. typhi, Ps. pseudomallei; variable against Shigella dysenteriae. **Other**: Mycobacterium marinum, Nocardia asteroides, Pneumocystis carinii. ***Note***: Pseudomonas aeruginosa, bacteroides, T. pallidum, Ureaplasma, enterococci NOT susceptible.			
TRIMETHOPRIM (Trimpex) (Prolomprim) (Metrima) (Syraprim) (Trimanyl)	<u>Urinary Tract Infections</u>: **PO**: 100 mg bid for 10 d. <u>Renal Impairment</u>: **PO**: 50 mg bid if creat. clearance = 15-30 ml/min; NOT recommended if < 15 ml/min.	PO (Tab's): 100, 200 mg	**SIDE EFFECTS**: Hematologic effects: leukopenia, neutropenia, megaloblastic anemia, decreased platelets and methemoglobinemia. GI effects in approximately 6% of patients: abdominal pain, nausea, vomiting, glossitis. Others: 5-7% have pruritis or exfoliative dermatitis, 10-25% on high doses develop a maculopapular and pruritic rash 1-2wks into therapy. **CAUTIONS**: Action of phenytoin may be increased by concurrent trimethoprim. **RECOMMEND**: Perform frequent CBCs; discontinue if blood changes occur. **CONTRAINDICATIONS**: Teratogenic in rats; NOT recommended for pregnant/lactating women.
FOR INDICATIONS IN ADDITION TO URINARY TRACT INFECTIONS			
TRIMETHOPRIM (TMP) + SULFAMETHOXAZOLE (SMX) (Bactrim) (Septra) (TMP/SMX) (Cotrim) (Sulfatrim) (Bethaprim) *Continued, next page*	<u>Bacterial Infections</u>: **PO**: 160 mg TMP + 800 mg SMX bid for 10-14 d. **Pediatric PO (≥ 40 kg)**: 4 mg/kg TMP + 20 mg/kg SMX bid (Otitis media and UTI, treat for 10d; Shigellosis, for 5d) maximum 160 mg TMP + 800 mg SMX bid. **IV**: 8-10 mg/kg/d TMP in 2-4 doses. <u>P. carinii Pneumonia</u>: **PO**: 5 mg/kg TMP + 25 mg/kg SMX qid for 14 d. **IV**: 15-20 mg/kg/d TMP in 3-4 doses for up to 14 d. *Continued, next page*	PO (Tab's): 80 mg TMP + 400 mg SMX; 160 mg TMP + 800 mg SMX PO (Liquid): 40 mg TMP + 200 mg SMX per 5 ml Infusion: 80mg TMP + 400 mg SMX per 5ml	**SPECTRUM OF ACTIVITY**: **Gram positive**: Most Streptococcus pneumoniae, Staphylococcus aureus, Streptococcus pyogenes, Nocardia. **Gram negative**: Most Enterobacteriaceae (including Acinetobacter, Enterobacter, E. coli, Klebsiella pneumoniae, P. mirabilis, Salmonella, Shigella), H. influenzae, H. ducreyi, N. gonorrhoeae, 70% of indole-positive proteus, 50% providencia and Serratia. **Anaerobes**: Most Bacteroides. *Continued, next page*

SULFONAMIDES AND URINARY TRACT AGENTS *Continued*

DRUG	INDICATIONS & DOSAGE	DOSE FORMS	REMARKS
TRIMETHOPRIM (TMP) + SULFAMETHOXAZOLE (SMX) (Continued)	**Penicillinase-producing N. gonorrhea (pharyngeal)**: **PO**: 9 tab's/d (80 mg TMP + 400 mg SMX) for 5 d. **P. carinii Prophylaxis**: **PO**: 10 mg/kg/d TMP + 50 mg/kg/d SMX or 150 mg/m^2/d TMP + 750 mg SMX/m^2/d in 2 doses. **Severe Infections or Shigellosis**: **IV**: 8-10 mg/kg/din 2-4 doses (14d for severe UTI; 5 d for Shigellosis). **In Renal Failure**: Reduce dose by 1/2 If creat. clearance = 15-30 cc/min; NOT recommended if < 15 cc/min.	See previous page.	**Protozoa**: Pneumocystis carinii. ***Note***: Some enterococci (including some S. faecalis), P. aeruginosa, Clostridium are NOT sensitive. - - - - - - - - - - **SIDE EFFECTS**: Side effects include: kernicterus in neonates, blood dyscrasias, crystalluria, glossitis, hemolysis in patients with G-6-PD deficiency. **CONTRAINDICATIONS**: Renal or hepatic disease, blood dyscrasias, pregnancy.
SULFADIAZINE	**Bacterial Infections**: **PO**: 2-4 gm initially, then 2-4 gm/d in 3-6 doses. **Pediatric PO**: 75 mg/kg or 2 gm/m^2 initially, then 50 mg/kg/d or 4 gm/m^2/d in 4-6 doses; maximum 6 gm/d. **Rheumatic Fever Prophylaxis**: **PO**: 1 gm/d. **Pediatric PO**: 500 mg/d.	PO (Tab's): 500 mg	**SIDE EFFECTS**: Crystalluria (maintain high urine output with alkaline pH), allergy (fever, rash, neutropenia, agranulocytosis, aplastic anemia, thrombocytopenia), hemolysis in patients with G-6-PD deficiency, Stevens-Johnson syndrome.
SULFASALAZINE (Azulfidine) (Azaline) (S.A.S.-500)	**Ulcerative Colitis**: **PO**: 3-4 gm/d in 3 doses. **Pediatric PO**: 40-60 mg/kg/d in 3-6 doses. **Maintenance Therapy**: **PO**: 500 mg q6h **Pediatric PO**: 30 mg/kg/d in 4 doses.	PO (Tab's): 500 mg PO (Liquid): 50 mg/m	To lessen adverse GI side effects, start therapy at 1-2 gm/d. Doses up to 8 gm/d may increase risk of adverse effects. Intervals between nighttime doses should not exceed 8 h. **SIDE EFFECTS**: Sulfasalazine has caused agranulocytosis; watch for sudden sore throat or infection. **RECOMMEND**: Use of enteric-coated tablets may reduce initial GI intolerance; reduce dose by 1/2 or discontinue drug for 5-7 d to decrease GI intolerance later in therapy (restart treatment at lower daily dose).
SULFADIAZINE + SULFAMERAZINE + SULFAMETHAZINE (Combination)	**Bacterial Infections**: **PO**: 2-4 gm initially, then 2-4 gm/d in 3-6 doses. **Pediatric PO**: 75 mg/kg or 2 gm/m^2 initially, then 150 mg/kg/d or 4 gm/m^2/d in 4-6 doses; maximum 6 gm/d.	PO (Tab's): 162 mg of each agent 167 mg of each agent PO (Liquid): 167 mg of each agent per 5 ml	**SIDE EFFECTS**: Similar to those for sulfadiazine, but risk of crystalluria is lower.

NON-SULFONAMIDE URINARY TRACT AGENTS

NOTE: Penicillins, cephalosporins and tetracyclines are all excreted in the urine in active form and are therefore effective urinary tract antibiotics. See the appropriate discussions for details of their use in urinary tract infections.

DRUG	INDICATIONS & DOSAGE	DOSE FORMS	REMARKS
CINOXACIN (Cinobac)	<u>Urinary Tract Infections</u>: **PO**: 1 gm/d in 2-4 doses for 7-14 d. <u>Renal Failure</u>: **PO**: 500 mg initially, then 500 mg q12h if creat. clearance > 80 cc/min; 250 mg q8h if 80-50 cc/min; 250 mg q12h if 50-20 cc/min; 250 mg q24h if < 20 cc/min.	PO (Cap's): 250, 500 mg	**SPECTRUM OF ACTIVITY**: **Gram negative**: E. coli, Proteus vulgaris and P. mirabilis, Klebsiella species, Enterobacter, Serratia species. **Note**: NOT effective against staphylococcus, enterococci or psuedomonas. - - - - - - - - - - A synthetic agent related to nalidixic acid. May be bacteriocidal when the concentration is doubled or quadrupled. Complete cross-reactivity with nalidixic acid. Bacterial resistance develops in 1% cases. **SIDE EFFECTS**: Common: nausea, dizziness, gastric discomfort (5%), dizziness, rashes and urticaria. Less frequent: diarrhea, vomiting, fatigue, tinnitus and photophobia. Symptoms often reverse quickly with interruption of treatment; discontinuance not usually required.
INDANYL CARBENICILLIN (Geocillin)	<u>Urinary Tract Infections</u>: **PO**: 382-764 mg q6h.	PO (Tab's): equivalent to 382 mg carbenicillin	**SPECTRUM OF ACTIVITY**: **Gram negative**: E. coli, Proteus species (mirabilis, vulgaris, rettgeri- including indole-positive forms), Morganella morganii, Pseudomonas species, Enterobacter and enterococci. **Note**: Recommended only for Pseudomonas aeruginosa. NOT effective for systemic infection. - - - - - - - - - - Penicillin Group Remarks apply. Limit in-hospital use; resistant strains may appear quickly. **SIDE EFFECTS**: Frequent: diarrhea, nausea, dysguesea and vomiting.
METHENAMINE **mandelate**: (Mandelamine) (Dannasol) (Uroquid) **hippurate**: (Hiprex) (Urex) *Continued, next page*	<u>Urinary Tract Infections</u>: **Mandelate**: **PO**: 1 gm q6h, after meals and at bedtime. **PO (6-12 y.o.)**: 500 mg q6h. **Hippurate**: **PO**: 1 gm q12h. **PO (6-12 y.o.)**: 0.5-1 gm q12h.	**Mandelate**: PO (Tab's): 0.5, 1 gm Tab's (enteric-coated): 0.25, 0.5, 1 gm PO (Liquid): 50, 100 mg/ml Granules: 0.5, 1 gm **Hippurate**: PO (Tab's): 1 gm	**SPECTRUM OF ACTIVITY**: **Gram positive**: Strptococcus faecalis, Staphylococcus aureus, S. epidermidis. **Gram negative**: E. coli, Klebsiella, Proteus, Pseudomonas aeruginosa. - - - - - - - - - - Methenamine forms formaldehyde in the urine, which inhibits bacterial growth. Development of resistance is unlikely. Effective only with an acidic urine (pH preferably about 5). Useful in suppressive therapy, especially after infecting organisms have been cleared. **SIDE EFFECTS**: Gastric irritation, nausea, vomiting, diarrhea, urinary tract inflammation (painful, *Continued, next page*

NON-SULFONAMIDE URINARY TRACT AGENTS *Continued*

DRUG	INDICATIONS & DOSAGE	DOSE FORMS	REMARKS
METHENAMINE *Continued*	See previous page.	See previous page.	frequent urination, albuminuria, hematuria-especially with high doses). Hypersensitivity reactions: rash, urticaria, stomatitis and pruritis.
			CAUTIONS: Hiprex tablets contain tartrazine dye (possible allergic reaction, especially in patients allergic to aspirin). Interferes with urine tests for catecholamines, vanilmandelic acid (VMA), 5-HIAA, 17 hydroxycorticosteroid and estriol. **RECOMMEND**: Perform periodic LFTs. AVOID in pyelonephritis. **CONTRAINDICATIONS**: Renal insufficiency, severe hepatic impairment or severe dehydration.
NALIDIXIC ACID (NegGram)	__Urinary Tract Infections__: **PO**: 1 gm q6h for 1-2 wk. **Pediatric PO**: 55 mg/kg/d in 4 doses.	PO (Tab's): 0.25, 0.5, 1 gm PO (Liquid): 50 mg/ml	**SPECTRUM OF ACTIVITY**: **Gram negative**: E. coli, Proteus species (mirabilis and indole-positive forms), Klebsiella, some strains of Salmonella and Shigella, Enterobacter and the majority of Enterobacteriaceae species. **Note**: NOT effective against Gram positive organisms.
			If bacterial resistance develops, it is usually apparent within 48 h of onset of therapy. Urinary pH does NOT usually affect the activity of nalidixic acid. In vitro: synergistic activity with kanamycin, gentamycin and colistin against most Enterobacteriaceae; NO synergism with penicillins or cephalosporins. Interferes with urine glucose and 17-ketosteroid tests. **SIDE EFFECTS**: Frequent: mild gastrointestinal upsets (nausea, vomiting, diarrhea). Less frequent: rash,, urticaria, fever, eosinophilia, photosensitivity headache, drowsiness, myalgia, weakness, visual changes, excitement, confusion, hallucinations, seizures, pseudotumor cerebri, metabolic acidosis. **CAUTIONS**: Displaces coumarin anticoagulants from plasma binding to increase their activity. May induce hemolysis in G-6-PD deficient patients. NOT for treatment of acute pyelonephritis or other systemic (especially intestinal) infections. **RECOMMEND**: AVOID prolonged exposure to sunlight (photosensitivity may occur). Perform periodic CBC, renal and liver functions tests with prolonged therapy. **CONTRAINDICATIONS**: History of convulsive disorders.
NITROFURANTOIN (Furadantin) (Cyantin) (Macrodantin) (Nitrex) (Trantoin) (Furadantin) (Nitrofan)	__Urinary Tract Infections__: **PO**: 50-100 mg q6h; maximum 400 mg/d. **Pediatric PO**: 5-7 mg/kg/d in 4 doses. **IV**: 180 mg bid. **Pediatric IV**: 3.3 mg/kg bid. __Long-Term Therapy__: **PO**: 25-50 mg q6h. **Pediatric PO**: 1-2 mg/kg/d in 4 doses.	PO (Tab's): 50, 100 mg PO (Cap's): 25, 50, 100 mg PO (Liquid): 5 mg/ml	**SPECTRUM OF ACTIVITY**: **Gram positive**: Staphylococcus aureus, S. epidermidis, Streptococcus faecalis. **Gram negative**: Citrobacter, Corynebacterium, Enterobacter, E. coli, Klebsiella, Neisseria, Salmonella and Shigella.
			Nitrofurantoin is a drug of second choice because of serious and potentially fatal side effects. Bactericidal at the higher concentrations achieved in urine; less active at alkaline pH. **SIDE EFFECTS**: Nausea, vomiting, diarrhea due to CNS action (15% patients receiving > 7 mg/kg). Allergic reactions frequent: fever, rash, urticaria, exzematoid eruption, pruritis and anaphylactic shock. Others: alcohol intolerance, cholestatic jaundice, chronic active hepatitis, headache, dizziness, drowsiness, polyneuropathy. Peripheral polyneuritis, with irreversible paralysis, can occur in renal failure (18% patients with BUN > 15 mmol/l), especially with large doses. Rare: allergic pneumonitis, asthma, pulmonary fibrosis, blood dyscrasias. **CAUTIONS**: NOT for use as a single agent in acute pyelonephritis or for infections other than of the urinary tract. Risk of hemolytic anemia attends use in newborns or pregnant women. Teratogenic/mutagenic in laboratory animals. **RECOMMEND**: Administer IV doses SLOWLY. Minimize GI side effects by frequent administration of small doses, with milk or food; also by use of macrocrystalline form (slow-release). **CONTRAINDICATIONS**: Anuria, oliguria, or significant renal impairment (creat. clearance < 40 cc/min) and pregnancy.

MISCELLANEOUS ANTIBACTERIAL AGENTS

DRUG	INDICATIONS & DOSAGE	DOSE FORMS	REMARKS
ERYTHROMYCIN			
ERYTHROMYCIN **base** (Eryc) (E-Mycin) (Ery-Tab) **stearate** (Erypar) (Ethril) **injection** (Erythrocin-lactobionate) (Ilotycin-glucephate) **estolate** (Ilosone)	<u>General</u>: **PO**: 1-2 gm/d in 3-4 doses; maximum 4 gm/d. **Pediatric PO**: 30-50 mg/kg/d in 4 doses; maximum 100 mg/kg/d. **IV**: 15-20 mg/kg/d; maximum 4 gm/d. **Pediatric IV**: 15-20 mg/kg/d in 4 doses. <u>Bacterial Endocarditis Prophylaxis</u>: **PO**: 1 gm 1-2 h prior to procedure, then 500 mg q6h for 8 doses. **Pediatric PO**: 20 mg/kg 1-2 h prior to procedure, then 10 mg/kg q6h for 8 doses. <u>Urethritis in Tetracycline Intolerant Males</u>: **PO**: 500 mg q6h for 7 d. <u>Lymphogranuloma Venereum</u>: **PO**: 500 mg q6h for 14 d. <u>Hemophilus Ducreyi (Chancroid)</u>: **PO**: 500 mg q6h for 10 d. <u>Epididymo-orchitis in Tetracycline Intolerant Patients</u>: **PO**: 500 mg q6h for 10 d. <u>Acute Gonorrheal Pelvic Inflammatory Disease</u>: **IV**: 500 mg q6h for 3d, then PO: 250 mg q6h for 7 d. <u>Legionnaire's Disease</u>: **PO, IV**: 1-4 gm/d. <u>Streptococcal Prophylaxis in Rheumatic Heart Disease (Continuous Therapy)</u>: **PO**: 250 mg q12h. <u>Dysenteric Amebiasis</u>: **PO**: 1 gm/d in 3-4 doses for 10-14 d. **Pediatric PO**: 30-50 mg/kg/d in 6 doses for 10-14 d. <u>Pertussis</u>: **Pediatric PO**: 40-50 mg/kg/d in 4 doses for 5-14 d. <u>Syphilis in Intolerant Patients</u>: **PO**: 500 mg q6h; 15 d course if < 1 year disease duration, 30d course if > 1 year duration. <u>Campylobacter Jejuni Enteric Infections</u>: **PO**: 500 mg q6h for 7 d.	**base**: PO (Cap's): 125, 250 mg PO (Tab's): 250, 333, 500 mg **stearate**: PO (Tab's): 250, 500 mg **estolate**: PO (Tab's): 125, 250, 500 mg PO (Cap's): 125, 250 mg PO (Liquid): 25, 50 mg/ml	**SPECTRUM OF ACTIVITY**: **Gram positive**: Staphylococci, Streptococci, Bacillus anthracis, Corynebacterium species, Clostridium species, Erysipelothrix species, and Listeria monocytogenes. **Gram negative**: Neisseria species, some strains of Haemophilus influenzae, Legionella pneumophila, Pasteurella, Brucella and Bordetella pertussis. **Others**: Chlamydiae and Actinomyces species, Mycoplasma pneumoniae, rickettsiae, treponema, trachoma, and lymphogranuloma inguinale. ***Note***: Spectrum of activity is broader than for penicillin G. Erythromycin inhibits bacterial protein synthesis. It is bacteriostatic at therapeutic concentrations; bacteriocidal only in higher concentrations. Base form is susceptible to inactivation by stomach acid; use enteric-coated preparations. Slightly higher PO doses needed for ethylsuccinate form. All doses expressed in terms of active base equivalent. **SIDE EFFECTS**: Dosage limited by occurrence of GI effects: abdominal pain, nausea, diarrhea, loose stools; especially with high PO doses. Allergic reactions (fever, eosinophilia, rashes) are rare. Estolate form causes cholestatic (obstructive) jaundice, but no liver damage. **CAUTIONS**: Some preparations contain tartrazine dye (potential for allergic reactions, especially in patients sensitive to aspirin). Penicillins, cephalosporins or tetracyclines generally act more rapidly and effectively. **CONTRAINDICATIONS**: Estolate form contraindicated in pre-existing liver disease.

MISCELLANEOUS ANTIBACTERIAL AGENTS *Continued*

INFREQUENTLY USED AGENTS

DRUG	INDICATIONS & DOSAGE	DOSE FORMS	REMARKS
CLINDAMYCIN (Cleocin) **LINCOMYCIN** (Lincocin)	**<u>Bacterial Infections</u>**: **<u>Clindamycin</u>**: **PO**: 150-300 mg q6h; maximum 450 mg q6h. **Pediatric PO**: <u>HCl</u>: 8-16 mg/kg/d in 3-4 doses (maximum 20 mg/kg/d) <u>palmitate HCl</u>: 8-12 mg/kg/d in 3-4 doses (maximum 25 mg/kg/d). **IM, IV**: 0.6-2.7 gm/d in 2-4 doses; maximum 4.8 gm/d. **Pediatric IM, IV**: 15-25 mg/kg/d in 3-4 doses; maximum 40 mg/kg/d. **<u>Lincomycin</u>**: **PO**: 500 mg q8h (maximum 500 mg q6h). **Pediatric PO**: 30 mg/kg/d in 3-4 doses; maximum 60 mg/kg/d. **IM**: 600 mg q24h (maximum 600 mg q12h). **IV**: 600-1000 mg q8-12h SLOWLY; maximum 8 gm/d. **Pediatric IV**: 10-20 mg/kg/d in 3-4 doses.	**Clindamycin**: PO (Cap's): 75, 150 mg Injection: 50 mg/ml Granules (for oral solution) **Lincomycin**: PO (Cap's): 250, 500 mg Injection: 300 mg/ml	**SPECTRUM OF ACTIVITY**: **Gram positive**: Staphylococcus aureus (S. epidermidis, S. pyognes), Streptococci (S. pneumoniae, ß-hemolytic streptococci, S. virians), Corynebacterium diphtheriae, Nocardia asteroides, some N. gonorrheae. **Gram negative**: Some H. influenzae. - - - - - - - - - - Generally equivalent to erythromycin but more toxic. Lincomycin is distributed better to bone; no clinical advantage established. **SIDE EFFECTS**: Potentially FATAL pseudomembranous colitis occurs in 0.1-10%. Others: rash, reversible elevation of LFTs, thrombophlebitis at infusion site, sterile abscesses at IM injection site, granulocytopenia, thrombocytopenia, eosinophilia, allergic reactions. Rare: polyarthritis and Stevens-Johnson syndrome. **CAUTIONS**: Rapid IV administration may precipitate circulatory collapse or cardiac arrest. Use cautiously in pre-existing GI disease, hepatic dysfunction, asthma or history of allergies. Some forms contain tartrazine dye (potential for allergic reactions, especially in patients sensitive to aspirin). May enhance the activity of neuromuscular blockers. **RECOMMENDATIONS**: Discontinue if severe diarrhea develops and evaluate patient for colitis. Vancomycin for treatment of pseudomembranous colitis due to Clostridium difficile.
VANCOMYCIN (Vancocin) *Continued, next page*	**<u>Bacterial Infections</u>**: **PO, IV**: 500 mg q6h or 1 gm q12h. **Pediatric PO, IV**: 44 mg/kg/d in 2-4 doses. **<u>Endocarditis Prophylaxis (Dental)</u>**: **IV**: 1 gm SLOWLY (over 30-60 min) 1 h prior to procedure; then erythromycin PO: 500 mg q6h for 8 doses. **Pediatric IV**: 20 mg/kg SLOWLY (over 30-60 min) 1 h prior to procedure; then erythromycin PO: 10 mg/kg q6h for 8 doses. **<u>Endocarditis Prophylaxis (GI/GU procedures)</u>**: **IV**: 1 gm SLOWLY (over 30-60 min) + streptomycin IM: 1 gm 1 h prior to procedure; then erythromycin PO: 500 mg q6h for 8 doses. **Pediatric IV**: 20 mg/kg SLOWLY (over 30-60 min) + streptomycin IM: 20 mg/kg 1 h prior to procedure; then erythromycin PO: 10 mg/kg q6h for 8 doses. *Continued, next page*	Powder for injection or oral suspension	**SPECTRUM OF ACTIVITY**: **Gram positive**: Staphylococci, Group A ß-hemolytic Streptococci, Pneumococci, Enterococci, Corynebacteria, and Clostridia. **Note**: NOT active against: Gram negative organisms, fungi, or yeast. Streptomycin or gentamicin may be synergistic against enterococci; questionable clinical because of additive toxicities. - - - - - - - - - - Vancomycin inhibits bacterial cell wall formation and is bactericidal. PO absorption poor (effectiveness and toxicity low). **SIDE EFFECTS**: Renal injury (elevated BUN, urinary casts, albuminuria) and ototoxicity (tinnitus, deafness) are the most severe; risk increases with high dose, *Continued, next page*

MISCELLANEOUS ANTIBACTERIAL AGENTS *Continued*

DRUG	INDICATIONS & DOSAGE	DOSE FORMS	REMARKS
VANCOMYCIN *Continued*	<u>**Renal Failure**</u>: **IV (dialysis patient)**: 15 mg/kg initially, then 1.9 mg/kg/d.	See previous page.	prolonged or IV therapy. Others: occasional thrombophlebitis, pain and flushing upon rapid IV administration. Hypersensitivity reactions (fever, chills, nausea, rash, transient leukopenia, eosinophilia and anaphylaxis) occur in 5-10% patients. **CAUTIONS**: NOT for IM injection (tissue irritation and necrosis). Use cautiously along with other neurotoxic, nephrotoxic or ototoxic agents (e.g., aminoglycosides, polymyxin B and colistin). **RECOMMENDATIONS**: Administer IV doses SLOWLY (over 30-60 min); dilute with saline, rotate sites. Perform periodic hematologic, liver and renal function tests in all patients; audiometric and serum level tests in patients > 60 y.o. or those with impaired renal function. Discontinue if tinnitus develops. Add steroids if rash, chills or fever occur during infusion. **CONTRAINDICATIONS**: Acute renal failure, preexisting deafness, pregnancy.
METRONIDAZOLE (Flagyl) *Continued, next page*	<u>**Anaerobic Bacterial Infections**</u>: **PO**: 7.5 mg/kg q6h; maximum 4 gm/d. **IV**: 15 mg/kg initially, then 7.5 mg/kg q6h for 5-10d; maximum 4 gm/d for 2-3 wk. Infuse dose over 1 h. <u>**Acute Pelvic Inflammatory Disease**</u>: **IV**: 1 gm q12h + doxycycline IV: 100 mg q12h (continue for 2 d after fever abates; minimum 4 d total); then PO: 1 gm + doxycycline PO: 100 mg q12h for 10-14 d total therapy. <u>**Prophylaxis for Surgery**</u>: **IV**: 0.5-1 gm SLOWLY (over 30-60 min) 1 h prior to surgery; 0.5 gm at 6 h and 12 h after first dose. <u>**Trichomoniasis**</u>: **PO**: 2 gm/d for 1 d or 250 mg q8h for 7 d. <u>**Amebiasis**</u>: **PO**: 750 mg q8h for 5-10 d. **Pediatric PO**: 35-50 mg/kg/d in 3 doses for 10 d. <u>**Amebic Liver Abscess**</u>: **PO**: 500-750 mg q8h for 5-10 d. <u>**Giardiasis**</u> (unlabeled use): **PO**: 250 mg q8h for 7 d.	PO (Tab's): 250, 500 mg Injection: 5 mg/ml	**SPECTRUM OF ACTIVITY**: **Gram positive**: Clostridium, peptococcus, and peptostreptococcus. **Gram negative**: Bacteroides (B. fragilis, B. melaninogenicus and others), Fusobacterium, Veillonella, Gardnerella vaginalis and Campylobacter fetus. **Others**: Entamoeba histolytica, Trichomonas vaginalis, Giardia lamblia, and Balantidium coli. Possibly effective against Dracunculus medinensis (guinea worm). ***Note***: Active against most obligately anaerobic bacteria and protozoa. Acts primarily against trophozoite forms of E. histolytica; limited activity against encysted forms. Inactive against fungi, viruses and most aerobic or facultatively anaerobic bacteria. - - - - - - - - - - See also Antiparasitic Agents. Metronidazole inhibits nucleic acid synthesis in anaerobic bacteria; strongly bactericidal. **SIDE EFFECTS**: GI effects (nausea, vomiting, diarrhea) occur in 3% patients. Others: headache, dry mouth and metalic taste. Rare: pseudomembranous colitis. Occasionally during prolonged, high dose therapy: CNS disorders (dizziness, ataxia, clouding of consciousness, seizures), paresthesias, glossitis, stomatitis, urticaria, rash, itching, dysuria, cystitis, reversible neutropenia, slight EKG changes and insomnia. Hypersensitivity reactions: rash, nasal *Continued, next page*

MISCELLANEOUS ANTIBACTERIAL AGENTS *Continued*

DRUG	INDICATIONS & DOSAGE	DOSE FORMS	REMARKS
METRONIDAZOLE *Continued*	See previous page	See previous page	congestion, fever, serum sickness-like joint pain. Produces a disulfuram type reaction with alcohol ingestion. **CAUTIONS**: May increase acitivity of oral anticoagulants. Carcinogenic in laboratory animals. **RECOMMENDATIONS**: In Trichomoniasis infections, treat sexual partner also. AVOID alcohol consumption for 24 h after dose. **CONTRAINDICATIONS**: First trimester of pregnancy, active CNS diseases and blood dyscrasias.
CHLORAMPHENICOL (Chloromycetin)	<u>**Bacterial Infections**</u>: **PO**: 50 mg/kg/d in 4 doses; maximum 100 mg/kg/d. **Pediatric PO** (immature hepatic/renal function): 50 mg/kg/d in 4 doses.	PO (Cap's): 250, 500 mg PO (Liquid): 30 mg/ml Powder for injection	**SPECTRUM OF ACTIVITY**: **Gram positive**: Streptococcus pneumoniae and many others. **Gram negative**: Salmonella, Haemophilus influenzae and Neisseria species. **Others**: Rickettsia, Vibrio cholera, Chlamydia (psittacosis-lymphogranuloma organisms), and Mycoplasma.

Drug of choice for S. typhi. NOT for treatment of trivial infections, for prophylaxis or for non-indicated uses; use ONLY when less toxic agents are not appropriate. Inhibits protein synthesis; bacteriostatic. **SIDE EFFECTS**: Potentially fatal blood dyscrasias (aplastic anemia, thrombocytopenia and granulocytopenia) have occurred after both short and long term use; 1-20 cases per 100,000 patients, fatal in 50%. Incidence increases with total dosage and length of therapy; most cases develop after 2-8 wk. Others: reversible bone marrow suppression associated with decreased hematocrit, pro-erythroblastic vacuole formation, leukocytopenia and increased serum iron; usually associated with serum levels > 25 mg/l. Common, although minor: flatulance, diarrhea, vomiting, stomatitis, glossitis. Allergic reactions (fever, rash) are rare. "Grey baby" syndrome: premature and newborn infants receiving doses > 25 mg/kg may develop grey skin coloration and vomiting, hypothermia, respiratory difficulty and circulatory collapse; often fatal within hours. The immature liver is unable to conjugate chloramphenicol for excretion. Very rare effects: optic and peripheral neuritis. **CAUTIONS**: Use only if essential and NOT near term or during labor or lactation. Use cautiously in patients with G-6-PD deficiency or acute intermittent porphyria. **RECOMMENDATIONS**: Restrict dosage and monitor carefully when used in neonates, especially if premature. Perform blood counts every 2 d during therapy; discontinue therapy if level of any formed element decreases. Note that irreversible marrow depression may develop in spite of these studies. Limit therapy to as short a duration as necessary. **CONTRAINDICATIONS**: History of toxicity from chloramphenicol; blood diseases (aplastic anaemia, pancytopenia); severe liver failure with jaundice. Do NOT use in combination with potentially haematotoxic agents (e.g., cytotoxic drugs, sulfonamides, phenothiazine, phenylbutazone, hydantoins).

DRUG INTERACTIONS:
<u>**Chloramphenicol**</u> inhibits the metabolism of ***dicoumarol***, ***phenobarbital***, ***diphenylhydantoin***, ***tolbutamide***, ***chlorpropamide*** and ***cyclophosphamide***; activity of these agents may be increased. It may also decrease the effect of ***penicillins***, ***aminoglycosides***, ***vitamin*** B_{12}, ***folic acid*** and ***iron salts***. ***Penicillin*** and ***acetaminophen*** may increase serum levels or half-life of <u>**chloramphenicol**</u>.

MISCELLANEOUS ANTIBACTERIAL AGENTS *Continued*

POLYMYXINS

SPECTRUM OF ACTIVITY:

Gram negative: Acinetobacter, Citrobacter, E. coli, Enterobacter, Haemophilus influenzae, Klebsiella pneumoniae, Pseudomonas aeruginosa, Salmonella, Shigella, and some strains of Bordetella and Vibrio.

Note: Most strains of Proteus, Providencia, Serratia, Neisseria gonorrhoeae, N. meningitidis, and Bacteroides fragilis are resistant to polymyxins.

GROUP REMARKS: The polymyxins act as cationic detergents and are bactericidal. Their action is mainly extracellular. They are used mainly by injection or topically. The polymyxins are too toxic for general use. **SIDE EFFECTS**: Neurotoxicity (headaches, lethargy, irritability, reversible paresthesias, ataxia, impaired vision/speech) and nephrotoxicity (reversible proteinuria, casts, hematuria, elevated BUN) may occur with high doses, prolonged treatment or accumulation due to renal impairment. Neuromuscular blockade and apnea have occurred in patients with renal impairment or on muscle relaxants; not antagonized by neostigmine. Allergic reactions (urticaria, rashes, fever) are rare. **CAUTIONS**: Polymyxins are additive with other nephrotoxic drugs (e.g., aminoglycosides). Additive neuromuscular blockade with: anesthetics, neuromuscular blocking agents, aminoglycosides and others. **RECOMMENDATIONS**: Monitor renal function; discontinue therapy upon elevation of BUN or creatinine, or if urine output decreases.

DRUG	INDICATIONS & DOSAGE	DOSE FORMS	REMARKS
COLISTIMETHATE (Coly-Mycin M)	**Bacterial Infections**: **IM, IV**: 2.5-5 mg/kg/d in 2-4 doses; maximum 5 mg/kg/d. **Renal Impairment**: **IM, IV**: 1.25-1.7 mg/kg q12h if serum creat. = 1.3-1.5 mg/dl; 2.5 mg/kg q24h if = 1.6-2.5 mg/dl; 1.5 mg/kg q36h if = 2.6-4 mg/dl.	Injection: 100, 150 mg	**CAUTIONS**: Teratogenic in laboratory animals. Use with extreme caution and reduce dosage in renal impairment. **RECOMMENDATIONS**: Administer injections SLOWLY, over 3-5 min.
COLISTIN (Coly-Mycin S)	**Bacterial Infections**: **PO**: 5-15 mg/kg/d in 3 doses.	PO (Liquid): 5 mg/ml	Diffuses poorly in agar; use other susceptibility tests. NOT absorbed systemically in measurable amounts. Cross-reactivity occurs between colistin and polymyxin-B. **SIDE EFFECTS**: None reported within the recommended dosage range. **CAUTIONS**: In azotemia, potential for renal toxicity exists due to absorption of small amounts. Suppression of intestinal bacteria (with concomitant overgrowth) may occur with prolonged use.
POLYMYXIN B (Aerosporin)	**Bacterial Infections**: **IM**: 25,000-30,000 units/kg/d in 3-6 doses. **IV**: 15,000-25,000 units/kg/d in 2 doses for < 5 d. **Intrathecal**: 50,000 units/d for 3-4 d, then 50,000 units q48h for ≥ 2 wk after CSF cultures are sterile and CSF glucose is normal.	Injection powder: 500,000 units (for 20 ml)	NOT absorbed after PO administration. Renal excretion is slow; repeated injections may lead to accumulation. Cross-reactivity occurs between colistin and polymyxin-B. Potential for renal injury is greater with polymyxin B than with colistin. **SIDE EFFECTS**: Intrathecal use can cause cramps and paralysis if doses are > 5 mg. Polymyxin-B sulphate **IM** injection causes pain at **IM** injection site; may cause thrombophlebitis at IV injection sites. Polymyxin-B releases histamine in the skin. **CAUTIONS**: Safe use during pregnancy has not been established. Use cautiously and reduce dose in renal failure.

ANTITUBERCULOUS AND RELATED AGENTS

GROUP REMARKS: Combinations of two or more antituberculous agents are always used in order to prevent the emergence of resistant strains and to increase effectiveness; an exception to this is the prophylactic use of isoniazid.

DRUG	INDICATIONS & DOSAGE	DOSE FORMS	REMARKS
		FIRST-CHOICE AGENTS	
ISONIAZID (Laniazid) (Niconyl) (Nydrazid) (Teebaconin)	<u>**Tuberculosis (Treatment)**</u>: **PO, IM**: 5-10 mg/kg/d (maximum 300 mg/d). **Intermittent therapy**: 15 mg/kg 2-3 doses/wk (maximum 900 mg/wk). **Pediatric PO, IM**: 10-20 mg/kg/d (maximum 300 mg/d). <u>**Tuberculosis (Prevention)**</u>: **PO, IM**: 300 mg/d. **Pediatric PO, IM**: 10 mg/kg/d (maximum 300 mg/d). Continue preventative therapy for 12 months.	PO (Tab's): 50, 100, 300 mg Injection: 100 mg/ml Syrup: 10 mg/ml	**SPECTRUM OF ACTIVITY**: **Mycobacterium**: M. tuberculosis, M. bovis, some strains of M. kansasii. Isoniazid inhibits bacterial nucleic acid and mycolic acid synthesis. Bacteriostatic to tubercle bacilli at concentrations of 0.05-0.2 mg/l; bactericidal at 4 to 5 times that concentration, during the phase of active bacterial growth. Give pyridoxine, 100-200 mg/d, for treatment of established neuropathy. **SIDE EFFECTS**: Hepatitis (potentially FATAL) occurs in 1% of patients (more frequent in combination with rifampicin than with ethambutol). Slight elevations (transient) of SGOT and SGPT noted in 10-20% of patients; usually occur within first 6 months of therapy. There is usually no need to discontinue therapy, although may progress to liver damage (rare < 20 y.o.; up to 2-3% > 50 y.o.). Side effects are rare with doses < 300 mg/d. CNS effects (dizziness, headaches, restlessness, psychological disorders) are most common; especially peripheral neuropathy (paresthesias), which is dose-related. Other side effects: nausea, vomiting, epigastric pain, cramps, muscle fibrillation, optic neuritis, seizures, encephalopathy, psychosis, liver damage (rare in children), blood dyscrasias. **CAUTIONS**: Isoniazid inhibits hepatic microsomal enzymes; may need to lower dose of phenytoin. Use with caution in alcoholics, epileptics, diabetics and patients with chronic liver disease or renal insufficiency. **RECOMMENDATIONS**: Pyridoxine 6-50 mg/d recommended in alcoholics, diabetics and others predisposed to neuropathy through malnutrition or disease. Take on an empty stomach ≥ 1 h before or 2 h after meals. Patient should minimize alcohol consumption because of increased risk of hepatitis. **CONTRAINDICATIONS**: Acute liver disease or a history of previous isoniazid-associated hepatic injury.
ETHAMBUTOL (Myambutol)	<u>**Tuberculosis (Initial Therapy)**</u>: **PO**: 15-25 mg/kg/d. <u>**Tuberculosis (with Previous Therapy)**</u>: **PO**: 25 mg/kg/d for 60 days or until smears and cultures become negative, then 15 mg/kg/d. <u>**Tuberculosis (Intermittent Therapy)**</u>: **PO**: 50 mg/kg 2-3 doses/wk.	PO (Tab's): 100, 400 mg	**SPECTRUM OF ACTIVITY**: **Myobacterium**: M. tuberculosis, M. bovis, M. marinum, and some strains of M. kansasii, M. acium, M. fortuitum, M. intracellulare. Absorption not significantly affected by food. **SIDE EFFECTS**: Optic neuritis (impaired vision and green sensitivity, later hemianopia and finally optic nerve atrophy); most commonly with doses > 25 mg/kg/d, prolonged treatment. Others: allergy (anaphylaxis, rash, pruritis), elevated uric acid levels, abnormal LFTs, fever, headache, nausea, vomiting, confusion, peripheral neuritis. **CAUTIONS**: Teratogenic in laboratory animals. Changes in color perception are early signs of toxicity. **RECOMMENDATIONS**: Monthly eye exams with doses ≥ 25 mg/kg/d. Reduce dose in renal failure. Perform periodic evaluation of hepatic, renal and hematologic function. Ethambutol NOT to be used as a single agent. **CONTRAINDICATIONS**: Optic neuritis; not recommended for use in children < 13 y.o.

ANTITUBERCULOUS AND RELATED AGENTS: FIRST-CHOICE AGENTS *Continued*

DRUG	INDICATIONS & DOSAGE	DOSE FORMS	REMARKS
RIFAMPIN (Rifadin) (Rifocin) (Rimactane)	**Pulmonary Tuberculosis**: **PO**: 600 mg q24h. **Pediatric PO (> 5 y.o.)**: 10-20 mg/kg/d; maximum 600 mg/d. **Meningitis (Prophylaxis or Asymptomatic Carrier)**: **PO**: 600 mg/d for 4 d. **Pediatric PO (1-12 y.o.)**: 10 mg/kg/d for 4 d (maximm: 600 mg/	PO (Cap's): 150, 300 mg Syrup: 10 mg/ml	**SPECTRUM OF ACTIVITY**: **Mycobacterium**: M. tuberculosis, M. bovis, M. marinum, M. kansasii, some strains of M. fortuitum, M. avium, M. intracellulare, dapsone-sensitive and dapsone-resistant M. leprae (experimental leprosy in mice). **Gram positive**: Staphylococcus aureus, **Gram negative**: Neisseria, Haemophilus influenzae, Legionella pneumophila. Others (very high concentrations): Chlamydia trachomatis, poxviruses, adenoviruses.
	Bactericidal on proliferating bacteria including tubercle bacilli. Resistant meningococcal organisms emerge rapidly. **SIDE EFFECTS**: Flu-like effects develop in 20-50% patients receiving > 25 mg/kg/wk. Transient increases in liver enzymes occur in 5-20% of patients. Others include: nausea, vomiting, cramps, diarrhea, headache, fatigue, elevated BUN or uric acid levels, ataxia, pain in extremities. Serious effects include hepatitis and blood dyscrasias (leukopenia, thrombocytopenia, hemolytic anemia). Therapy may cause an orange discoloration of urine, tears, sweat and saliva. A hypersensitivity reaction producing interstitial nephritis, acute tubular necrosis or severe cortical necrosis can occur with the interruption and subsequent resumption of rifampin therapy. **CAUTIONS**: Carcinogenic (at 2-10 times maximum clinical dosages) and teratogenic in laboratory animals. Serum folate and vitamin B_{12} assays are inhibited by rifampin. **RECOMMENDATIONS**: Discontinue rifampin therapy immediately if SGOT or SGPT levels exceed 100 IU/litre or if serum bilirubin increases (hepatitis due to rifampin can be FATAL). Not for intermittent use, because of rare renal hypersensitivity reactions. Patients should NOT use oral contraceptives for birth control. In patients receiving warfarin, monitor protime and adjust dose accordingly. Take on empty stomach ≥ 1 h before or > 2 h after meals. **CONTRAINDICATIONS**: Acute hepatitis, obstructive jaundice, other severe liver diseases, pregnancy.		
	DRUG INTERACTIONS: **Rifampin** induces the metabolism, and decreases the action, of: ***beta-Blockers, Oral Contraceptives, Oral Anticoagulants, Oral Antidiabetics, Progestins, Corticosteroids, Quinidine*** and ***Methadone***. ***P-aminosalicylic acid*** may decrease **Rifampin** serum levels; give these drugs ≥ 8 h apart.		
STREPTOMYCIN (Strycin)	See Aminoglycosides and Related Agents.		
	SECOND-LINE AGENTS		
PYRAZINAMIDE (PZA) (Aldinamide) *Continued, next page*	**Tuberculosis**: **PO**: 15-30 mg/kg/d in 3-4 doses; maximum 3 gm/d. **Alternate Dosage**: PO: 50-70 mg/kg for 2 doses/wk.	PO (Tab's): 500 mg	**SPECTRUM OF ACTIVITY**: **Mycobacterium**: Mycobacterium tuberculosis. **Note**: Pyrazinamide is ineffective against other microorganisms. *Continued, next page*

ANTITUBERCULOUS AND RELATED AGENTS: SECOND-LINE AGENTS *Continued*

DRUG	INDICATIONS & DOSAGE	DOSE FORMS	REMARKS
PYRAZINAMIDE (PZA) *Continued*	See previous page.	See previous page.	Use ONLY when first-line drugs are ineffective and NEVER alone. No reliable test for pyrazinamide resistance exists. Bactericidal on human tubercle bacilli, but NOT usually on atypical mycobacteria. More active at acid pH; especially good in caseous necrosis. No cross-resistance with other antituberculous agents. **SIDE EFFECTS**: Hepatotoxicity develops in 2-20% of patients; ranging from elevated LFTs through minor fever, malaise and anorexia to fulminant hepatitis, hepatic necrosis and death; incidence increased at higher doses and may be associated with administration of PAS. Other effects: hyperuricemia, gouty attacks, hyperglycemia, sideroblastic anemia, thrombocytopenia, rashes, photosensitivity, nausea, vomiting, diarrhea. **CAUTIONS**: Use with caution in diabetes, history of gout, acute intermittent porphyria. Safe use in pregnancy has not been established. **RECOMMENDATIONS**: Perform baseline LFTs and serum uric acid determinations; repeat q2-4wk during treatment. Discontinue use if signs of hepatic damage develop. Reduce dose in renal impairment. **CONTRAINDICATIONS**: Severe hepatic damage, severe liver damage and gout.
CAPREOMYCIN (Capastat sulfate)	<u>**Tuberculosis**</u>: **IM**: 1 gm/d for 2-3 months, then 1 gm 2-3 doses/wk for 18-24 months; maximum 20 mg/kg/d.	Injection: 1 gm (powder for reconstitution)	**SPECTRUM OF ACTIVITY**: **Mycobacterium**: M. tuberculosis, M. bovis, M. kansasii, and some M. avium and M. intracellulare. M. lepare in mice. Resistance develops rapidly during treatment; partial cross-resistance with kanamycin. **SIDE EFFECTS**: Superficial injections may cause pain and sterile absesses. Most patients develop eosinophil count > 5%. Common effects: rash, urticaria, fever, renal injury (BUN elevations in 33% patients), uremia, proteinuria, neutropenia, leukopenia, eosinophilia, impaired BSP excretion without transaminase elevation, impaired hearing. Ototoxicity (less than with streptomycin and kanamycin) occurs subclinically in 11% and clinically in 3% of patients; also tinnitus and vertigo. **CAUTIONS**: Large IV doses have been associated with peripheral neuromuscular blockade; reversed by neostigmine. **RECOMMENDATIONS**: Give by deep IM injection into large muscle. **CONTRAINDICATIONS**: Renal insufficiency, preexisting middle ear damage, pregnancy.
ETHIONAMIDE (Trecator SC) *Continued, next page*	<u>**Tuberculosis**</u>: **PO**: 0.5-1 gm/d in 1-3 doses; maximum 1 gm/d. **Pediatric PO**: 12-15 mg/kg/d in 3-4 doses; maximum 750 mg/d.	PO (Tab's): 250 mg	**SPECTRUM OF ACTIVITY**: **Mycobacterium**: M. tuberculosis, M. bovis, M. kansasii and some strains of M. avium and M. intracellulare. M. leprae in mice. Bacteriostatic at therapeutic levels; bactericidal at higher concentrations. **SIDE EFFECTS**: Half of patients receiving > 500 mg/d develop anorexia, nausea and vomiting; 5% develop diarrhea, metallic taste, hepatitis and elevated LFTs (particularly diabetics). Drowsiness and depression are common. Others: sleep disturbances, peripheral neuropathy, stomatitis, impotence, gynecomastia, postural hypotension, headache, rash, weight loss, jaundice, thrombocytopenia, pellagra-like syndrome, difficulty managing diabetes mellitus (hypoglycemia), hypothyroidism, eosinophilia, leucocytopenia, and *Continued, next page*

ANTITUBERCULOUS AND RELATED AGENTS: SECOND-LINE AGENTS *Continued*

DRUG	INDICATIONS & DOSAGE	DOSE FORMS	REMARKS
ETHIONAMIDE *Continued*	See previous page.	See previous page.	menstrual disorders. Also, seizures in epileptics, acne and photosensitization. **CAUTIONS**: Teratogenic in laboratory animals. Caution when co-administering ethionamide with cycloserine and other antituberculous drugs due to possible seizures. Use with care in epileptic and psychotic patients. AVOID alcohol. **RECOMMENDATIONS**: Begin with 250 mg bid and increase by 125 mg/d at intervals of 5 d until maximum dose achieved. Use ONLY with other antituberculous agents. Administer pyridoxine (50-150 mg/d) for prophylaxis and treatment of side effects. Evaluate baseline LFTs and monitor q2-4wk during therapy. **CONTRAINDICATIONS**: Severe hepatic impairment, early pregnancy, gastric complaints.
AMINOSALICYLIC ACID (p-aminosalicylic acid) (PAS) (Pamisyl) (Parasal) (Teebacin)	<u>**Tuberculosis**</u>: **PO**: 14-16 gm/d in 2-4 doses. **Pediatric PO**: 275-420 mg/kg/d in 3-4 doses.	PO (Tab's): 0.5, 1 gm	**SPECTRUM OF ACTIVITY**: **Mycobacterium**: M. tuberculosis. Contains 54.5 mg Na^+/500 mg tablet. Relatively weak bacteriostatic action. **SIDE EFFECTS**: Common: hematuria, leukocyturia, casts, albuminuria, GI disturbances (very frequent), hypersensitivity, hepatotoxicity, eosinophilia, fever, rashes. Rare: leuckcytopenia, hepatotoxicity and hypothyroidism. Goiter and myxedema occur occasionally. **CAUTIONS**: May precipitate fluid overload due to high Na^+ content; use cautiously in patients with CHF, hypertension or edema. Absorption/effects of rifampin oral folic acid and vitamin B_{12} are inhibited; may require parenteral B_{12} or folic acid. **RECOMMENDATIONS**: Maintain neutral/basic urine pH to prevent crystalluria. **CONTRAINDICATIONS**: Hypersensitivity to aminosalicyclic acids, severe liver damage or renal failure, gastritis, gastric or duodenal ulcer.
CYCLOSERINE (Seromycin)	<u>**Tuberculosis**</u>: **PO**: 250 mg bid initially; then increase by 250 mg q2d up to 1000 mg/d at 1 wk (maximum 1000 mg/d).	PO (Cap's): 250 mg	**SPECTRUM OF ACTIVITY**: **Gram positive**: Staphylococcus aureus **Gram negative**: Enterobacter, Escherichia coli. **Mycobacterium**: M. tuberculosis, M. bovis, and some strains of M. kansasii, M. marinum, M. ulcerans, M. avium, M. smegmatis, M. intracellulare. Bacteriostatic action. **SIDE EFFECTS**: Side effects prominent at doses > 1 gm/d or upon rapid dose increase early in treatment. Also early in treatment, transient increases in temperature, leukocytosis, ESR, and sputum production. Others: rash, drowsiness, agitation, visual disturbances, tremor, vertigo, confusion, psychosis, character changes, paresis, coma, elevated LFTs, deficiency of vit. B_{12} or folate. **LEVELS**: Toxicity greatly increased at levels > 30 µg/ml. **CAUTIONS**: Toxicity increased by excessive alcohol ingestion, seizure disorders, severe depression, anxiety or psychosis, renal insufficiency. Isoniazid may increase CNS toxicity. **RECOMMENDATIONS**: Determine drug levels weekly in patients with renal impairment and those receiving > 500 mg/d or with symptoms of toxicity. If CNS toxicity or rash develops, discontinue or reduce dosage. **CONTRAINDICATIONS**: Excessive alcohol ingestion, seizure disorders, severe depression, anxiety or psychosis, renal insufficiency.

ANTIFUNGAL AGENTS

DRUG	INDICATIONS & DOSAGE	DOSE FORMS	REMARKS
AMPHOTERICIN B (Fungizone) (Mysteclin-F; combination with tetracycline)	<u>**Fungal Infections**</u>: **IV**: 0.25 mg/kg initially, increase by 5-10 mg/d; maintenance 0.5-1 mg/kg/d (maximum 1 mg/kg/d <u>or</u> 1.5 mg/kg qod). Infuse over 3-6h. Treatment may require several months; continue until a total dose = 1-3 gm is given.	Injection: 50 mg (powder) PO (Cap's): 50 mg Amphotericin B + 250 mg tetracycline PO (Liquid): 5 mg Amphotericin B + 25 mg tetracycline/ml	**SPECTRUM OF ACTIVITY**: **Fungi**: Aspergillus fumigatus, Paracoccidioides brasiliensis, Coccidioides immitis, Cryptococcus neoformans, Histoplasma capsulatum, Mucor mucedo, Rhodotorula species, Sporothrix schenckii, Blastomyces dermatitidis. Amebae: Naegleria fowleri, Acanthamoeba polyphaga, A. castellanii. ***Note***: NOT effective against bacteria, rickettsiae, viruses. Recommended in systemic infections with moniliasis, histoplasmosis, coccidioidomycosis, cryptococcosis (torulosis), North American blastomycosis, mucormycosis (phycomycosis), aspergillosis (A. fumigatus), sporotrichosis (S. schenckii).
	NOT for use in common clinically inapparent forms of fungal infection. Alters fungal membrane permeability. Efficacy of oral forms (amphotericin + tetracycline) NOT established. **SIDE EFFECTS**: Permanent renal damage associated with a total dose > 5 gm; symptoms are hematuria, proteinuria, hyposthenuria, azotemia, hyperkaliuria, hypokalemia, hypomagnesemia, renal tubular acidosis. Common side effects: fever, headache, malaise, anorexia, nausea, vomiting, myalgias, phlebitis and pain at injection site. Uncommon, severe side effects: arrhythmias, cardiac arrest, anaphylaxis, coagulation disorders, blood dyscrasias, liver failure, GI bleeding, hypo/hypertension. **CAUTIONS**: Hypokalemia may precipitate digitalis or skeletal muscle relaxant toxicity. Safety for use during pregnancy has not been established. Do NOT reconstitute with saline; discard if any evidence of precipitation or foreign material. **RECOMMENDATIONS**: Blastomyces dermatitides may require higher drug concentrations. Serum concentrations should be maintained at twice the in vitro MIC for the infecting fungus. Administer by slow IV drip (6 h); concentration < 0.1 mg/ml. Use only in hospitalized or closely supervised patients. Measure serum creatinine (or clearance), BUN and liver function weekly; discontinue if creat. > 3 mg/dl, if BUN > 40 mg/dl or if LFTs become abnormal; wait for improvement before resuming. Acute reactions to amphotericin administration may be inhibited by use of antihistamines, antiemetics, aspirin or steroids (use minimal steroid doses). **CONTRAINDICATIONS**: In life-threatening conditions, drug hypersensitivity might NOT preclude cautious use. Impending renal failure.		
KETOCONAZOLE (Nizoral) *Continued, next page*	<u>**Fungal Infections**</u>: **PO**: 200 mg/d (maximum 400 mg/d). **Pediatric PO (> 2 y.o.)**: 3.3-6.6 mg/kg/d.	PO (Tab's): 200 mg	**SPECTRUM OF ACTIVITY**: **Gram positive**: Nocardia, actinomadura. **Fungi**: Petriellidium boydii, Aspergillus fumigatus, Actinomadura madurae, Nocardia, Sporothrix schenckii, Torulopsis glabrata, Candida albicans, Blastomyces dermatitidis, Coccidioides immitis, Cryptococcus neoformans, Epidermophyton floccosum, Histoplasma capsulatum, Malassezia furfur (formerly Pityrosporum orbiculare), Microsporum canis, Trichophyton mentagrophytes, T. rubrum, T. tonsurans. **Note**: Some activity in vitro against Leishmania and chloroquine-sensitive/resistant Plasmodium falciparum. Some strains of Candida albicans and Paracoccidioides brasiliensis are inhibited by > 25 µg/ml in vitro. *Continued, next page*

ANTIFUNGAL AGENTS *Continued*

DRUG	INDICATIONS & DOSAGE	DOSE FORMS	REMARKS
KETOCONAZOLE *Continued*	See previous page.	See previous page.	Results of in vitro susceptibility tests are method-dependent and may not accurately reflect the in vivo susceptibility of some fungi (especially Candida). **SIDE EFFECTS**: GI effects (nausea, vomiting, diarrhea) in 10-20% of patients; gynecomastia in 3-8%; itching in 1-2%. Dizziness, headaches, liver damage and rashes are less frequent. Hepatotoxicity occurs in 1 of 10,000 patients, usually reversible with discontinuance; several cases reported in pediatric patients and some fatalities have occurred. **CAUTIONS**: Teratogenic in laboratory animals; excreted in breast milk. Requires acid pH for proper dissolution; antacids, H_2-blockers, anticholinergics and achlorhydria will inhibit absorption. **RECOMMENDATIONS**: Administer with meals. Perform baseline and monthly LFTs during treatment; especially in patients receiving other potentially hepatotoxic drugs. Mothers should NOT breast feed their children. **CONTRAINDICATIONS**: Pregnancy.
GRISEOFULVIN (Fulvicin U/F) (Grifulvin) (Grisactin) (Gris-PEG)	<u>**Fungal Infections**</u>: **PO**: 0.5-1 gm/d microsize crystals <u>OR</u> 250-660 mg/d ultramicrosize in 1-2 doses. **Pediatric PO (> 23 kg)**: 250-500 mg/d microsize in 1-2 doses. **Pediatric PO (13.5-23 kg)**: 125-250 mg/d microsize in 1-2 doses.	**Microsize**: PO (Cap's): 125, 250 mg PO (Tab's): 250, 500 mg PO (Liquid): 25 mg/ml **Ultramicrosize**: PO (Tab's): 125, 165, 250, 330 mg	**SPECTRUM OF ACTIVITY**: **Fungi**: Trichophyton rubrum, T. tonsurans, T. mentagrophytes, T. verrucosum, T. megninii, T. gallinae, and T. schoenleinii, Microsporum audouinii, M. canis, M. gypseum, Epidermophyton floccosum. ***Note***: NOT active against bacteria, Candida, Actinomyces, Aspergillus, Blastomyces, Cryptococcus, Coccidioides, Geotrichum, Histoplasma, Nocardia, Saccharomyces, Sporotrichum, Pityrosporum orbiculare, chromoblastomycosis, tinea versicolor. Fungistatic; no antibacterial activity. Ultramicrosize form has 1.5 times the biological activity of microsize forms (330 mg ultramicrosize = 500 mg microsize). Treatment may take from 2-4 weeks (tinea pedis) to 4-6 months (tinea unguium). **SIDE EFFECTS**: Side effects are rare despite prolonged administration. Most common: allergy (rash, urticaria). Less frequent: paresthesias, nausea, vomiting, diarrhea, GI upset, headache, fatigue, dizziness, confusion, psychological disturbances, impaired vision. Also: alcohol intolerance, impaired judgment or ability to perform routine activities, photosensitivity, insomnia, proteinuria, leukopenia, reversible leukocytopenia, monocytosis, granulocytopenia, transient albuminuria, lupus, erythematosus-like syndromes have been reported. May precipitate acute intermittent porphyria. **CAUTIONS**: Carcinogenic, embryotoxic and teratogenic in laboratory animals. Theoretical cross-sensitivity may exist with penicillin-allergic patients. Decreases the activity of warfarin-type coagulants; may potentiate the effects of alcohol. **RECOMMENDATIONS**: Periodically evaluate liver, kidney and blood function; discontinue if granulocytopenia occurs. **CONTRAINDICATIONS**: Porphyria, pregnancy, severe liver disease, hepatocellular failure.
MICONAZOLE (Monistat) *Continued, next page*	<u>**Fungal Infections**</u>: **IV**: 0.2-3.6 gm/d in 3 doses for 1-20 wk. **Pediatric IV**: 20-40 mg/kg/d in 3 doses; maximum:15 mg/kg/dose. <u>**Coccidioidomycosis**</u>: **IV**: 0.6-1.2 gm q8h for 3-20 wk. <u>**Petriellidiosis**</u>: **IV**: 0.2-1 gm q8h for 5-20 wk. *Continued, next page*	Injection: 10 mg/ml Topical: 2% cream, lotion or powder	**SPECTRUM OF ACTIVITY**: **Gram positive**: Staphylococcus aureus. **Fungi**: Candida albicans, Epidermophyton floccosum, Trichophyton mentagrophytes, T. rubrum, Microsporum canis, C. guilliermondi, C. tropicalis. Cremophor, a proprietary solvent in the IV preparation, can cause hyperlipemia and changes in the CBC. **SIDE EFFECTS**: Generally well tolerated. GI effects in 5-20% of patients: anorexia, nausea, vomiting, diarrhea. Other common effects: flushes, fever, drowsiness. Also: pruritis, rash, *Continued, next page*

ANTIFUNGAL AGENTS *Continued*

DRUG	INDICATIONS & DOSAGE	DOSE FORMS	REMARKS
MICONAZOLE *Continued*	**Candidiasis**: **IV**: 0.2-0.6 gm q8h for 1-20 wk. **Cryptococcosis**: **IV**: 0.4-0.8 gm q8h for 3-12 wk. **Paracoccidiomycosis**: **IV**: 0.06-0.4 gm q8h for 2-16 wk.	See previous page. **Dermal Fungal Infections**: **Topical**: Apply bid for 2-4 wk. Cover affected areas.	allergic reactions, phlebitis, transient fall in serum sodium, hematocrit or platelets; lipemia. Thrombophlebitis can complicate administration. Tachycardia and arrhythmias can follow rapid injection. **CAUTIONS**: Initial treatment with miconazole IV should be done in a hospital. May potentiate effects of coumarin anticoagulants; may antagonize antifungal activity of amphotericin B. **RECOMMENDATIONS**: Perform baseline and periodic CBC, electrolytes and lipid levels.
FLUCYTOSINE (Ancobon) (5-FC)	**Fungal Infections**: **PO**: 50-150 mg/kg/d in 4 doses.	PO (Cap's): 250, 500 mg	**SPECTRUM OF ACTIVITY**: **Fungi**: Cryptococcus species, Candida species, Toruloposis glabrata, Sporothrix schenckii and some Aspergillus, Cladosphorium, Phialophora. **NOTE**: Little or no activity against Coccidioides immitis, Paracoccidioides brasilkiensis, Histoplasma capsulatum, Blastomyces dermatidis, Madurella species, phycomycetes, dermatophytes, or bacteria. Flucytosine and amphotericin B exhibit in vitro synergistic inhibition of Cryptococcus neoformans, Candida albicans, Candida tropicalis. ***Note***: Resistance frequently develops in Cryptococcus; less frequently in Candida, Torulopsis, Cladosporium. Any Cryptococcus strain requiring > 12.5-16 µg/ml for inhibition and any Candida strain requiring > 100 µg/ml is considered resistant (≤ 25% of pretreatment clinical isolates of Candida may be resistant to flucytosine). Concurrent use with amphotericin B may increase toxicity of flucytosine. Therapy may need to be continued for up to 4-6wks. **SIDE EFFECTS**: Reversible blood dyscrasias (anemia, leukopenia, thrombocytopenia) occur in 10% of patients; fatal cases of agranulocytosis have occurred. Common: nausea, vomiting, diarrhea, rash, increased BUN or creatinine, elevated liver enzymes. Rare: dizziness, headache, fatigue, GI upset, hallucinations and fatal hepatic necrosis. **CAUTIONS**: Teratogenic in laboratory animals. Safe use in pregnancy has not been established. Use extreme caution and monitor blood levels in patients with renal impairment; maintain blood levels of flucytosine < 100 µg/ml. Use with great caution in renal failure, liver damage and bone-marrow suppression due to malignancy. **RECOMMENDATIONS**: GI upset can be minimized by taking capsules over a 15 min period. Evaluate baseline hepatic, hematologic and renal function; monitor hepatic function frequently. **CONTRAINDICATIONS**: Pregnancy.
NYSTATIN (Mycostatin) *Continued, next page*	**Intestinal Candidiasis**: **PO**: 500,000-1 million units q8h; continue ≥ 48h after symptoms have disappeared. *Continued, next page*	PO (Tab's): 100,000, 500,000 units PO (Liquid): 100,000 units/ml Intravaginal (Tab's): 100,000 units	**SPECTRUM OF ACTIVITY**: **Fungi**: Candida albicans, C. guilliermondi, C. krusei, Geotrichum lactis. *Continued, next page*

ANTIFUNGAL AGENTS *Continued*

DRUG	INDICATIONS & DOSAGE	DOSE FORMS	REMARKS
NYSTATIN *Continued*	<u>**Oral Candida Infections**</u>: **PO**: 400,000-600,000 units q6h (retain in mouth). **Pediatric PO**: 200,000 units q6h. <u>**Vaginal Candidiasis**</u>: **Intravaginal**:1-2 tablets/d for 2 wk.	See previous page.	Not appreciably absorbed with PO administration; used for treatment of GI candida infections. **SIDE EFFECTS**: Nausea, vomiting and loose stools may follow a large oral dose. **RECOMMENDATIONS**: Continue use for at least 2 d after symptoms have subsided. Keep in mouth as long as possible.
CLOTRIMAZOLE (Mycelex)	<u>**Oral Candida Infections**</u>: **PO**: 1 troche q3h for 2 wk.	Troche: 10 mg	**SPECTRUM OF ACTIVITY**: **Fungi**: Candida species, including Candida albicans. - - - - - - - - - - Fungicidal. **SIDE EFFECTS**: Elevates SGOT in 15% of patients; produces nausea and vomiting in 5%. **CAUTIONS**: Safe use in pregnancy or children < 3 y.o. has not been established. **RECOMMENDATIONS**: Allow troche to slowly dissolve in mouth.

ANTIPARASITIC AGENTS

DRUG	INDICATIONS & DOSAGE	DOSE FORMS	REMARKS
CHLOROQUINE (Aralen) (Nivaquine) (Roquine)	***Note***: Doses expressed as chloroquine base; 500 mg phosphate = 300 mg base, 50 mg parenteral HCl salt = 40 mg base. **Malaria Chemoprophylaxis**: **PO**: 300 mg once/wk. **Pediatric PO**: 5 mg/kg once/wk; maximum 300 mg/wk. **Acute Malaria**: **IM**: 160-200 mg, repeat at 6 h (maximum 800 mg on1st day); then adjust doses for days 2 & 3 so that total dose for 1st 3 d is ≤ 1.5 gm. Start PO therapy ASAP. **Pediatric IM**: 5 mg/kg, repeat at 6 h (maximum 10 mg/kg on 1st day). Start PO therapy ASAP (PO: 5 mg/kg 18 h after last IM dose; then 5 mg/kg at 24 h. **Extraintestinal Amebiasis**: **PO**: 600 mg/d for 2 d, then 300 mg/d for 2-3 wk. **IM**: 160-200 mg for 10-12 d; then PO. **Rheumatoid Arthritis**: **PO**: 200 mg/d. **Lupus Erythematosus**: **PO**: 200 mg/d. **Clonorchis sinensis (liver fluke)**: **PO**: 150 mg q8h for 6 wk.	PO (Tab's): 250 mg (= 150 mg base), 500 mg (= 300 mg base) as phospate Injection: 50 mg/ml (= 40 base) HCl	**SPECTRUM OF ACTIVITY**: **Effective against**: asexual erythrocytic forms of most strains of Plasmodium malariae, P. ovale, P. vivax, many strains of P. falciparum; gametocyticidal for P. malariae and P. vivax, trophozoite form of Entamoeba histolytica. ***Note***: NOT active against preerythrocytic or exoerythrocytic forms of plasmodia. NO direct activity against the gametocytes of P. falciparum. Use in rheumatoid arthritis is investigational. **SIDE EFFECTS**: Cardiovascular effects: hypotension, EKG changes (T-wave inversion, widened QRS complexes). Common: Headaches, agitation, nausea, vomiting, diarrhea, cramps, anorexia. Nerve-type deafness reported in rare cases (associated with high doses and long treatment). Reversible blurring of vision, difficulty in focusing, corneal changes may occur. Irreversible retinal changes have occurred with evidence of loss of foveal reflex, macular lesions, optic disk pallor, optic atrophy, patchy retinal pigmentation and arteriolar narrowing; nyctalopia, scotomas, halos may be signs of ocular damage. Others: pruritis, depigmentation of hair, rash, weight loss, alopecia, extraocular palsies and rare discoloration of nails or oral mucosa. **CAUTIONS**: Chloroquine concentrates in the liver; use with caution in alcoholics or hepatic disease. May induce hemolysis in G-6-PD deficient patients. Infants and children particularly sensitive to overdose. **RECOMMENDATIONS**: For prophylaxis of malaria, start therapy 2 wk prior to entering malaria-endemic area; continue through 8 wk after leaving area. Use in conjunction with pyramethamine-sulfadoxine in areas endemic for chloroquine-resistant malaria. Perform baseline and periodic CBCs, ophthalmalogic and neurologic exams. Discontinue if any severe blood disorder (not attributable to disease) appears. Measure G-6-PD in susceptible individuals prior to therapy. **CONTRAINDICATIONS**: Drug hypersensitivity to 4-aminoquinoline derivatives, psoriasis, G-6-PD deficiency, patients with 4-aminoquinoline-induced retinal or visual field changes.
HYDROXYCHLORO-QUINE (Plaquenil)	***Note***: Doses are expressed as hydroxychloroquine base; 400 mg sulfate = 310 mg base. **Malaria Chemoprophylaxis**: **PO**: 310 mg once/wk. **Pediatric PO**: 5 mg/kg once/wk; maximum 310 mg/wk. ***Note***: Start 2 wk prior to exposure. **Acute Malaria**: **PO**: 620 mg initially; then 310 mg at 6 h; then 310 mg/d for 2 d. **Pediatric PO**: 10 mg/kg initially; then 5 mg/kg at 6 h; then 5 mg/kg/d for 2 d.	PO (Tab's): 200 mg (=155 base)	Hydroxylated derivative of chloroquine; agent of second choice for malaria. 400 mg hydroxychloroquine is equivalent to 500 mg chloroquine. Otherwise, the drugs are very similar, especially in side effects and cautions.

DRUG	INDICATIONS & DOSAGE	DOSE FORMS	REMARKS
IODOQUINOL (DIIODOHYDROXY-QUIN) (Mobequin) (Yodoxin)	<u>**Parasitic Infections**</u>: **PO**: 630-650 mg q8-12h for 20 d. **Pediatric PO**: 10-13 mg/kg q8h for 20 d.	PO (Tab's): 210, 650 mg Powder	**SPECTRUM OF ACTIVITY**: **Effective against**: trophozoite and insisted forms of Entamoeba histolytica.
		SIDE EFFECTS: Common: rash, acne, slight thyromegaly, nausea, vomiting, diarrhea, cramps, anal pruritis, skin eruptions, urticaria, fever, chills, headache, vertigo. Optic neuritis and peripheral neuropathy associated with high dose, prolonged therapy. Rare: optic atrophy and visual impairment after prolonged use in children. **CAUTIONS**: Use cautiously in patients with thyroid disease. **RECOMMENDATIONS**: Avoid long-term therapy when possible. **CONTRAINDICATIONS**: Hypersensitivity to iodine or 8-hydroxyquinolines, hepatic or renal disease, pre-existing optic neuropathy.	
QUINACRINE HYDROCHLORIDE (Atabrine)	<u>**Acute Malaria**</u>: **PO**: 200 mg with 1 gm Na+ bicarbonate q6h for 5 doses; then 100 mg tid for 6 d. **Pediatric PO (4-8 y.o.)**: 200 mg tid for 1 d; then 100 mg bid for 6 d. **Pediatric PO (1-4 y.o.)**: 100 mg tid for 1 d; then 100 mg/d for 6 d. <u>**Malaria Suppression**</u>: **PO**: 100 mg/d for 3 months. **Pediatric PO**: 50 mg/d for 3 months. <u>**Giardiasis**</u>: **PO**: 100 mg q8h for 5-7 d. **Pediatric PO**: 7 mg/kg/d in 3 doses for 5 d; maximum 300 mg/d. <u>**Beef, Pork or Fish Tapeworm**</u>: **PO**: 200 mg with 600 mg Na+ bicrbonate, for 4 doses. **Pediatric PO**: 200 mg with 600 mg Na+ bicrbonate.	PO (Tab's): 100 mg	**SPECTRUM OF ACTIVITY**: **Effective against**: intra-erythrocytic trophozoites of vivax, falciparum, quartan malaria, Giardia lamblia, Taenia saginata, Taenia solium, Hymenolepsis nana, Hymenolepsis dimunita, Diphyllobothrium latum, Dipylidium caninum. ***Note***: NOT effective against the gametocytes and sporozoites of all forms of malaria. Cross-resistance between chloroquine and quinacrine may occur.
		Take after meals with large quantities of water. **SIDE EFFECTS**: Common: diarrhea, anorexia, nausea, abdominal cramps, headache, vomiting. Rare: skin eruptions (exfoliative or contact dermatitis) vertigo, irritability, emotional change, nightmares, transient psychosis. Aplastic anemia, hepatitis, lichen planus-like eruptions, corneal deposits, corneal edema, retinopathy noted after prolonged therapy. Temporary yellow skin and urine color (not jaundice). **CAUTIONS**: Instruct patients on prolonged therapy to report any visual disturbances. May precipitate attacks in patients with porphyria or psoriasis. Administer cautiously to patients with G-6-PD deficiency. **RECOMMENDATIONS**: Perform periodic CBC for patients on prolonged therapy. Discontinue if any severe blood disorder (not attributable to disease) appears. **CONTRAINDICATIONS**: Concurrent administration of primaquine. ***Note***: For children 11-14 y.o., repeat q10min for 3 doses; for children 5-10 y.o., repeat q10min for 2 doses only.	
PRIMAQUINE PHOSPHATE *Continued, next page*	<u>**Acute Malaria**</u>: **PO**: 15 mg/d for 14 d <u>or</u> 45 mg once/wk for 8 wk. **Pediatric PO**: 0.3 mg/kg/d for 14 d <u>or</u> 0.9 mg/kg once/wk for 8 wk. *Continued, next page*	PO (Tab's): 26.3 mg (=15 mg base) as phosphate	**SPECTRUM OF ACTIVITY**: **Effective against**: preerythrocytic and exoerythrocytic forms of Plasmodium falciparum, P. malariae, P. ovale, P. vivax; gametocytes of P. falciparum and other plasmodia. ***Note***: NOT active against the erythrocytic forms of plasmodia. *Continued, next page*

ANTIPARASITIC AGENTS *Continued*

DRUG	INDICATIONS & DOSAGE	DOSE FORMS	REMARKS
PRIMAQUINE PHOSPHATE *Continued*	***Dosing Notes***: Use 2 wk prior to, or imediately following cessation of chloroquine (prophylaxis after departure from endemic area; P. vivax and P. ovale only). Doses are expressed as primaquine base; 26.5 mg phosphate = 15 mg base (0.53 mg phosphate = 0.3 mg base).	**Chloroquine + Primaquine**: PO (Tab's): 500 mg (300 mg base) chloroquine phosphate + 79 mg (45 mg base) primaquine phosphate	Primaquine phosphate 26.3 mg = primaquine base 15 mg. May be taken with food if GI upset occurs. **SIDE EFFECTS**: Common: nausea, vomiting, abdominal cramps, epigastric distress, methemoglobinemia, cyanosis, leukopenia. Hemolytic reactions (moderate to severe) may occur in: G-6-PD deficient patients, preexisting hemolytic anemia, methemoglobinemia, leukopenia or NADH-methemoglobin reductase deficient patients. May cause mental depression and confusion. Anemia, methemoglobinemia and leukopenia have followed large doses. **RECOMMENDATIONS**: Do not exceed recommended dose. Perform periodic CBC and hemoglobin determinations during pregnancy. Discontinue if urine darkens or hemoglobin concentration or leukocyte counts decrease. **CONTRAINDICATIONS**: Acute diseases with a tendency to granulocytopenia (e.g., rheumatoid arthritis, lupus erythematosus); concurrent administraton of quinacrine or other potentially hemolytic drugs or bone marrow depressants.
QUININE SULFATE (Quinine acid sulfate)	<u>**Chloroquine-resistant Malaria**</u>: **PO**: 650 mg q8h for 10-14 d. **Pediatric PO**: 25 mg/kg q8h for 10-14 d. <u>**Nocturnal Leg Cramps**</u>: **PO**: 260-300 mg at bedtime.	PO (Cap's): 130,195, 200, 300, 325 mg PO (Tab's): 260, 325 mg PO (Liquid): 110 mg/5 ml	**SPECTRUM OF ACTIVITY**: **Effective against**: asexual erythrocytic forms of Plasmodium falciparum, P. malariae, P. ovale, P. vivax; gametocyticidal for P. malariae and P. vivax. ***Note***: NOT active against sporozoites or preerythrocytic or exoerythrocytic forms of plasmodia and no direct activity against the gametocytes of P. falciparum.
		SIDE EFFECTS: Cinchonism, hemolysis (especially in G-6-PD deficient patients), agranulocytosis, thrombocytopenic purpura, hypoprothrombinemia, photophobia, blurred vision with scotomata, nyctopelopia, diplopia, amblyopia, altered color vision, tinnitus, deafness, vertigo, headache, fever, apprehension, delirium, convulsions, GI upset, hepatitis, hypersensitivity, rashes, flushing, sweating, edema. Idiosyncratic asthma and angina. Slightly disturbed vision, headache, tinnitus usually subside rapidly with discontinuation of therapy. **CAUTIONS**: Quinine is an isomer of quinidine; use with caution in patients with conduction defects or cardiac arrhythmias. Excreted in breast milk. **RECOMMENDATIONS**: Discontinue immediately upon any evidence of hypersensitivity or hemolysis. **CONTRAINDICATIONS**: G-6-PD deficiency, optic neuritis; tinnitus; history of blackwater fever and thrombocytopenic purpura associated with previous quinine ingestion. Contraindicated in pregnancy; quinine has an oxytocic action and passes the placental barrier and congenital malformations have been reportedly associated with large doses.	

ANTIPARASITIC AGENTS *Continued*

DRUG	INDICATIONS & DOSAGE	DOSE FORMS	REMARKS
PRAZIQUANTEL (Biltricide)	<u>Parasitic Infections</u>: **PO**: 20 mg/kg in 3 doses 4-6 h apart, for 1 d.	PO (Tab's): 600 mg	**SPECTRUM OF ACTIVITY:** **Effective against**: Schistosoma mekongi, S. japonicum, S. mansoni, S. hematobium.
	Parasite destruction within the eyes may cause irreparable lesions. **SIDE EFFECTS**: Praziquantel is well tolerated. Side effects may be more serious in patients with a heavy worm burden. Drowsiness on day of treatment and the following day. Minimal increases in liver enzymes, malaise, headache, dizziness, abdominal discomfort, fever, urticaria (rare). **CAUTIONS**: Safe use in pregnancy and children < 4 y.o. has not been established. **RECOMMENDATIONS**: Hospitalize patient for the duration of treatment when schistosomiasis or fluke infection is found to be associated with cerebral csyticercosis. Mothers are not to nurse on day of therapy or for next 4 d. Tablets should be swallowed unchewed with liquid during meals. **CONTRAINDICATIONS**: NOT for treatment of ocular cysticercosis.		
MEBENDAZOLE (Vermox)	<u>Trichuriasis, Ascariasis and Hookworm Infection</u>: **PO**: 100 mg bid for 3 d. <u>Enterobius vermicularis (pinworm)</u>: **PO**:100 mg (single dose), repeat in 2 wk.	Chewable Tab's: 100 mg	**SPECTRUM OF ACTIVITY:** **Effective against**: Enterobius vermicularis, Ascaris lumbricoides, Ancylostoma duodenale, Necator americanus, Trichuris trichiura. ***Note***: NOT effective in hydatid disease. **SIDE EFFECTS**: Diarrhea, abdominal pain, fever; rare neutropenia has been seen. **CAUTIONS**: Embryotoxic and teratogenic in laboratory animals at single doses as low as 10 mg/kg. **RECOMMENDATIONS**: Treat all family members in cases of pinworm infection; change and launder undergarments, bed linens, towels and night clothes daily. **CONTRAINDICATIONS**: Pregnancy.
THIABENDAZOLE (Mintezol) *Continued, next page*	<u>Intestinal Strongyloides stercoralis, Cutaneous larva migrans, Necator americanus (hookworm) or Trichostrongylus species</u>: **PO (> 70 kg)**: 1.5 gm bid for 2 d; maximum 3 gm/d. **PO (13.6-70 kg)**: 22 mg/kg bid for 2 d; maximum 3 gm/d. *Continued, next page*	Chewable Tab's: 500 mg PO (Liquid): 100 mg/ml	**SPECTRUM OF ACTIVITY:** **Effective against**: Enterobius vermicularis, Ascaris lumbricoides, Ancyclostoma duodenale, Necator americanus, Strongyloides stercoralis, Dracunculus medinesis, Capillaria philippenensis, Trichostrongylus species, larvae of Ancyclostoma braziliense and Ancyclostoma caninum. ***Note***: Larvicidal against Trichinella spiralis in pig muscle; effectiveness in humans has NOT been established. Variable effect on trichuris trichiura. Appears to be fungicidal in animals and in vitro, particularly against Trichophyton and Microsporum species. *Continued, next page*

ANTIPARASITIC AGENTS *Continued*

DRUG	INDICATIONS & DOSAGE	DOSE FORMS	REMARKS
THIABENDAZOLE *Continued*	<u>**Trichinella spiralis (Trichinosis).**</u> <u>**Disseminated Strongyloides stercoralis**</u>: **PO (> 70 kg)**: 1.5 gm bid for 2-4 d (maximum 3 gm/d). **PO (13.6-70 kg)**: 22 mg/kg bid for 2-4 d (maximum 3 gm/d). ***Note***: Extend treatment to 7 d for severe visceral larva migrans.	See previous page.	Appearance of live Ascaris in the mouth and nose sometimes occurs with therapy. **SIDE EFFECTS**: Anorexia, nausea, vomiting, vertigo (3-4 h after ingestion), diarrhea, enuresis, pruritis, fatigue, drowsiness, headache, tinnitus, abnormal ocular sensations, olfactory disturbances, numbness, collapse, hyperglycemia, bradycardia, hypotension, transient elevation of SGOT, jaundice, cholestrasis and parenchymal liver damage, rash, crystalluria, hallucinations, Stevens-Johnson syndrome, erythema multiforme, angioedema, anaphylaxis, transient leukopenia, lymphadenopathy. **CAUTIONS**: Safe use during pregnancy and lactation have not been established. Use with caution in renal or hepatic failure. **RECOMMENDATIONS**: Prior to initiating therapy, correct problems of anemia, dehydration or malnourishment. Monitor patients with hepatic or renal dysfunction carefully. Discontinue therapy immediately if hypersensitivity reactions occur.
LINDANE (1% GAMMA-BENZENEHEXA-CHLORIDE) (Kwell) (G-well) (Kwildane) (Scabene)	<u>**Scabies**</u>: **Lotion**: Apply to entire skin surface, leave on for 12 h; remove by thorough washing. Repeat after 7 d if needed. <u>**Pediculosis pubis and Pediculosis capitis**</u>: **Lotion and cream**: Rub into skin and hair, leave on for 8-12 h; remove by thorough washing. Repeat after 7 d if necessary. Treat sexual contacts at same time. **Shampoo**: Apply 1-2 oz, massage thoroughly into hair, leave for 4min; remove by rinsing thoroughly. Use fine-tooth comb or tweezers to remove remaining nits.	Cream: 1% Lotion: 1% Shampoo: 1%	**SPECTRUM OF ACTIVITY**: **Effective against**: Sarcoptes scabiei (scabies) and their eggs; Pediculus capitis (head louse), Pediculus corporis (body louse), Phthirus pubis (crab louse). ***Note***: Resistance may develop in strains of Pediculus capitis. - - - - - - - - - - Simultaneous use of creams, ointments or oils may enhance absorption. **SIDE EFFECTS**: Adverse reactions occur in < 0.001% of patients; rash, dizziness; convulsions and aplastic anemia. Seizures associated with excessive use/ingestion of lindane. **CAUTIONS**: Use cautiously in infants and children. If eye contact occurs, immediately flush eyes with water. Carcinogenic in laboratory animals. Skin penetration with inflammation, maceration or other lack of integrity; potential exists for CNS toxicity. **RECOMMENDATIONS**: Do not exceed the recommended dose or apply to inflamed, raw or weeping skin. Do not use prophylactically. Treat no more than twice during pregnancy. **CONTRAINDICATIONS**: Premature neonates, seizure disorders, hypersensitivity to lindane components.
CROTAMITON (Eurax)	<u>**Scabes**</u>: **Lotion and cream**: Apply to all skin surfaces and repeat at 24 h; remove at 48 h by thorough washing. Repeat in 7-10 d if necessary. Change bed clothing and linen in the morning after the first application.	Cream: 10% Lotion: 10%	**SPECTRUM OF ACTIVITY**: **Effective against**: Sarcoptes scabiei. - - - - - - - - - - Scabicidal and antipruritic. **SIDE EFFECTS**: Mild irritation or allergic sensitivity may occur. **CAUTIONS**: Safe use in pregnancy and children has not been established. **RECOMMENDATIONS**: Do NOT apply to raw or weeping skin, or near eyes or mouth. Discontinue immediately if severe irritation or sensitization develops.
METRONIDAZOLE (Flagyl)	See section: Miscellaneous Agents; Frequently Used Agents.		

ANTIVIRAL AGENTS

<table>
<tr><th>DRUG</th><th>INDICATIONS & DOSAGE</th><th>DOSE FORMS</th><th>REMARKS</th></tr>
<tr><td rowspan="2">ACYCLOVIR
(Zovirax)</td><td rowspan="2"><u>Immunocompromised Patients</u>:
IV: 5 mg/kg (over 1 h) q8h for 7 d.
Pediatric IV (< 12 y.o.): 250 mg/m^2 (over 1 h) q8h for 7 d.

<u>Initial Genital Herpes</u>:
PO: 200 mg q4h (while awake) for 10 d; maximum 1 gm/d.

<u>Chronic Suppressive Therapy for Recurrent Herpes</u>:
PO: 200 mg tid (while awake) for 6 months (maximum 1000 mg/d).

<u>Intermittent Therapy</u>:
PO: 200 mg q4h (while awake) for 5 d; reinitiate at first sign of recurrence.

<u>Renal Failure</u>:
PO: 200 mg q12h if creatinine clearance ≤10 cc/min/1.73 m^2.
IV: 5 mg/kg q8h if creat. clearance > 50 cc/min/1.73 m^2; q12h if 25-50 cc/min/1.73 m^2; q24h if 10-25 cc/min/1.73 m^2; 2.5 mg/kg q24h if < 10 cc/min/1.73 m^2. Administer a dose after hemodialysis.

<u>Ointment</u>:
Apply 1.25 cm ribbon/2.5 cm^2 area q3-6h for 7 d.</td><td>PO (Cap's): 200 mg
Injection: 50 mg/ml
Ointment: 5%</td><td>SPECTRUM OF ACTIVITY:
Effective against: herpes simplex virus types 1 and 2 (HSV-1 and HSV-2), varicella-zostervirus, Epstein-Barr virus, herpesvirus simiae, cytomegalovirus.
Note: In vitro susceptibility testing of viruses to acyclovir antiviral activity has not been standardized.</td></tr>
<tr><td colspan="2">SIDE EFFECTS: Renal dysfunction occurs in 10% patients receiving a bolus injection; administer SLOWLY. Encephalopathic changes occur in 1% of patients receiving IV acyclovir: lethargy, obtundation, tremors, confusion, hallucinations, agitation, seizures or coma. Inflammation of phlebitis may occur at IV injection site. Others: nausea, vomiting, diarrhea, headache, lymphadenopathy, dysgeusia, arthralgia, palpitation, muscle cramps, menstrual abnormalities, transient elevations of serum creatinine, rashes, hives, diaphoresis, hematuria, hypotension, thrombocytosis. CAUTIONS: Crystals can precipitate in renal tubules if the dose is greater than the maximum recommended dose or is administered by bolus injection. Additive renal damage possible with other nephrotoxic drugs, preexisting renal disease and dehydration. Prolonged or repeated courses of therapy may induce resistant viruses. Testicular atrophy has occurred in laboratory animals. Use with caution in those patients who have underlying neurologic abnormalities, serious renal, hepatic or electrolyte abnormalities or significant hypoxia, and those with prior neurologic reactions to cytotoxic drugs. RECOMMENDATIONS: Accompany IV infusion by adequate hydration.</td></tr>
<tr><td>AMANTADINE
(Symmetrel)
Continued, next page</td><td><u>Influenza A</u>:
<u>Symptoms</u>:
PO: 100 mg bid (100 mg/d if > 65 y.o.).
Pediatric PO (1-9 y.o.): 4.4-8.8 mg/kg /d in 2-3 doses; maximum 150 mg/d.
<u>Prophylaxis</u>:
PO: 100 mg bid for ≥ 10d after exposure (up to 90d).
Continued, next page</td><td>PO (Cap's): 100 mg
PO (Liquid): 10 mg/ml</td><td>SPECTRUM OF ACTIVITY:
Effective against: several strains of influenza A [including HONI, HINI, H2N2 (Asian type), H3N2 (Hong Kong type) and Hsw1N1 (Fort Dix)] virus, influenza C virus.
Note: NOT effective aginst influenza B, parainfluenza types 1, 2 and 3, rhinoviruses, adenoviruses, respiratory syncytial viruses.
Continued, next page</td></tr>
</table>

ANTIVIRAL AGENTS *Continued*

DRUG	INDICATIONS & DOSAGE	DOSE FORMS	REMARKS
AMANTADINE *Continued*	**<u>Renal Impairment</u>**: **PO**: 100 mg q12h if creat. clearance > 80 cc/min/1.73 m^2; 300 mg over 2 d if 60-80 cc/min/1.73 m^2; 100 mg q24h if 40-60 cc/min/1.73 m^2; 400 mg/wk in 2 doses if 30-40 cc/min/1.73 m^2; 300 mg/wk in 3 doses if 20-30 cc/min/1.73 m^2; 150 mg/wk if 10-20 cc/min/1.73 m^2. **<u>Parkinson's Disease</u>**: **PO**: 100 mg bid (maximum 400 mg/d). Lower doses may suffice when used in combination with other agents.	See previous page.	**SIDE EFFECTS**: Depression, CHF, orthostatic hypotension, psychosis, urinary retention are commonly seen. Other side effects include: hallucinations, confusion, anxiety, irritability, anorexia, nausea, constipation, ataxia, dizziness, livedo reticularis, peripheral edema, vomiting, dry mouth, dyspnea, fatigue, insomnia. Skin rash, slurred speech, visual disturbances, seizures, leukopenia, neutropenia, eczematoid dermatitis, oculogyric episodes are rare. **CAUTIONS**: Teratogenic in animals; excreted in breast milk. Use cautiously in patients with liver disease, psychosis, severe psychoneurosis or a history of recurrent eczematoid rash. **RECOMMENDATIONS**: Do NOT discontinue abruptly; some Parkinson's patients have experienced a parkinsonian crisis with sudden discontinuation. Adjust the dose carefully in renal impairment, peripheral edema or orthostatic hypotension. Closely observe and titrate dosage in patients with a history of seizures, CHF or peripheral edema.
VIDARABINE (Vira A) (Ara-A) (Adenine Arabinoside)	**<u>Herpes Simplex Encephalitis</u>**: **IV**: 15 mg/kg/d for 10 d (infuse the daily dose over 12-24 h). **<u>Herpes Zoster</u>**: **IV**: 10 mg/kg/d for 5 d.	Injection: 200 mg/ml	**SPECTRUM OF ACTIVITY**: **Effective against**: herpes simplex virus types 1 and 2, varicella-zoster, cytomegalovirus, vaccinia, hepatitis B virus, Epstein-Barr virus, various animal DNA viruses, rhabdoviruses, oncornaviruses. ***Note***: NOT effective against adenovirus, other DNA or RNA viruses, bacteria, fungi. **SIDE EFFECTS**: Anorexia, nausea, vomiting, hematemesis, diarrhea are usually mild. SGOT and total bilirubin may be elevated. Fatal metabolic encephalopathy can occur. Also, tremor, dizziness, malaise, hallucinations, confusion, psychosis, ataxia. Decreased reticulocytes, hemoglobin or hematocrit, WBC and platelet count. Others: weight loss, pruritus, rash, pain at injection site. **CAUTIONS**: Doses > 20 mg/kg/d can produce bone marrow depression. Do not administer in biological or colloidal fluids. Carcinogenic and teratogenic in laboratory animals. Carefully maintain fluid balance in patients susceptible to fluid overloading or cerebral edema. Renal impairment may slow excretion; observe closely for toxicity. **RECOMMENDATIONS**: Monitor hematologic status during therapy.

Section 3: CENTRAL AND AUTONOMIC NERVOUS SYSTEM AGENTS

Table of Contents

NARCOTIC ANALGESICS

GROUP REMARKS: Analgesic strength (most important property) closely parallels addictive potential. **SIDE EFFECTS**: **Therapeutic doses**: Euphoria and/or dysphoria. Sedation, inattention, confusion, dizziness. Nausea, vomiting (usually only with initial doses - decreased by recumbancy). Hyperglycemia, miosis, pylorospasm, some antidiuretic effect. Postural hypotension (with fainting). Pruritis, urticaria, flush & tearing (may be related to histamine release). Elevated amylase & lipase (secondary to biliary sphincter contraction). May prolong labor (esp. if cervix < 4-5 cm). **Chronic use**: Altered menses, constipation, urinary retention, atelectasis, tolerance. **Toxic doses**: Above effects plus increased intracranial pressure (secondary to increased P_aCO_2). Bradycardia, mydriasis, ileus. Profound respiratory depression, hypothermia, shock, respiratory & cardiac arrest, coma. **WITHDRAWAL SYMPTOMS** (develop within 8-16 h after last dose and intensify over 72 h; effects persist for > 4 wks - chronic effects can occur): Insomnia, autonomic hyperactivity, hyperexcitability, rare convulsions, dehydration (can precipitate CV collapse), leukocytosis, muscle & joint pain, anxiety. Opiate antagonists can precipitate withdrawal effects in minutes and reach maximum intensity in 30 min. Withdrawal decreases cardiac preload and increases venous pooling. Withdrawal prolonged in hepatic/renal dysfunction, septic shock, ascites and eclampsia. **CAUTIONS**: Increased ICP most likely following IV injection. Toxic colonic dilation can occur in acute ulcerative colitis. Decreased P_aCO_2 sensitivity (solerespiratory drive is hypoxia), caution with increasing F_IO_2. May potentiate hypothyroidism. Concurrent phenothiazines may increase postural hypotension, sedation. Vasopressin release can increase post-op risk of water intoxication. Tolerance can develop in a few days with q4-6h dosing (as in constant/severe pain). **RECOMMENDATIONS**: **Pain management**: Mild, acute: codeine, oxycodone. Short duration: meperidine, alaphradine, fentanyl. Acute/severe: IV adminst. (can exceed maximum doses). Pre/post-op, labor: IM, SC adminst. **Other recommendations**: Slow IV adminst. may decrease toxicity. Correct fluid volume prior to narcotic adminst. Atropine to treat bradycardia. IM, SC adminst. may delay effects of toxicity (delayed onset). Reduce dose in: Very old or very young patients with concurrent CNS depressants. **Treatment of toxicity**: Gastric lavage effective for hours after ingestion (delayed gastric emptying). Opiate antagonists & respiratory support. **CONTRAINDICATIONS**: Conditions in which hypercapnia especially dangerous (increased ICP, COPD), end-stage liver disease. **NOTE**: Potency defined in terms of intensity of pain relieved (drugs equally efficacious only within categories - no amount of codeine will relieve severe pain).

DRUG	ANALGESIA DOSAGE	ONSET (min)	DURATION (hours)	EQUIVALENT DOSES	REMARKS
HIGH POTENCY *(Withdrawal severity: Minimal if < 80 mg/d for < 30 d; Severe if > 240 mg/d for > 30d).*					
MORPHINE SULFATE (M.S.)	**IV**: 2.5-15 mg q3-4h (inject SLOWLY over 4-5 min).	5-10		IM, SC: 10 mg PO: 60 mg	Drug of first choice in pulmonary edema. In labor: 10 mg, IM, SC. In MI: 8-15 mg, with additional, smaller doses q3h PRN.
	IM, SC: 5-20 mg q4h.	30-90	4-5		
	Rectal: 10-20 mg q4h.				
	PO: 10-30 mg q4h.				
HYDROMORPHONE (Dilaudid) (Dihydromorphone)	**IV**: 2-4 mg (> 1 mg/min) q4-6h.			IM, SC: 1.5-2 mg PO: 7.5 mg	More rapid onset and shorter duration than MS, also more effective after PO adminst.
	PO, IM, SC: 2-4 mg q4-6h.	15-30	4-5		
LEVORPHANOL (Levodromoran)	**IV**: See Remarks.	<20		IM, SC: 2 mg PO: 4 mg	Equivalent to morphine. To prevent respiratory depression, adminst. Levorphanol:Levallorphan (10:1 ratio) by slow IV.
	PO, SC: 2-3 mg.	60-90			

NARCOTIC ANALGESICS: HIGH POTENCY *Continued*

DRUG	ANALGESIA DOSAGE	ONSET (min)	DURATION (hours)	EQUIVALENT DOSES	REMARKS
METHADONE (Dolophine)	**PO, IM, SC**: 2.5-10 mg q3-4h.	10-15	4-6	IM, SC: 10 mg PO: 20 mg	Relative to MS: Less euphoria & sedation, better GI absorption. Withdrawal prolonged, but of lesser intensity (onset 3-4 d, peak 6 d, duration 10-14 d). Detox treatment: 20 mg/d bid until symptoms subside, then taper q1-2d over 3 wk. Maintenance: 40-100 mg/d (exceed maximum dose if tolerance or intractable pain).
	PO: 5-20 mg q6-8h (maximum 40 mg/dose, 120 mg/d).				
OXYMORPHONE (Numorphan)	**IV**: 0.5 mg initially; increase PRN.	5-10	3-6	IM, SC: 1 mg PO: 6 mg	Dose in labor: 0.5-1 mg IM.
	IM, SC: 1-1.5 mg q4-6h.				
	Rectal: 5 mg q4-6h.	5-10	3-6		
FENTANYL (Sublimase)	**IV (low dose)**: 2 µg/kg. **IV (mod dose)**: 2-20 µg/kg, then 25-100 µg PRN. **IV (high dose)**: 20-50 µg/kg, then 25 µg PRN.	0.5-1		IM, SC: 100-200 µg	Group Remarks EXCEPT: Nausea less frequent, chest wall rigidity more frequent than with MS. Accumulation with frequent dosing. Respiratory depressant effects may outlast analgesia. Reduce dose in geriatrics, poor risk patients. Decrease dose by 25-35% if concurrent other CNS depressants. Low dose for minor surgery, moderate dose for major surgery, high dose for open heart surgery.
	IV, IM (pre-op): 50-100 µg (over 1-2 min, 0.5-1 h pre-op.	5-15	1-2		
MODERATE POTENCY					
MEPERIDINE (Demerol) (Isonipecaine) (Pethidine)	**PO, IM, SC**: 50-150 mg q3-4h. **Pediatric PO**: 1.8 mg/kg q3-4h.	10-15	2-4	IM, SC: 75-100 mg PO: 300 mg	Group Remarks EXCEPT: Excitement in some patients, mydriasis, minimal constipation. Withdrawal: onset 3-4 h, peak 8-12 h, duration 4-5 d. Action decreased with PO adminst. Addiction potential & biliary sphincter effects same as other intermediate opiates. Potential interactions with MAO Inhibitors. Anesthesia: Administer 30-90 min pre-op. Labor: 50-100 mg IM or SC. Often administered with antihistamine to potentiate effect.
OXYCODONE (in Percodan) (in Tylox) (in Percocet)	**PO**: 5 mg q6h.	10-15	3-6	IM, SC: 15-20 mg PO: 30 mg	Not recommended for use in children.

NARCOTIC ANALGESICS *Continued*

DRUG	ANALGESIA DOSAGE	ONSET (min)	DURATION (hours)	EQUIVALENT DOSES	REMARKS
INTERMEDIATE POTENCY *(Agonists with weak antagonist acitivity)*					
BUTORPHANOL (Stadol)	**IV**: 0.5-2 mg q3-4h.	1-2	2-4	IV, IM: 2-3 mg	Group Remarks EXCEPT: Possibly less addicting than MS. After 2 mg, additional drug only prolongs (does not increase) respiratory depression. Limited abuse potential (see Nalbuphine Remarks).
	IM: 1-4 mg q3-4h.	5-30	3-4		
NALBUPHINE (Nubain)	**IV**: 10-20 mg q3-6h.	2-3	3-6	IV, IM: 10 mg	Limited abuse potential due to mixed agonist & antagonist properties. Respiratory depression plateaus after 30 mg (10 mg/h) - additional drug only prolongs effect. Withdrawal symptoms not suppressed (may precipitate withdrawal in opiate-dependent patients).
	IM: 10-20 mg q3-6h.	<15	3-6		
	SC: 10-20 mg q3-6h.				
	Maximum: 160 mg/d IV, IM, SC.				
PENTAZOCINE (Talwin) (in Talacen)	**IV**: 30 mg q3-4h (max. 360 mg/d).	2-3	3	IV, IM: 20-60 mg	Group Remarks EXCEPT: Higher doses (30-45 mg) may increase GI motility. Antagonist activity only 2% that of nalorphine. IM adminst. is 3-4 times more potent than PO. Large IV doses may precipitate seizures. Compounded with naloxone to discourage IV abuse (no naloxone effect if administered PO).
	IM, SC: 30-60 mg q3-4h (maximum 360 mg/d).	15-20	3		
	PO: 50-100 mg q3-6h (maximum 600 mg/d).	15-30	3		
LOWEST POTENCY					
CODEINE (Methylmorphine)	**Analgesia**: **PO, IM, IV, SC**: 15-60 mg q4-6h. **Antitussive**: **PO**: 10-20 mg q4-6h (maximum 120 mg/d). **Pediatric PO**: **6-12 y.o.**: 5-10 mg q4-6h (maximum 60 mg/d). **2-6 y.o.**: 2.5-5 mg q4-6h (maximum 30 mg/d).	15-30	4-6	IM: 120 mg PO: 300 mg	Group Remarks EXCEPT: Occasional excitement rather than sedation (rarely convulsions). PO analgesic potency approximately 66% of parenteral. Usual dose: 30 mg q4h.

NARCOTIC ANALGESICS: LOWEST POTENCY *Continued*

DRUG	ANALGESIA DOSAGE	ONSET (min)	DURATION (hours)	EQUIVALENT DOSES	REMARKS
HYDROCODONE (in Hycodan)	**Analgesia**: **PO**: 5 mg q4-6h.	4-8			Used mainly as an antitussive.
	Antitussive: **PO**: 5 mg q4-6h (maximum 15 mg/dose).				
DIHYDROCODEINE (in Compal) (in Synalgos-DC)					Both combinations have 10 mg/tablet. Dihydrocodeine is equivalent to codeine, except that recommended doses are lower.
PROPOXYPHENE (Darvon, HCl) (Profene, HCl) (Darvon-N, napsylate)	**PO (HCl)**: 65 mg q4h (maximum 390 mg/d). **PO (napsylate)**: 100 mg q4h (maximum 600 mg/d).	15-60	4-6		Occasional excitement rather than sedation (rarely convulsions). Napsylate 100 mg corresponds to HCl 65 mg. Not classified as a narcotic. Overdose may precipitate heart block, seizures, rapid death. Little/no antitussive activity. NOT effective in treatment of withdrawal from other narcotics. Minimum lethal dose: 9-19 mg/kg. Serum concentrations: toxic = 0.6-10 μg/ml; lethal > 10 μg/ml.

NARCOTIC ANTAGONISTS

GROUP REMARKS: Narcotic antagonists are used to dramatically reverse narcotic-induced respiratory depression. Pure antagonists are preferred because of their lack of depressant agonist properties and their efficacy. The antagonists are not effective against non-opiate respiratory depression. Although opiate depressant effects are reversed, opiate stimulant actions (convulsions & excitement) are unaffected. Naltrexone, the one antagonist that is active when given orally, is used in the treatment of narcotic dependence. **SIDE EFFECTS**: Nausea and vomiting may occur in post-operative patients. Reversal of analgesia may occur in patients receiving antagonists after surgery. **NOTES**: Narcotic antagonists should be used with caution in patients suspected of opiate dependence; sudden precipitation of withdrawal (by a large antagonist dose) can be dangerous. Withdrawal appears in 5-15 min, peaks in 30-45 min, and lasts only a few hours; the opiate effect may return as the antagonist is eliminated. Use during delivery: In cases of anticipated neonatal respiratory depression due to use of narcotics in labor, the mother should receive the antagonist approximately 15 min prior to delivery. Subsequent antagonist can be administered via the umbilical vein.

DRUG	INDICATIONS & DOSAGE	DOSE FORMS	REMARKS
NALOXONE (Narcan)	**Partial Post-operative Narcotic Reversal**: **IV**: 0.1-0.2 mg q2-3min PRN. **Pediatric IV**: 0.01 mg/kg initially; then 0.1 mg/kg PRN. **Opiate Overdosage**: **IV**: 0.4-2.0 mg q2-3min PRN (observe after 10 mg administered).	Injection: 0.4 mg/ml Injection (neonatal): 0.02 mg/ml	Pure narcotic antagonist; no respiratory depression. Minimally effective when given orally. Short duration of action (1-4 h); observe patient closely for signs of recurrent narcotic effects (many narcotics have longer duration of action). **SIDE EFFECTS**: Hypotension, hypertension, ventricular arrhythmias and pulmonary edema occur rarely in post-operative patients; use cautiously in patients with cardiovascular disease. Hypersensitivity to naloxone can develop. **CAUTION**: Do NOT mix with bisulfites or large anions.
NALTREXONE (Trexan)	**Opiate Maintenance**: **PO**: 50 mg/d (initiate slowly and only if opioid-free).	PO: 50 mg	Only use is to aid maintenance of non-narcotic state in former addicts. Concurrent narcotic use will be without effect. Do NOT administer to a patient failing a naloxone challenge to confirm narcotic-free state. **SIDE EFFECTS**: GI upset, nervousness, headache, malaise. Rare hepatic injury. Hypersensitivity may develop. **CAUTION**: Use cautiously in pre-existing hepatic disease. **RECOMMEND**: Perform baseline and periodic LFTs.

NON-NARCOTIC ANALGESICS

GROUP REMARKS: Also known as Non-Steroidal Anti-Inflammatory Drugs (NSAIDs); although technically incorrect for acetaminophen. All of these drugs have analgesic (against mild-moderate pain) and antipyretic (against elevated body temperature) activity. Most also have anti-inflammatory activity at much higher doses and are useful in arthritic conditions such as rheumatoid, juvenile and osteo- arthritis; many are also effective in gout and ankylosing spondylitis. Acetaminophen is NOT anti-inflammatory. Most of the newer NSAIDs are also effective in treating dysmenorrhea. A few agents possess additional properties. Newer NSAIDs are comparable, but NOT superior, to aspirin for analgesic, antipyretic and anti-inflammatory effects; they should be used only after an aspirin trial proves ineffective. Considerable interpatient variability exists and trials of many different NSAIDs may be necessary. Maximal effects may require 1-4 weeks to develop. NSAIDs do NOT alter the course of disease. **NOTES**: Combinations of NSAIDs are no more effective than single agents alone and may interfere with each other's bioavailability. **SIDE EFFECTS**: Gastric irritation (nausea, vomiting, epigastric discomfort) occurs with all NSAIDs, but is more common with aspirin; minimize by administration with meals or fluids. NSAIDs may produce or reactivate ulcers and should be used cautiously in patients with a history of GI lesions. Other GI effects: diarrhea, constipation, irritation. Incidence of gastric upset is greater with high-dose regimens, but tolerance appears to develop. NSAIDs which MAY cause less gastric irritation are naproxen (< 750 mg/d), ibuprofen (< 400 mg qid), sulindac; others (esp. acetic acid derivatives) are more likely to cause bleeding along the entire length of the GI tract. CNS effects are also common; headache, dizziness, lightheadedness, drowsiness and confusion are the most frequent and may occur in 5-15% patients. Tinnitus and visual disturbances occur to varying degrees with the different NSAIDs. Auditory or ophthalmic examinations should be performed upon signs or symptoms from any NSAID. NSAIDs produce borderline elevations of liver function tests (LFTs), SGPT (ALT) and SGOT (AST), in 10-15% patients (significant elevations occur in < 1%). Elevated LFTs may persist, progress or revert with time; consider withdrawal of drug if LFTs acheive > 3 times the upper limit of normal range. Hepatitis, jaundice or other severe hepatotoxicities occur rarely. Closely evaluate patients who develop signs. Discontinue drug upon evidence of significant hepatic dysfunction: persistent or worsening abnormal LFTs, clinical signs and symptoms consistent with liver disease, systemic manifestations (eosinophilia, rash, etc.). Occult bleeding occurs with most of the NSAIDs; usually due to gastric irritation. Decreases in hematocrit or hemoglobin concentration develop occasionally. Anemias and blood dyscrasias occur rarely, but are a major cause of fatalities. NSAIDs inhibit platelet function to a lesser extent than does aspirin; bleeding time may be prolonged but bleeding at surgery (dental, hip replacement) is NOT increased. Significant renal toxicity occurs rarely: papillary necrosis (most common), interstitial or glomerular nephritis, nephrotic syndrome and acute renal failure. Rare urinary abnormalities: hematuria, dysuria, oliguria. NSAIDs may cause fluid and sodium retention. **CAUTIONS**: Patients who are receiving diuretics, especially those causing potassium retention, may be especially sensitive to the renal effects of NSAIDs. Use any NSAID cautiously in patients with previous hypersensitivity reaction (urticaria, bronchospasm, shock) to any other NSAID (including aspirin) or history of nasal polyps and asthma. Use cautiously in patients with active or historical GI lesions, hepatic, renal, cardiovascular or coagulation dysfunction. Use cautiously in patients on concurrent anticoagulant therapy; NSAIDs themselves inhibit coagulation (inhibit platelet aggregation) and many can displace anticoagulants from plasma protein binding sites. **RECOMMENDATIONS**: Some NSAIDs have produced ocular changes (blurred vision, corneal and retinal alterations, loss of color vision); perform ophthalmologic examination if visual disturbances occur. Minimize risk for patients on long-term therapy by adjusting dose to the lowest possible effective level. Periodic WBC counts and LFTs should be performed during chronic therapy. **CONTRAINDICATIONS**: Pregnancy and ulcerative gastrointestinal disease are both contraindications. NSAIDs should be avoided in patients with history of adverse renal reactions to any NSAID or pre-existing renal dysfunction.

DRUG	INDICATIONS & DOSAGE	DOSE FORMS	REMARKS
ASPIRIN & RELATED AGENTS			
ASPIRIN (Acetysalicylic acid) (ASA) Various Trade Names *Continued, next page*	**Pain, Fever**: **PO**: 325-650 mg q4-6h; maximum 4 gm/d. **Pediatric PO**: 10-15 mg/kg q4-6h; maximum 3.6 gm/d. If aspirin alone is ineffective, add acetaminophen q4-6h; NO advantage in alternating the two drugs. *Continued, next page*	PO (Cap's): 325 mg PO (Tab's): 325, 500, 650 mg	May protect against myocardial infarction in men with unstable angina. Anti-thrombotic effect may be limited to males and is NOT shared by other salicylates. No significant differences in time to onset between different preparations of aspirin. **SIDE EFFECTS**: GI upset is the major side effect; *Continued, next page*

NON-NARCOTIC ANALGESICS: ASPIRIN & RELATED AGENTS *Continued*

DRUG	INDICATIONS & DOSAGE	DOSE FORMS	REMARKS
ASPIRIN *Continued*	<u>**Arthritic Conditions**</u>: **PO**: 2.4-3.6 gm/d initially, increase by 0.325-1.2 gm/d q1wk; maintenance 3.6-5.4 gm/d in 4-6 doses. **Juvenile PO**: 60-90 mg/kg/d initially, increase by 10 mg/kg/d q1wk; maintenance 80-100 mg/kg/d in 4-6 doses. Maintain serum salicylate levels = 0.2-0.3 μg/ml. <u>**Rheumatic Fever**</u>: **PO**: 4.9-7.8 gm/d in 4-6 doses. **Juvenile PO**: 90-130 mg/kg/d in 4-6 doses. <u>**Transient Ischemic Attacks (Men)**</u>: **PO**: 150-1300 mg/d in 2-4 doses.	Enteric Tablets: 325, 650, 972 mg PO (Ext'd release): 650, 800 mg Suppositories: 60, 125, 150, 325, 650, 1200 mg	may be lessened with enteric-coating. Occult blood loss (> 10 ml/d in 10-15% of patients) occurs from the GI tract (prothrombin time rarely increases); increases with dose, tolerance does NOT develop and iron-deficiency anemia may result from long-term therapy. Overdosage ("salicylism"): tinnitus, headache, dizziness, confusion, fever, hyperventilation, respiratory alkalosis then metabolic acidosis. Overdosage usually > 150 mg/kg. Hepatotoxicity may develop in patients with rheumatic disease, especially at serum levels > 0.2-0.25 mg/ml. Allergic reactions: rash, urticaria, bronchospasm. Cross-sensitivity with tartrazine dye (FD&C Yellow 5) in 10% of allergic patients. **LEVELS**: Useful only in evaluation of acute overdosage; must be correlated with time since ingestion. **CONTRAINDICATIONS**: Use of salicylates (esp. aspirin) during chickenpox or influenza in children is suspected to precipitate Reye's syndrome (vomiting, lethargy, delirium and coma with a 20-30% mortality rate). **DRUG INTERACTIONS**: ***Heparin/Oral Anticoagulants***: increased bleeding tendency via additional anticoagulation and displacement of coumarins from plasma protein binding. ***Probenecid/Sulfinpyrazone***: inhibition of uricosuric effect. ***Methotrexate***: increased toxicity (blood dyscrasias) via binding displacement and decreased renal secretion.
SALSALATE (Disalcid)	<u>**Pain**</u>: **PO**: 3000 mg/d in 2-4 doses.	PO (Cap's): 500 mg PO (Tab's): 500, 750 mg	Parent drug; hydrolyzed to two molecules of salicylic acid in the GI tract and at the liver. Administer with food or liquid. May be useful in patients with gastric intolerance to aspirin.
DIFLUNISAL (Dolobid)	<u>**Pain**</u>: **PO**: 1000 mg initially, then 500 mg q8-12h; maximum 1500 mg/d. <u>**Arthritic Conditions**</u>: **PO**: 250-500 mg q12h; maximum 1500 mg/d.	PO (Tab's): 250, 500 mg	Salicylic acid derivative; comparable in effectiveness but longer-acting than aspirin. May cause less GI irritation than other NSAIDs.

NON-NARCOTIC ANALGESICS: PROPIONIC ACID DERIVATIVES

DRUG	INDICATIONS & DOSAGE	DOSE FORMS	REMARKS
PROPIONIC ACID DERIVATIVES			
GROUP NOTES: The propionic acid derivatives are pharmacologically very similar to aspirin or the other salicylates and distinctly less toxic than the acetic acid derivatives or the pyrazolones.			
NAPROXEN (Naprosyn) **NAPROXEN SODIUM** (Anaprox)	**Arthritic Conditions**: **PO**: 250-375 mg naproxen q12h; maximum 1250 mg/d. **PO**: 275 mg qAM, 550 mg qPM N-sodium; maximum 1375 mg/d. **Acute Gout**: **PO**: 750 mg naproxen initially, then 250 mg q8h. **PO**: 825 mg N-sodium initially, then 275 mg q8h. **Pain/Dysmenorrhea**: **PO**: 500 mg naproxen initially, then 250 mg q6-8h; maximum 1250 mg/d. **PO**: 550 mg N-sodium initially; then 275 mg q6-8h; maximum 1375 mg/d.	PO (Tab's): 250, 275 (N-sodium), 375, 500 mg	Naproxen 250 mg = naproxen sodium 275 mg. Naproxen sodium contains 1 mEq sodium in each 275 mg dose. **SIDE EFFECTS**: GI effects (discomfort, constipation, nausea) and irritation are the primary side effects; CNS effects (headache, dizziness) occur less frequently than with aspirin. Other adverse effects: tinnitus, urinary abnormalities, blood dyscrasias, rashes and rare hepatic dysfunction. Better tolerated than Indomethacin.
IBUPROFEN (Motrin) (OTC: Advil, Susprin)	**Arthritic Conditions**: **PO**: 300-600 mg q6-8h; maximum 2400 mg/d. **Dysmenorrhea**: **PO**: 400 mg q4h PRN. **Pain**: **PO**: 200-400 mg q4-6h.	PO (Tab's): 300, 400, 600 mg	**SIDE EFFECTS**: Generally well tolerated. Headache, dizziness or tinnitus are relatively common. Rare visual disturbances, rashes. **CONTRAINDICATIONS**: History of sensitivity to any other NSAID.
FENOPROFEN (Nalfon)	**Arthritic Conditions**: **PO**: 300-600 mg q6-8h; maximum 3200 mg/d. **Pain**: **PO**: 200 mg q4-6h.	PO (Cap's): 200, 300 mg PO (Tab's): 600 mg	**SIDE EFFECTS**: CNS effects occur regularly: headache, tiredness. Other adverse reactions: tinnitus, urinary abnormalities, purpura, blood dyscrasias and rare hepatic dysfunction. **CAUTIONS**: Caution in renal impairment; evidence of glomerulonephritis, renal papillary necrosis, hepatocellular hypertrophy in rats. **CONTRAINDICATIONS**: Sensitivity to any NSAID, including aspirin.

NON-NARCOTIC ANALGESICS: ACETIC ACID DERIVATIVES

DRUG	INDICATIONS & DOSAGE	DOSE FORMS	REMARKS
ACETIC ACID DERIVATIVES			
GROUP NOTES: In general the acetic acid derivatives are similar to the other NSAIDs. They are somewhat more effective but produce a higher incidence and severity of adverse effects.			
INDOMETHACIN (Indocin)	<u>**Arthritic Conditions**</u>: **PO**: 25 mg q8-12h initially, increase 25-50 mg/d; maximum 200 mg/d. **PO (Ext'd release)**: 75 mg/d initially, increase to 75 mg bid.	PO (Cap's): 25, 50 mg PO (Ext'd release): 75 mg	Due to high incidence of severe adverse effects, use ONLY as second-tier drug in patients unresponsive to other NSAIDs. **SIDE EFFECTS**: Higher incidence than other NSAIDs (30-60% of patients, esp. geriatrics); CNS effects (headache, dizziness, incoordination) most common. Psychotic episodes may occur. Frequent GI irritation and bleeding along the entire GI tract. Anemias and blood dyscrasias may also occur. Corneal or retinal changes may occur. **CAUTIONS**: Use cautiously when renal or hepatic dysfunction exists; discontinue if elevated LFTs persist or other signs develop. May produce more cross-hypersensitivity than other NSAIDs. **RECOMMEND**: Decrease dose or discontinue if adverse effects develop, esp. if ocular. Perform yearly ophthamologic exams. **CONTRAINDICATIONS**: AVOID in children < 14 y.o. Epilepsy, Parkinson's disease, psychosis, renal disease.
SULINDAC (Clinoril)	<u>**Pain**</u>: **PO**: 150-200 mg bid; maximum 400 mg/d. <u>**Acute Gout**</u>: **PO**: 200 mg bid for 7 d.	PO (Tab's): 150, 200 mg	Similar to indomethacin. Sulindac is a pro-drug; largely inactive until absorbed (causes less GI upset) and metabolized by the liver. Administer with food. **SIDE EFFECTS**: GI effects (discomfort, nausea, vomiting, diarrhea, constipation) are common. CNS effects (headache, dizziness) are also frequent; tinnitus occurs less often than with aspirin. Rash occurs frequently. Cross-reactivity to other NSAIDs is common. **CAUTIONS**: Use cautiously if concurrent anticoagulants or history of GI bleeding/ulcer.
TOLMETIN (Tolectin)	<u>**Pain**</u>: **PO**: 400 mg tid initially; maintenance 600-1800 mg/d in 3-4 doses. **Pediatric PO**: 5 mg/kg tid initially; maintenance 15-30 mg/kg/d in 3 doses.	PO (Tab's): 200 mg PO (Cap's): 400 mg	**SIDE EFFECTS**: GI effects common (nausea); ulcers may occur/reactivate; give with milk/food. CNS effects (headache, dizziness, nervousness) also common. Rarely: anemia, urinary abnormalities, hepatic dysfunction, edema or skin reactions. **CAUTIONS**: AVOID in pregnancy. Use cautiously in ocular, renal, hepatic or cardiovascular dysfunction. **RECOMMEND**: Periodic ophthalmologic exams.

DRUG	INDICATIONS & DOSAGE	DOSE FORMS	REMARKS
	MISCELLANEOUS ORGANIC ACIDS		
MEFENAMIC ACID (Ponstel)	**Pain/Dysmenorrhea**: **PO**: 500 mg initially, then 250 mg q6h.	PO (Cap's): 250 mg	For short-term use, NOT > 1 week. **SIDE EFFECTS**: GI effects prominent: diarrhea, nausea, vomiting and discomfort. Diarrhea may be severe and is dose-related; decrease dose or discontinue. Renal failure, nephritis and papillary necrosis occur rarely, as does hepatotoxicity. Other adverse reactions: visual disturbances (including loss of color perception), anemia, skin reactions. **CAUTIONS**: Discontinue drug if: severe diarrhea, rash, signs of renal dysfunction or severe hepatic dysfunction. **CONTRAINDICATIONS**: Renal disease, current or historical GI lesions, hypersensitivity to any NSAID.
MECLOFENAMATE (Meclomen)	**Arthritic Conditions**: **PO**: 50-100 mg q6-8h; maximum 400 mg/d.	PO (Cap's): 50, 100 mg	Sodium content: 0.34 mEq sodium in each 100 mg dose. Enhances warfarin activity. **SIDE EFFECTS**: Most frequent side effects are GI related: diarrhea, nausea, vomiting; diarrhea may be severe enough to discontinue drug. Headaches and dizziness are also common, as is rash. Decreased hematocrit or hemoglobin concentration may occur, but are rarely serious. Tinnitus occurs less often than with aspirin.
PIROXICAM (Feldene)	**Arthritic Conditions**: **PO**: 20 mg/d in 1-2 doses.	PO (Cap's): 10, 20 mg	Due to a long half-life, blood levels increase over several days; allow 2 wks to assess therapeutic effect. **SIDE EFFECTS**: GI effects (nausea, abdominal discomfort) are more common (20% patients) than with other NSAIDs. Dizziness, edema, headache, hematological changes and rash are the next most common. **CAUTIONS**: Use cautiously in patients with bleeding disorders or impending surgery; prolonged increased bleeding tendency due to long half-life, inhibition of platelet aggregation. Use cautiously in patients with compromised cardiovascular function.

NON-NARCOTIC ANALGESICS: ACETAMINOPHEN

DRUG	INDICATIONS & DOSAGE	DOSE FORMS	REMARKS
ACETAMINOPHEN			
ACETAMINOPHEN (APAP) Various Trade Names	<u>Fever, Pain</u>: **PO**: 325-650 mg q4-6h; maximum 4.0 gm/d. **Pediatric PO**: 10 mg/kg q4h; maximum 2.6 gm/d.	PO (Tab's): 325, 500, 650 mg Liquid: 120 mg/5 ml, 500 mg/15 ml Drops: 48 mg/ml, 100 mg/m Suppositories: 125, 325, 600, 650 mg	NO anti-inflammatory activity; antipyretic and analgesic effects comparable to aspirin. **SIDE EFFECTS**: No side effects if used as directed. Allergic reactions: rash, bronchospasm. Acute overdosage: GI upset, fever, hepatotoxicity (jaundice), blood dyscrasias, delirium then depression, collapse; N-acetylcysteine is antidote. **CAUTIONS**: May be hepatotoxic with chronic use or with large single doses.
PHENOTHIAZINE			
METHOTRIMEPRAZINE (Levomepromazine) (Levoprome)	<u>Pain</u>: **IM**: 5-10 mg q4-6h initially; maintenance 5-40 mg q1-24h. <u>Preoperative</u>: **IM**: 2-20 mg q45-180 min (decrease if concurrent atropine or scopolamine is being used). <u>Obstetric Analgesia</u>: **IM**: 15-20 mg.	Injection: 20 mg/ml	Phenothiazine sedative & analgesic. Administer ONLY by IM injection. Non-addicting. **SIDE EFFECTS**: Orthostatic hypotension, dizziness; confine patient to bed following initial doses or until tolerance develops. Excess sedation, dizziness nausea, difficult urination, dry mouth. Local inflammation at injection site may occur. **CAUTIONS**: Use cautiously in elderly patients with cardiovascular disease.

SEDATIVE-HYPNOTICS AND ANXIOLYTICS

GROUP REMARKS: Sedative-hypnotics produce generalized depression of the CNS; extent of depression varies with dose and ranges from relief of anxiety (low doses) to general anesthesia (high doses). There are two major chemical classes of sedative-hypnotics, the Barbiturates and the Benzodiazepines; pharmacologic differences between the two have less therapeutic significance than pharmacokinetic properties of their individual members. Many other chemical classes are also sedative-hypnotics, most notably ethanol. Actions of all of sedative-hypnotics (with increasing dose): sedation (loss of anxiety), excitement (disinhibition), hypnosis (induction of sleep), general anesthesia and medullary depression leading to death. With chronic use: anticonvulsant action, habituation with physical dependence (withdrawal state upon cessation) and relaxation of voluntary muscle (depression of spinal reflexes). Among the various sedative-hypnotics, differences in pharmacokinetic properties and recommended doses are exploited to establish different drugs for different clinical conditions. Short-acting agents are recommended for hypnosis (to minimize "hangover") and longer-acting agents are recommended for sedation or treatment of seizures. **NOTES**: All are equivalent to, and additive with, alcohol in their effects; and with all other CNS depressants. Sedative-hypnotics reduce rapid eye movement (REM) and stage 4 sleep; partial tolerance develops to REM sleep reduction, but rebound dreaming and nightmares often occur upon discontinuance. **SIDE EFFECTS**: Drowsiness and impairment of motor performance/judgement are very common. Morning "hangover" is common, especially with longer-acting agents. Some reduction of tone and motility of the GI tract occurs. Disinhibition ("paradoxical excitement") may occur; often as euphoria and impairment of self-control and judgement. Children, the elderly and patients in pain are most prone to disinhibition; elderly patients are also prone to confusion. **Overdosage**: Anesthetic-level depression of the CNS occurs; medullary depression produces respiratory depression and shock. Treatment is conservative; given symptomatic treatment, only 2-3% patients die. **WITHDRAWAL**: Sedative-hypnotics induce a severe psychological and physical dependence; characterized by: sleep disturbances (REM sleep rebound, nightmares), anxiety, weakness, agitation, tremors, elevated blood pressure, excitement and seizures. Following use of short- or intermediate-acting sedative-hypnotics, symptoms begin within 18-24 h and peak at 2-3 d; the reaction is dose-related; mild effects (insomnia) may occur even after the usual bedtime dose. With long-acting agents, symptoms may not appear for a week (being slowly eliminated, these compounds taper their own offset). Sedative-hypnotics, or metabolites, cross the placenta and neonates may experience withdrawal. **CAUTIONS**: Elderly or debilitated patients are more prone to side effects and may NOT tolerate usual doses. **RECOMMENDATIONS**: Reduce dosage in hepatic disease (NOT usually a contraindication). Patients hypersensitive to one sedative-hypnotic should receive an agent of a different chemical type.

BENZODIAZEPINE GROUP REMARKS

The benzodiazepines are the newest chemical class of the sedative-hypnotics; substituent diversity yields many agents with different pharmacokinetic properties (onset/duration) and hence different clinical recommendations. **NOTES**: Benzodiazepines are alleged to produce less sedation at anxiolytic doses and be less toxic with overdosage; these conclusions are based on studies in which pharmacokinetic differences may have been confounding factors. Benzodiazepines do not induce hepatic enzymes; they do NOT produce changes in prothrombin time or oral anticoagulant dosage requirements. Other effects (e.g. respiratory depression, abuse withdrawal) are as described in Group Remarks. As anxiolytics, the benzodiazepines are more effective than the barbiturates or meprobamate. They have NO specific action in acute musculoskeletal conditions and behave like other sedative-hypnotics. Oral administration produces more rapid and complete absorption than IM route.

BARBITURATE GROUP REMARKS

Barbiturates are derivatives of barbituric acid; their pharmacokinetics (rapid onset with short duration OR slow onset with long duration) are determined by the lipid solubility of their different substituents **NOTES**: Although all are anticonvulsants, only phenobarbital, metharbital and mephobarbital are effective at doses NOT markedly sedating. Some loss of efficacy at inducing and maintaining sleep occurs after 2 wks of therapy. **LEVELS**: Overdose blood levels correlate poorly with mortality rates; begin treatment prior to receiving results. **CAUTIONS**: Liver microsomal enzymes and metabolic activity are increased by barbiturates; may affect levels of concurrent medications; inactivation of coumarin anticoagulants is stimulated (their dosage must be increased; then reduced upon cessation of the barbiturate). Rapid IV administration may cause respiratory depression, laryngospasm, vasodilation and lowered blood pressure. **RECOMMENDATIONS**: Hypersensitivity reactions are usually rashes or cutaneous lesions (fatal in rare cases). Discontinue at the first sign of a skin reaction. **CONTRAINDICATIONS**: Acute intermittent porphyria or familial history of porphyria.

NOTE: Potential adverse drug interactions between the benzodiazepines/barbiturates and other therapeutic agents are described in Anticonvulsant Group Remarks.

SEDATIVE-HYPNOTICS AND ANXIOLYTICS *Continued*

DRUG	INDICATIONS & DOSAGE	DOSE FORMS	REMARKS
ULTRASHORT-ACTING (Anesthetic Induction) BARBITURATES			
These highly lipid-soluble barbiturates are used chiefly for the induction of anesthesia. They are rapidly absorbed by the CNS (producing rapid onset) and then quickly redistributed out of the CNS (yielding short duration of action). In all other respects they share the common properties of the barbiturates. **CAUTION**: Respiratory depression, hypotension and laryngospasm may develop suddenly during induction of anesthesia. Sln = solution.			
THIOPENTAL (Pentothal)	**Test Dose**: **IV**: 25-75 mg, wait 1 min; observe for adverse effects. **Anesthesia**: **IV**: 50-75 mg SLOWLY (q20-40sec) for induction; maintenance 25-50 mg PRN. **Convulsions**: **IV**: 75-125 mg SLOWLY (< 250 mg over 10 min if due to local anesthetics).	Injection: 250, 400, 500 mg syringes; 0.5, 1, 2.5, 5 gm vials/kits	Dosage must be titrated for each individual patient. **CONTRAINDICATIONS**: Status asthmaticus.
THIAMYLAL (Surital)	**Anesthesia**: **IV**: 1 ml (2.5% sln) q5sec for induction (3-6 ml usually sufficient); maintenance 0.3% sln drip.	Injection: 1, 5, 10 g	For IV administration ONLY; dosage must be titrated for each individual patient. Injection of 3-6 ml (2.5% sln) is usually adequate for short periods of surgical anesthesia.
SHORT-ACTING (Hypnotic) BENZODIAZEPINES			
FLURAZEPAM (Dalmane)	**Hypnotic**: **PO**: 15-30 mg at hs. (Initiate at lower doses in geriatric and debilitated pts.)	PO (Cap's): 15, 30 mg	Approved only for use as a hypnotic for ≤ 4 wks duration. Peak plasma levels at 0.5-1 h, half-life = 50-100 h (active metabolite), duration = 7-8 h. Sleep onset at 15-45 min. Decrease dose in geriatric patients; long-acting metabolites may accumulate.
TEMAZEPAM (Restoril)	**Hypnotic**: **PO**: 15-30 mg at hs. (Initiate at lower doses in geriatric and debilitated pts.	PO (Cap's): 15, 30 mg	Approved only for use as a hypnotic for ≤ 5 wks duration. Peak plasma levels at 2-3 h, half-life = 10-12 h.
TRIAZOLAM (Halcion)	**Hypnotic**: **PO**: 0.25-0.5 mg. **Geriatric PO**: 0.125 mg initially; maximum 0.25 mg.	PO (Tab's): 0.25, 0.5 mg	Approved only for use as a hypnotic for ≤ 6 wks duration. Peak plasma levels at about 1.5 h, half-life = 1.5-3 h. Very short-acting; may produce less "hangover" (but more night-time waking) than other hypnotics.

DRUG	INDICATIONS & DOSAGE	DOSE FORMS	REMARKS
SHORT-ACTING (Hypnotic) BARBITURATES AND RELATED AGENTS			
PENTOBARBITAL (Nembutal)	**Hypnotic**: **PO**: 100 mg. **Rectal**: 120-200 mg. **IM**: 150-200 mg. **Pediatric Rectal**: 60 or 120 mg for 1-12 y.o. **Daytime Sedation**: **PO**: 30 mg tid or qid. **Pediatric PO**: 6 mg/kg/d in 2-3 doses (maximum 100 mg/d). **Convulsive Emergencies**: **IV**: 100 mg (≤ 50 mg/min) initially (maximum 200-500 mg).	PO (Cap's): 30, 50, 100 mg Injection: 50 mg/ml Rectal: 30, 60, 120, 200 mg Elixer: 18.2 mg/5 ml	Often prescribed in hospitals for hypnosis as: 100 mg h.s. & may repeat 1x before 2AM. Onset at 10-15 min, peak plasma levels at 3-4 h, half-life = 15-20 h. Plasma levels > 30 µg/ml are potentially lethal. Hypnotic usefulness > 2 wks NOT proven. Nembutal 30 and 100 mg capsules contain tartrazine dye (potential for allergic reactions, esp. in patients hypersensitive to aspirin).
SECOBARBITAL (Seconal)	**Hypnotic**: **PO, IM**: 100-200 mg. **IV**: 50-250 mg (NOT > 50 mg/15 sec). **Pediatric IM**: 3-5 mg/kg. **Pre-Surgical Sedation**: **PO**: 200-300 mg 2-3 h before surgery. **Pediatric PO**: 50-100 mg 2-3 h before surgery. **Pediatric Rectal**: 4-5 mg/kg. **Convulsive Emergencies**: **IV**: 5.5 mg/kg (NOT > 50 mg/15 sec) q3-4h PRN.	PO (Cap's): 50, 60,100 mg PO (Tab's): 100 mg Injection: 50 mg/ml Rectal: 30, 60, 120, 200 mg	Onset at 10-15 min, peak plasma levels at 3-4 h, half-life = 15-40 h. Hypnotic usefulness > 2 wks NOT proven. Taper discontinuance over 5-6 d to prevent rebound in REM sleep. NOT recommended for routine sedation.
METHYPRYLON (Noludar)	**Hypnotic**: **PO**: 200-400 mg at hs. **Pediatric PO**: 50-200 mg (> 12 y.o.).	PO (Tab's): 50 mg PO (Cap's): 300 mg	Similar to Barbiturates. Onset about 60min, peak plasma levels at 1-2 h, half-life = 3-6 h. Taper withdrawal after chronic use to avoid nightmares. NOT recommended for routine sedation.

SEDATIVE-HYPNOTICS AND ANXIOLYTICS: SHORT-ACTING (Hypnotic) BARBITURATES AND RELATED AGENTS *Cont'd*

DRUG	INDICATIONS & DOSAGE	DOSE FORMS	REMARKS
ETHCHLORVYNOL (Placidyl)	Hypnotic: **PO**: 500-750 mg (100-200 mg to reinstitute sleep upon early morning insomnia); maximum 1000 mg/d.	PO (Cap's): 100, 200, 500, 750 mg	Onset at about 30 min, peak plasma levels at 1-2 h, half-life = 10-20 h. NOT recommended for routine sedation. 750 mg tablets contain tartrazine dye (potential for allergic reactions, esp. in patients hypersensitive to aspirin). **SIDE EFFECTS**: Similar to Barbiturates. Rare amblyopia.
PARALDEHYDE (Paral)	Hypnotic: **PO**:4-8 ml. **IM**: 10 ml. Alcohol Withdrawal: **PO**: 10-35 ml. **Rectal**: 10-20 ml (as 50% mixture in olive oil).	Injection: 1 g/ml Oral Liquid	There is no basis for the continued use of this agent. Dilute liquid prior to administration (ice and juice). Onset about 5-15 min, peak plasma levels at 20-60 min, half-life = 3-10 h following oral administration. **SIDE EFFECTS**: Characteristic taste and odor on breath. GI irritation and rash are also common. IM administration is painful; may produce sterile abscess or injury to adjacent nerves. Hepatitis and nephrosis have occurred rarely. **CAUTIONS**: Disulfiram may inhibit metabolism and increase plasma levels. **CONTRA-INDICATIONS**: Bronchopulmonary or hepatic disease.
CHLORAL HYDRATE (Noctec)	Hypnotic: **PO**: 500-1000 mg (maximum 2 gm/d). **Pediatric PO**: 20-40 mg/kg (maximum 50 mg/kg/d, 1 gm/dose or 2 gm/d).	PO (Cap's): 250, 500 mg Syrup: 100 mg/ml Elixir: 100 mg/ml	**SIDE EFFECTS**: Same as for Barbiturates, also GI irritation.
METHAQUALONE (Quaalude)			Included for identification purposes only, Methaqualone is no longer manufactured for use in the U.S., although it is still sometimes encountered as a "street drug." It is equivalent to the above sedative-hypnotics, but with an undeserved reputation "on the street" as an aphrodisiac.

INTERMEDIATE-ACTING (Hypnotic/Sedative) BENZODIAZEPINE

DRUG	INDICATIONS & DOSAGE	DOSE FORMS	REMARKS
DIAZEPAM (Valium)	Sedation: **PO**: 2-10 mg q6-12h. **PO (Ext'd release)**: 15-30 mg/d. **Pediatric PO**: 1-2.5 mg q6-8h. **IV**: 2-10 mg q3-4h PRN. Alcohol Withdrawal: **PO**: 10 mg, 3-4 doses over 24 h, then 5 mg q6-8h PRN. **IV, IM**: 10 mg, repeat q3-4h (once). Muscle Spasms: **IV, IM**: 5-10 mg, repeat q3-4h (once). **PO**: 2-10 mg q6-8h (maximum 30 mg/d).	PO (Tab's): 2, 5, 10 mg PO (Ext'd release): 15 mg Injection: 5 mg/ml Seizures: **IV, IM**: 5-10 mg initially, repeat q10-15min PRN (maximum 30 mg). **PO**: 2-10 mg q6-12h.	Peak plasma levels at 0.5-2 h, half-life = 30-120 h (active metabolite). Rapid onset. IM use NOT recommended due to slow and erratic absorption. Administer IV doses ≤ 5 mg/min. Decrease doses in geriatric or debilitated patients. Pre-operative use to sedate the patient and produce some anterograde amnesia, but note additive effects with narcotics and other sedatives. Pre-Operative Sedation: **IV**: 5-20 mg 5-60min prior to procedure. **IM**: 5-10 mg 30min prior to procedure.

DRUG	INDICATIONS & DOSAGE	DOSE FORMS	REMARKS
	INTERMEDIATE-ACTING (Hypnotic/Sedative) BARBITURATES AND RELATED AGENTS		
AMOBARBITAL (Amytal)	**Hypnotic**: **PO**: 100-200 mg. **Sedation**: **PO**: 30-50 mg (maximum 120 mg) bid-tid. **Pre-Surgical Sedation**: **PO**: 200 mg 1-2 h prior to surgery.	PO (Tab's): 15, 30, 50, 100 mg PO (Cap's): 65, 200 mg Generic powder **Sedation**: **IV, IM**: 65-500 mg	Barbiturate Group Remarks. Onset at 45-60 min, peak plasma levels at 6-8 h, half-life = 16-40 h. With IV administration, do NOT exceed 1 cc/min infusion.
BUTABARBITAL (Butisol) (Butatran)	**Sedation**: **PO**: 15-30 mg tid-qid. **Pediatric PO**: 7.5 to 30 mg. **Hypnotic**: **PO**: 50-100 mg.	PO (Tab's): 5, 30, 50, 100 mg PO (Cap's): 15, 30 mg	Barbiturate Group Remarks. Onset at 45-60 min, peak plasma levels at 6-8 h, half-life = 16-14 h.
TALBUTAL (Lotusate)	**Hypnotic**: **PO**: 120 mg at hs.	PO (Tab's): 120 mg	Barbiturate Group Remarks. Onset at 45-60 min, peak plasma levels at 6-8 h, half-life = 15 h.
GLUTETHIMIDE (Doriden)	**Hypnotic**: **PO**: 250-500 mg at hs.	PO (Tab's): 250, 500 mg	Similar to the Barbiturates. Should be used only for 3-7 d. **SIDE EFFECTS**: Typical sedative-hypnotic side effects; also, rare skin rash, nausea.
MEPROBAMATE (Miltown) (Equanil)	**Sedation**: **PO**: 1200-1600 mg/d in 3-4 doses; maximum 2400 mg/d.	PO (Tab's): 200, 400, 600 mg PO (Cap's): 400 mg PO (Ext'd release): 200, 400 mg	Barbiturate Group Remarks. Onset at 45-60 min, peak plasma levels at 6-8 h, half-life = 15 h. The selective muscle relaxant activity claimed for meprobamate has never been proven. Habituation/withdrawal as with other sedative-hypnotics; more toxic psychosis and hallucinations have been reported.
CARISOPRODOL (Soma) (Soprodol) (Rela)	See Muscle Relaxants.		

SEDATIVE-HYPNOTICS AND ANXIOLYTICS *Continued*

DRUG	INDICATIONS & DOSAGE	DOSE FORMS	REMARKS
LONG-ACTING (Anxiolytic) BENZODIAZEPINES			
CHLORDIAZEPOXIDE (Librium) (Libritabs) (A-poxide) (Lipoxide)	**Sedation**: **PO**: 15-40 mg/d in 3-4 doses (maximum 100 mg/d). **IV**:25-100 mg initially, then 25-50 mg q6-8h PRN; maximum 300 mg/d. **Alcohol Withdrawal**: **IV, IM**: 50-100 mg initially, repeat q2-4h PRN. **Pre-Operative Sedation**: **IM**: 50-100 mg 1 h before surgery.	PO (Cap's): 5, 10, 25 mg Injection: 100 mg	Peak plasma levels at 0.5-4 h, half-life = 5-30 h. IM use NOT recommended due to slow and erratic absorption. Administer IV doses over > 1 min.
LORAZEPAM (Ativan)	**Sedation**: **PO**: 2-3 mg/d initially; maintenance 1-10 mg/d in 2-3 doses. **Pre-Operative Sedation**: **IM**: 0.05 mg/kg, ≥ 2 h before surgery. **IV**: 0.044-0.05 mg/kg, 15-20 min before surgery (maximum 2 gm total). **Hypnotic**: **PO**: 2-6 mg/d in 2-3 doses (largest at bedtime).	PO (Tab's): 0.5, 1, 2 mg Injection: 2, 4 mg/ml	Pre-operative use to sedate the patient and produce some anterograde amnesia. Peak plasma levels at 1-6 h, half-life = 10-18 h (PO). Do NOT administer by intra-arterial injection; gangrene may result from arteriospasm.
OXAZEPAM (Serax)	**Sedation**: **PO**: 30-120 mg/d in 3-4 doses. **Geriatic PO**: 30 mg/d in 3 doses (maximum 60 mg/d).	PO (Cap's): 10, 15, 30 mg PO (Tab's): 15 mg	Peak plasma levels at 1-4 h, half-life = 3-13 h. Clearance independent of age or liver disease. Short-acting; may produce less "hangover" (but more nighttime waking) than other hypnotics. Oxazepam is an active metabolite of: diazepam, temazepam, prazepam, clorazepate and halazepam.
ALPRAZOLAM (Xanax)	**Sedation**: **PO**: 0.25-0.5 mg/d in 3 doses (maximum 4 mg/d).	PO (Tab's): 0.25, 0.5, 1 mg	Peak plasma levels at 1-2 h, half-life = 12-15 h. Anxiety associated with depression also resonds to alprazolam.
HALAZEPAM (Paxipam)	**Sedation**: **PO**: 20-40 mg/d in 3-4 doses initially; maintenance 80-160 mg/d in 3-4 doses.	PO (Tab's): 20, 40 mg	Major activity due to metabolism to desmethyldiazepam (active metabolite of diazepam). Peak plasma levels at 1-3 h, half-life = 30-120 h (active metabolite).

SEDATIVE-HYPNOTICS AND ANXIOLYTICS: LONG-ACTING (Anxiolytic) BENZODIAZEPINES *Continued*

DRUG	INDICATIONS & DOSAGE	DOSE FORMS	REMARKS
PRAZEPAM (Centrax)	<u>**Sedation**</u>: **PO**: 20-60 mg/d. **Geriatric PO**: 10-15 mg/d initially, increase SLOWLY PRN.	PO (Tab's): 10 mg PO (Cap's): 5, 10, 20 mg	Major activity due to metabolism to desmethyldiazepam (active metabolite of diazepam). Peak plasma levels at 1.5-6 h, half-life = 30-120 h (active metabolite). Very slow onset.
CLORAZEPATE (Tranxene)	<u>**Sedation**</u>: **PO**: 15-60 mg/d in 1-4 doses. <u>**Partial Seizures**</u>: **PO**: 7.5 mg tid initially; incremental increase = 7.5 mg/week (maximum 90 mg/d).	PO (Tab's): 3.75, 7.5, 11.25, 15, 22.5 mg PO (Cap's): 3.75, 7.5, 15 mg	Major activity due to metabolism to desmethyldiazepam (active metabolite of diazepam). Peak plasma levels at 1-2 h, half-life = 30-120 h (active metabolite). Fast onset. Use in seizures is adjunctive to Anticonvulsants.
	LONG-ACTING (Anxiolytic) BARBITURATES		
PHENOBARBITAL (Luminal) (Solfoton)	<u>**Sedation**</u>: **PO**: 30-120 mg/d in 2-3 doses. **PO (Ext'd release)**: 65 mg q12h. IV, IM: 100-300 mg/d (maximum 600 mg/d). **Pediatric IM**: 16-100 mg.	PO (Tab's): 8, 16, 32, 65, 100 mg PO (Ext'd release): 65 mg Elixir: 4 mg/ ml Injection: 30, 60, 65, 130, 325 mg Generic powder	See Anticonvulsants for a more complete discussion Due to long half-life, divided dosage not necessary. Peak plasma levels at 8-12 h, half-life = 2-6 d. **RECOMMENDATIONS**: Administer IV doses SLOWLY. **CONTRAINDICATIONS**: Acute intermittent porphyria.
MEPHOBARBITAL (Mebaral)	<u>**Sedation**</u>: **PO**: 32-100 (often 50) mg tid-qid.	PO (Tab's): 32, 50, 100, 200 mg	Prodrug; demethylated to phenobarbital, therefore similar side effects, etc.

MUSCLE RELAXANTS

GROUP REMARKS: Centrally-acting muscle relaxants are CNS depressants purported to inhibit muscle spasm by selective inhibition of spinal reflexes. Although these sedative-hypnotics and related agents inhibit spinal polysynaptic reflexes in the laboratory, their clinical efficacy as muscle relaxants is due primarily to the relief of situational anxiety. The drugs currently promoted as muscle relaxants can be split into two categories on the basis of use; sedative-hypnotics (chiefly carbamates) are used to treat muscle spasm associated with tension and the others are used to treat spasticity. Although controlled clinical trials have NOT established any usefulness, these central muscle relaxants are often used to treat muscle spasm associated with sprains, bursitis, arthritis, etc. Since these agents are all general CNS depressants, the Group Remarks made for the sedative-hypnotics apply for these as well (esp. Side Effects; after very large doses depression comparable to that caused by the sedative-hypnotics appears).

DRUG	INDICATIONS & DOSAGE	DOSE FORMS	REMARKS
CARBAMATE SEDATIVE-HYPNOTICS			
MEPROBAMATE (Miltown) (Equanil)	<u>**Muscle Relaxation/Sedation**</u>: **PO**: 1200-1600 mg/d in 3-4 doses (maximum 2400 mg/d).	PO (Tab's): 200, 400, 600 mg PO (Cap's): 400 mg PO (Ext'd release): 200, 400 mg	Group Remarks as for Barbiturate Sedative-Hypnotics. Indicated for the treatment of acute, painful musculoskeletal conditions; ineffective in spasticity states. The selective muscle relaxant activity claimed for meprobamate has never been proven. Severe habituation/withdrawal potential.
CARISOPRODOL (Soma) (Soprodol) (Rela)	<u>**Muscle Relaxation/Sedation**</u>: **PO**: 350 mg qid.	PO (Tab's): 350 mg	Structurally and functionally similar to meprobamate. Indicated for the treatment of acute, painful musculoskeletal conditions; ineffective in spasticity states. Onset at 30 min, duration = 4-6 h. Dependence may develop with chronic use. **SIDE EFFECTS**: Similar to Barbiturate Sedative-Hypnotics, especially drowsiness and dizziness. Hypersensitivity reactions include weakness, ataxia, temporary quadriplegia and loss of vision. **CONTRAINDICATIONS**: Porphyria, hypersensitivity to meprobamate.
METHOCARBAMOL (Robamol) (Robaxin)	<u>**Muscle Relaxation/Sedation**</u>: **IM**: 500 mg tid. **IV**: 1-3 gm/d; maximum 3 ml/min. **PO**: 1.5-2 gm qid initially (2-3 d), then 1 gm qid. **Pediatric IV**: 60 mg/kg/d in 4 doses.	Injection: 100 mg/ml PO (Tab's): 500, 750 mg	Indicated for the treatment of acute, painful musculoskeletal conditions; ineffective in spasticity states. Use in children is recommended only for tetanus. Administer IV injections SLOWLY. Maximum daily dose = 3 gm (except in tetanus). Vehicle contains polyethylene glycol 300. **SIDE EFFECTS**: Similar to Barbiturate Sedative-Hypnotics, especially drowsiness and dizziness.
CHLORPHENESIN CARBAMATE (Maolate)	<u>**Muscle Relaxation/Sedation**</u>: **PO**: 800 mg tid initially; 400 mg qid maintenance.	PO (Tab's): 400 mg	Structurally and functionally related to methocarbamol. Indicated for the treatment of acute, painful musculoskeletal conditions; ineffective in spasticity states. Contains tartrazine dye. **SIDE EFFECTS**: Similar to Barbiturate Sedative-Hypnotics, especially drowsiness and dizziness.

DRUG	INDICATIONS & DOSAGE	DOSE FORMS	REMARKS
OTHER SEDATIVE-HYPNOTICS			
DIAZEPAM (Valium)	**Muscle Relaxation/Sedation**: **IV, IM**: 5-10 mg, repeat q3-4h (once). **PO**: 2-10 mg q6-8h.	PO (Tab's): 2, 5, 10 mg Injection: 5 mg/ml	See section: Sedative-Hypnotics: Benzodiazepines.
CHLORZOXAZONE (Paraflex) (in Parafon Forte)	**Muscle Relaxation/Sedation**: **PO**: 250-750 mg tid-qid. **Pediatric PO**: 125-500 mg tid or qid.	PO (Tab's): 250 mg	Chlorzoxazone is a CNS depressant; clinical effect probably due to sedative action. Indicated for the treatment of acute, painful musculoskeletal conditions; ineffective in spasticity states. Chlorzoxazone is a metabolite of zoxazolamine, which was removed from the market because of hepatotoxicity (hepatitis has developed coincident with chlorzoxazone therapy). **SIDE EFFECTS**: Drowsiness and dizziness most common, but generally well tolerated. **RECOMMENDATIONS**: Periodic LFTs; discontinue therapy at first sign of hepatic dysfunction.
METAXALONE (Skelaxin)	**Muscle Relaxation/Sedation**: **PO**: 800 mg tid-qid.	PO (Tab's): 400 mg	Metaxalone is a CNS depressant; clinical effect probably due to sedative action. Indicated for the treatment of acute, painful musculoskeletal conditions; ineffective in spasticity states. **SIDE EFFECTS**: Drowsiness, dizziness and nausea most common, but generally well tolerated.
CHLORMEZANONE (Chlormethazanone) (Trancopal)	**Muscle Relaxation/Sedation**: **PO**: 100-200 mg tid-qid. **Pediatric (5-12 y.o.) PO**: 50-100 mg tid-qid.	PO (Tab's): 100, 200 mg	Chlormezanone is a CNS depressant; clinical effect is questionable and probably due to sedative action. Indicated for the treatment of acute, painful musculoskeletal conditions; ineffective in spasticity states. Chlormezanone is also indicated for anxiety. **SIDE EFFECTS**: Drowsiness and dizziness most common.
TRICYCLIC COMPOUND			
CYCLOBENZAPRINE (Flexeril)	**Muscle Relaxation/Sedation**: **PO**: 10-20 mg tid.	PO (Tab's): 10 mg	Structurally and functionally related to the tricyclic antidepressants; see appropriate Group Remarks. Indicated for the treatment of acute, painful musculoskeletal conditions; ineffective in spasticity states. Restrict use to 2 wks duration. **SIDE EFFECTS**: Similar to the tricyclic antidepressants, especially drowsiness, dry mouth and dizziness (10-40% patients). Prominent anticholinergic effects.

DRUG	INDICATIONS & DOSAGE	DOSE FORMS	REMARKS
MISCELLANEOUS			
DANTROLENE (Dantrium)	**Spasticity**: **PO**: 25 mg/d initially, incremental increase = 25 mg/d q4-7d; 100 mg bid-qid maintenance (use LOWEST effective dose). **Pediatric PO**: 0.5 mg/kg bod initially, incremental increase = 0.5 mg/kg q4-7d; 3 mg/kg bid-qid maintenance (maximum 100 mg qid). **Malignant Hyperpyrexia**: **PO**: 4-8 mg/kg/d in 3-4 doses for 1-2 d before surgery (or 1-3d after hyperpyrexic episode). **IV**: 1 mg/kg initially, repeat PRN (IV maximum 10 mg/kg).	PO (Cap's): 25, 50, 100 mg Injection: 20 mg	Some usefulness in spasticity due to upper motor neuron disorders; otherwise NOT indicated. Therapeutic effect may require 1 wk to develop; discontinue therapy if no positive response within 45 d (not all patients respond). **CAUTIONS**: Potentially fatal hepatotoxicity occurs most frequently with dosage > 300 mg/d for > 2 months or with ≥ 800 mg/d intermittently. Hepatotoxocity is often preceded by GI distress. Patients at greater risk: female, > 35 y.o., concurrent additional medication (esp. estrogens). **SIDE EFFECTS**: Adverse effects are common. Muscle weakness may produce slurred speech, drooling, enuresis. Also drowsiness, dizziness, diarrhea, nausea, malaise and photosensitivity. Tolerance may develop to side effects; if not, lower dosage. If diarrhea persists after decreasing dosage, discontinue therapy. **RECOMMENDATIONS**: Periodic LFTs; discontinue therapy if abnormal LFTs or signs of hepatitis.
ORPHENADRINE (Norflex)	**Parkinsonism**: **PO**: 50 mg tid initially; 150-250 mg/d maintenance. **Muscle Relaxation**: **PO**: 100 mg bid. **IM, IV**: 60 mg bid.	PO (Tab's): 50 mg (HCl); 100 mg (citrate) Injection: 30 mg/ml	Orphenadrine is an antihistamine-like agent with atropinic actions and is used in the treatment of Parkinsonism and muscle tension. See Atropine. **SIDE EFFECTS**: Mainly due to anticholinergic action: dry mouth, urinary retention, dizziness, blurred vision, mydriasis, elevated intraocular pressure and tachycardia.
BACLOFEN (Lioresal)	**Spastic Disorders**: **PO**: 5 mg tid initially, increase 15 mg/d q3d; maintenance 40-80 mg/d in 3-4 doses.	PO (Tab's): 10, 20 mg	Analog of gamma-aminobutyric acid (GABA), an inhibitory transmitter. Inhibits polysynaptic and monosynaptic reflexes and is a depressant at supraspinal sites (may be basis of clinical action). Useful in spasticity in multiple sclerosis and possibly in other spinal cord lesions. NOT indicated for muscle spasms in rheumatic disorders. **SIDE EFFECTS**: Drowsiness common, also dizziness, weakness, nausea and hypotension. **RECOMMENDATIONS**: Slow withdrawal (possible hallucinations, exacerbation of spasticity with abrupt discontinuation). Allow 1-2 months to evaluate effectiveness of therapy.

NEUROMUSCULAR BLOCKING AGENTS

GROUP REMARKS: These agents paralyze skeletal muscle by interfering with nerve impulse transmission at the neuromuscular junction. They are used as adjuncts to anesthesia (to facilitate intubation, block laryngospasm and relax skeletal muscle) or to control convulsions. Neuromuscular blockers do NOT affect pain perception or consciousness. There are two classes of neuromuscular blockers: Depolarizing and Non-depolarizing (Competitive) agents. **CAUTIONS**: All of these agents can produce respiratory depression; they should be used ONLY when the experience and equipment for RAPID INTUBATION and MECHANICAL RESPIRATION is present. Safe use in pregnancy and lactating mothers has not been established. Newborns and patients with myasthenia gravis are especially sensitive to these agents. **SIDE EFFECTS**: Hypotension, bradycardia/tachycardia and bronchospasm.

DRUG INTERACTIONS:
Actions of all **neuromuscular blockers** may be potentiated by ***inhalation anesthetics, quinidine, aminoglycosides (esp. IV), polymyxins, ß-blockers*** and ***magnesium***. Concurrent or sequential administration of **depolarizing** and **non-depolarizing neuromuscular blockers** may produce **synergistic** or **antagonistic** results.

DRUG	INDICATIONS & DOSAGE	DOSE FORMS	REMARKS
	NON-DEPOLARIZING (COMPETITIVE) NEUROMUSCULAR BLOCKERS		
GROUP NOTES: Non-depolarizing agents block the ACh receptor, preventing the stimulation of muscle contraction by ACh released from the associated nerve. Because this blockade is competitive, it is reversible, in part, by cholinesterase inhibitors (e.g., neostigmine, pyridostigmine) which prolong the presence of ACh at the motor end-plate. Non-depolarizing blockers also release histamine, which is responsible for bronchiolar constriction and some of the fall in blood pressure.			
DRUG INTERACTIONS: Actions of the **non-depolarizing NM blockers** may be potentiated by ***succinylcholine, bacitracin, tetracyclines, diazepam, and hypokalemia (diuretics, corticosteroids)***, in addition to the agents listed in the general Group Remarks. Their actions may be diminished by ***cholinesterase inhibitors***.			
TUBOCURARINE (Delacurarine)	**Surgery**: **IV**: 40-60 units initially, then 20-30 units in 3-5 min PRN. Alternate dosage: 1.1 units/kg.	Injection: 3 mg/ml (10, 20 ml)	May also be given IM. **SIDE EFFECTS**: Allergic reactions. **RECOMMENDATIONS**: Administer IV injections over 1-2 min. **CONTRAINDICATIONS**: Hypersensitivity.
PANCURONIUM (Pavulon)	**Endotracheal Intubation**: **IV**: 0.06-0.1 mg/kg initially; effect should be seen in 2-3 min. If additional effect required give 0.01 mg/kg. ***Note***: Additional maintenance doses may markedly prolong the period of paralysis while increasing the intensity of paralysis only slightly to moderately.	Injection: 1 mg/ml (10 ml), 2 mg/ml (2, 5 ml)	**SIDE EFFECTS**: Allergic reactions, rash, mild salivation. **RECOMMENDATIONS**: Administer IV injections over 1-2 min. **CONTRAINDICATIONS**: Hypersensitivity.
METOCURINE (Metubine)	**Surgery**: **IV**: 0.2-0.4 mg/kg initially, then 0.5-1 mg PRN. **Electroconvulsive Therapy**: **IV**: 1.75-5.5 mg; administ. SLOWLY, until head-drop is produced.	Injection: 2 mg/ml	Administer IV injections over 30-60 sec. Reduce dosage by 1/3-1/2 if concurrent strong anesthetics are to be used.

NEUROMUSCULAR BLOCKING AGENTS *Continued*

DRUG	INDICATIONS & DOSAGE	DOSE FORMS	REMARKS
ATRACURIUM (Tracrium)	Surgery: **IV**: 0.4-0.5 mg/kg initially, expect effect in 2-5 min; 0.08-0.1 mg/kg maintenance dose PRN (usually at 15-40 min).	Injection: 10 mg/ml	May release less histamine than other non-depolarizing blockers. Reduce dose by ≤ 1/3 if inhalation anesthetics or succinylcholine are used.
VECURONIUM (Norcuron)	Surgery: **IV**: 0.08-0.1 mg/kg initially, 0.01-0.015 mg/kg maintenance PRN (usually at 15-30 min).	Powder: 10 mg/5 ml vial	For IV use only.

DEPOLARIZING NEUROMUSCULAR BLOCKER

GROUP NOTES: Depolarizing agents, of which succinylcholine is the only one used clinically to any extent, initially stimulate the muscle's ACh receptors, producing fasciculations. A flacid paralysis (phase 1) ensues as the motor end-plate's ability to respond is exhausted. Cholinesterase inhibitors may prolong/intensify the action of succinylcholine. Repeated administration may induce a non-depolarizing type of blockade (phase 2). Phase 2 blockade may elicit prolonged respiratory depression which may be reversed by neostigmine (after confirmation of phase 2 state by peripheral nerve stimulation).

DRUG INTERACTIONS:
Actions of **succinylcholine** may be potentiated by ***local anesthetics, cholinesterase inhibitors, cyclophosphamide, phenothiazines*** and ***phenelzine***. Its actions may be diminished by ***diazepam***.

DRUG	INDICATIONS & DOSAGE	DOSE FORMS	REMARKS
SUCCINYLCHOLINE (Anectin) (Quelicin) (Sucostrin) (Suxinyl)	Surgery and Anesthesia: **IV**: 0.3-1.1 mg/kg (over 10-30 sec); effect should be seen within 1 min. Prolonged Muscular Relaxation: **IV**: 0.3-1.1 mg/kg (over 10-30 sec) initially, then 0.04-0.07 mg/kg PRN.	Injection: 20, 50, 100 mg/ml (5, 10, 20 ml) Powder for Injection: 0.1, 0.5, 1 g/vial	Blockade is short-lived; onset is 30-60 sec (IV), 1-3 min (IM); duration of action after IV administration is 4-6 min. **SIDE EFFECTS**: Fever, arrhythmias, myoglobinemia, muscle fasciculations which also cause post-paralysis myalgias, and increased salivation. Malignant hyperthermia, increased intraocular pressure, rash, and hyperkalemia. **CAUTIONS**: Use with caution in patients with history of glaucoma or cardiovascular impairment. If patient recently digitalized or has digitalis toxicity, LETHAL arrhythmias may occur. Prolonged apnea is possible in rare patients with familial defects in pseudocholinesterase. Pseudocholinesterase may also be reduced in hepatocellular disease, dehydration, burns, collagen disorders, myxedema and pregnancy. **RECOMMENDATIONS**: Post-paralysis myalgias may be reduced by a small dose of pancuronium given prior to starting therapy. **CONTRAINDICATIONS**: History of febrile reaction to anesthesia in patient or family, myopathies with elevated CPK and hypersensitivity.

ANTICONVULSANTS

GROUP REMARKS: Epilepsy is the major indication for these drugs, but other convulsive states (e.g, intracranial tumor, trauma, uremia) are also treated effectively. The various anticonvulsants are effective in different types of seizures: drugs active against tonic-clonic seizures are sometimes useful in partial seizures, but often ineffective in absence, akinetic or myoclonic seizures; drugs active in the latter types are usually inactive in the former. Combined seizures can be treated with combinations of anticonvulsants. Anticonvulsants are specific CNS depressants and act by directly suppressing the seizure focus and/or interfering with the spread of seizure activity. Because of the long-term use of anticonvulsants for many patients, chronic toxicity is a major concern in their use. Long-acting agents are preferred due to the relative ease of maintaining consistent plasma levels. Fluctuating levels (or withdrawal) may precipitate seizures. If toxicity specific for one compound appears (especially drug rash or other allergic reaction) substitute another anticonvulsant. **SIDE EFFECTS**: Side effects due to CNS depression are common: drowsiness, irritability, dizziness, confusion, nystagmus, ataxia and slurred speech. Some tolerance usually develops. GI disturbances (nausea, vomiting, diarrhea, constipation, anorexia) are also fairly common.

ANTICONVULSANT DRUG INTERACTIONS:

Phenytoin: conversion of ***Primidone*** to phenobarbital enhanced (phenobarbital levels increased); displaces ***Dicoumarol*** from plasma protein binding and enhances metabolism (phenytoin metabolism inhibited), do NOT use concurrently; metabolism of phenytoin inhibited by ***Isoniazid*** (phenytoin toxicity possible); may decrease half-life of ***Doxycycline***; enhanced metabolism of ***Digitoxin*** (monitor and adjust Digitoxin levels); ***Disulfiram*** inhibits phenytoin metabolism (possible phenytoin toxicity).

Phenobarbital (induces liver enzymes and enhances metabolism of many other drugs): ***Coumarin Anticoagulant*** levels decreased (risk of hemorrhage upon discontinuance of phenobarbital if coumarin dosage increased to compensate); ***Phenytoin*** metabolism enhanced or inhibited producing an increase, decrease or no effect on phenytoin blood levels (monitor serum levels); decreases effectiveness of ***Oral Contraceptives*** (advise alternate contraception); potentiates adverse reactions to ***Tricyclic Antidepressants***; metabolism of phenobarbital inhibited by ***Monoamine Oxidase Inhibitors*** (adjust dosage); may decrease half-life of ***Doxycycline***; enhanced metabolism of ***Digitoxin*** (monitor and adjust Digitoxin levels).

Valproic Acid: plasma levels of ***Phenobarbital*** (either alone or as metabolite of primidone) increased; ***Phenytoin*** plasma levels decreased (seizures may result).

Anticonvulsants (in general): ***Tricyclic Antidepressants*** induce seizures (anticonvulsant dosage may require adjustment upward); will have additive effects with any other ***CNS depressants*** (e.g., ***alcohol***).

GRAND MAL & COMPLEX PARTIAL SEIZURES

HYDANTOINS

Hydantoins control convulsions without producing sedation. Primary action of the hydantoins is to limit the spread of seizure activity. Hydantoins are useful in grand mal and psychomotor epilepsy, also in symptomatic convulsions; they may worsen mixed epilepsy. **SIDE EFFECTS**: Vestibulocerebellar side effects (ataxia, nystagmus and slurred speech) are the most common. Nervousness and tremors or fatigue and drowsiness are also relatively common combination side effects. **ADVERSE EFFECTS-CHRONIC THERAPY**: Phenytoin alone causes irreversible gingival hypertrophy in 20% of patients (regular brushing may minimize development; gum excision may be necessary). Prolonged use of phenytoin or phenytoin-phenobarbital mixtures: coarsened facies, altered vitamine D metabolism (increased alkaline phosphatase, decreased serum 25-hydroxycalciferol, decreased bone mass and rarely osteomalacia), failure of folate absorption with macrocystosis or megaloblastic anemia. Allergic morbilliform rash occurs in 2-10% patients (occasionally accompanied by pyrexia, eosinophilia, and lymphadenopathy); discontinue therapy if exfoliative, purpuric or bullous rash develops (rare). Lymphadenopathy and blood dyscrasias occur rarely. A teratogenic effect of hydantoins (above that of epilepsy) is NOT established. A specific dysmorphism (fetal phenytoin syndrome) is suggested by clinical evidence. Thyroid function tests depressed. **RECOMMENDATIONS**: Reduced dosage in small decrements; allow intervals of several weeks between adjustments (risk of precipitating seizures).

ANTICONVULSANTS: GRAND MAL & COMPLEX PARTIAL SEIZURES - HYDANTOINS *Continued*

DRUG	INDICATIONS & DOSAGE	DOSE FORMS	REMARKS
PHENYTOIN (Dilantin) (DPH) (Diphenylhydantoin)	<u>**Seizure Disorders**</u>: **PO**: 100 mg tid initially, increase by 100 mg/d q2-4wk; maintenance 300-600 mg/d (day 1 loading dose = 1000 mg in 3 doses). **Pediatric PO**: 5 mg/kg/d in 2-3 doses (day 1 loading dose = 500-600 mg in 3 doses); maintenance 4-8 mg/kg (maximum 300 mg/d). **IM**: 50% > established PO dosage; 1 wk course only (reduce subsequent PO dose by 50% for 1 wk following IM regimen). <u>**Status Epilepticus**</u>: **IV**: 150-250 mg initially, then 100-150 mg in 30 min PRN. **Pediatric IV**: 10-15 mg/kg (divided into 5-10 mg/kg doses).	PO (Cap's): 30, 100 mg Injection: 50 mg/ml Oral Suspension: 6, 25 mg/ml	Maximal anticonvulsant effect at 5-10 d. Also used as an antiarrhythmic (see Antiarrhythmics). **SIDE EFFECTS**: Usual anticonvulsant side effects and adverse reactions. GI irritation common; minimize by administration with or following meals or divided dosing. Hirsutism (esp. of the extremities) often develops in girls. **LEVELS**: 10-20 µg/ml are usually therapeutic. Nystagmus, diplopia and ataxia may occur at serum levels > 20 µg/ml. **CAUTIONS**: As dose is increased, metabolism saturates and sudden rapid rise in blood levels can occur. Bioavailability varies between different manufacturers' products; switch brands cautiously. **RECOMMENDATIONS**: Administer IV doses SLOWLY, to avoid serious CVS/CNS depression.
MEPHENYTOIN (Mesantoin)	<u>**Seizure Disorders**</u>: **PO**: 50-100 mg/d initially, increase by 50-100 mg/d q1wk; maintenance 200-600 mg/d in 3 doses (maximum 800 mg/d). **Pediatric PO**: 50-100 mg/d initially, increase by 50-100 mg/d q1wk; maintenance 100-400 mg/d in 3 doses.	PO (Tab's): 100 mg	Use only in patients/conditions refractory to Phenytoin. **SIDE EFFECTS**: See Remarks for phenytoin. Mephenytoin produces much less gingival hypertrophy, but more drowsiness and serious toxic reactions (e.g., blood dyscrasias), than phenytoin. Frequent rash and neutropenia. Rare aplastic anemia, pancytopenia, and liver damage (more than with phenytoin). **LEVELS**: 25-40 µg/ml are usually therapeutic. **RECOMMENDATIONS**: Pre-therapy and periodic CBC and WBC.
ETHOTOIN (Peganone)	<u>**Seizure Disorders**</u>: **PO**: ≤ 1000 mg/d initially in 4-6 doses; maintenance 2000-3000 mg/d. **Pediatric PO**: ≤ 750 mg/d initially; maintenance 500-2000 mg/d (maximum 3000 mg/d).	PO (Tab's): 250, 500 mg	In general, is less effective than phenytoin and is NOT antiarrhythmic. **SIDE EFFECTS**: See comments for phenytoin. Produces less gingival hypertrophy and hirsutism than phenytoin. **CONTRAINDICATIONS**: Hepatic or hematologic disorders.

BARBITURATES & DERIVATIVES

All barbiturates are anticonvulsant; only 4 (Phenobarbital, Mephobarbital, Metharibital and Primidone) are used clinically - because of their long duration of action and because their anticonvulsant effect may be obtained without hypnotic action. These barbiturates and related drugs are useful in grand mal epilepsy and symptomatic convulsions; they are less effective for psychomotor and petit mal epilepsy. **SIDE EFFECTS**: Most side effects are related to sedation or disinhibition, but barbiturates are generally well tolerated. In addition to side effects shared by all anticonvulsants, diplopia, and personality changes are common and mental dulling may occur. See also Group Remarks for barbiturates in Sedative-Hypnotics. Minimize side effects by combining different anticonvulsants. Tendency to hyperexcitable withdrawal state (from discontinuing or rapidly reducing dosage). Chronic phenobarbital therapy is neither dangerous nor habituating.

ANTICONVULSANTS: GRAND MAL & COMPLEX PARTIAL SEIZURES - BARBITURATES *Continued*

DRUG	INDICATIONS & DOSAGE	DOSE FORMS	REMARKS
PHENOBARBITAL (Luminal) (Solfoton)	**Seizure Disorders**: **PO**: 100-300 mg/d in 2-3 doses (maximum 600 mg/d). **Pediatric PO**: 4-6 mg/kg/d for 7-10 d; maintenance 10-15 mg/kg/d. **Status Epilepticus**: **IV**: 200-300 mg, allow 30 min for full effect; repeat at 6 h PRN. **Pediatric IV**: 3-5 mg/kg.	PO (Tab's): 8, 16, 32, 65, 100 mg Elixir: 4 mg/ ml Injection: 30, 60, 65, 130, 325 mg units	**SIDE EFFECTS**: Generally well tolerated. Drowsiness is the most common side effect. **NOTES**: Due to long half-life: divided dosage NOT necessary, 3-4wk required to attain steady-state plasma levels. Effectiveness in status epilepticus limited by slow onset, even after IV administration. **LEVELS**: Therapeutic: 15-40 μg/ml. **CAUTIONS**: Administer IV doses SLOWLY. **RECOMMEND**: When changing dosage in patients on concurrent coumarin anticoagulants, monitor prothtrombin times. **CONTRAINDICATIONS**: Acute intermittent porphyria.
PRIMIDONE (Mysoline) (Primaclone) (Desoxyphenobarbital)	**Seizure Disorders**: **PO**: 100-125 mg qd for 3 d, then bid for 3 d, then tid for 3 d; 250 mg tid-qid maintenance (maximum 2000 mg/d). **Pediatric (< 8 y.o.) PO**: 50 mg qd for 3 d, then bid for 3 d, then 100 mg bid for 3 d; 125-250 mg tid maintenance.	PO (Tab's): 50, 250 mg Suspension: 250 mg/5 ml	Prodrug; oxidized to phenobarbital and phenylethylmalonamide (has weak anticonvulsant activity). **SIDE EFFECTS**: See Remarks for phenobarbital. Severe reactions are rare, but an acute psychosis-like reaction has been reported. **LEVELS**: Therapeutic: 7-15 μg/ml primidone or 20-40 μg/ml phenobarbital (attained in 4 d). **CAUTIONS**: Inhibits folic acid absorption; may produce macrocytosis (less likely than with hydantoins).
METHARBITAL (Gemonil)	**Seizure Disorders**: **PO**: 100 mg 1-3 times/d, 100-800 mg/d maintenance. **Pediatric PO**: 5-15 mg/kg/d in 1-3 doses; increase PRN (maximum 600-800 mg/d).	PO (Tab's): 100 mg	Prodrug; demethylated to barbital, a long-acting barbiturate. May be especially effective in petit mal variant epilepsy. **SIDE EFFECTS**: See Remarks for phenobarbital, but may produce less drowsiness.
MEPHOBARBITAL (Mebaral)	**Seizure Disorders**: **PO**: 400-600 mg/d. **Pediatric (> 5 y.o.) PO**: 32-64 mg tid-qid. **Pediatric (< 5 y.o.) PO**: 16-32 mg tid-qid.	PO (Tab's): 32, 50, 100, 200 mg	Prodrug; demethylated to phenobarbital. **SIDE EFFECTS**: See Remarks for phenobarbital, with less hyperactivity. **LEVELS**: Measure phenobarbital levels; maintain in range of 15-40 μg/ml.
MISCELLANEOUS			
DIAZEPAM (Valium)	**Seizure Disorders**: **IV, IM**: 5-10 mg initially, repeat q10-15min PRN (maximum 30 mg total dose). **PO**: 2-10 mg bid-qid (Ext'd release: 15-30 mg/d). **Pediatric PO**:1-2.5 mg tid-qid.	PO (Tab's): 2, 5, 10 mg PO (extended release): 15 mg Injection: 5 mg/ml	See Benzodiazepine Sedative-Hypnotics. Main use: reverse status epilepticus (IV); some oral use as adjunct agent, but efficacy alone unproven. Administer IV doses ≤ 5 mg/min; give IM if IV not possible. **SIDE EFFECTS**: Drowsiness is major side effect.

ANTICONVULSANTS: GRAND MAL & COMPLEX PARTIAL SEIZURES - MISCELLANEOUS *Continued*

DRUG	INDICATIONS & DOSAGE	DOSE FORMS	REMARKS
CARBAMAZEPINE (Tegretol)	**Seizure Disorders**: **PO**: 200 mg bid initially, increase by ≤ 200 mg/d (to maximum 1000-1200 mg/d) in 3-4 doses. **Pediatric PO**: 100 mg bid initially, increase by 100 mg/d to maximum 1000 mg/d in 3-4 doses when > 200 mg/d. **Trigeminal Neuralgia**: **PO**: 100 mg bid for 1 d, increase by 100 mg q12h; usual maintenance 400-800 mg/d (maximum 1200 mg/d).	PO (Tab's): 200 mg	Exhibits significant sedative, anticholinergic and antidiuretic properties. **SIDE EFFECTS**: Sedation, ataxia. Serious (life-threatening) adverse reactions have occurred: aplastic anemia, blood dyscrasias, congestive heart failure. Other serious reactions: peripheral neuritis, paresthesias, paralysis, depression, agitation, SLE-like syndrome, urinary retention, cataracts, tinnitus. **LEVELS**: Steady-state plasma levels attained in 2-4 d. Therapeutic: 4-12 µg/ml. **CAUTIONS**: A small group of patients develop life-threatening reactions to carbamazepine. It is used as a "first-line" agent for trigeminal neuralgia, it is NOT a "first-line" anticonvulsant. **RECOMMEND**: Baseline and periodic CBC, WBC, serum iron, LFTs, BUN and urinalysis. Discontinue therapy at first sign of hematologic problem: altered blood counts or syndrome of fever, sore throat, oral ulcers, bruising, petechial/purpuric hemorrhage. **CONTRAINDICATIONS**: Bone marrow suppression, concurrent MAO inhibitor (allow 14 d interval after MAO Inhibitor).

PETIT MAL SEIZURES - CLASSIC TYPE

SUCCINIMIDES

Succinimides are used primarily to treat petit mal epilepsy (absence seizures). The succinimides suppress the characteristic spike and wave EEG pattern of this type of seizure. When used in mixed forms of epilepsy, the succinimides may increase the incidence of tonic-clonic seizures (other anticonvulsants should be added to the regimen to counter this effect).

DRUG	INDICATIONS & DOSAGE	DOSE FORMS	REMARKS
ETHOSUXIMIDE (Zarontin)	**Seizure Disorders**: **PO**: 500 mg/d initially in 1-2 doses, increase 250 mg/d q4-7d (maximum 1500 mg/d). **Pediatric PO**: 250 mg/d initially; 20 mg/kg/d maintenance (strict supervision for doses ≥ 1500 mg/d).	PO (Cap's): 250 mg Syrup: 50 mg/ml	Drug of choice for absence seizures. **SIDE EFFECTS**: Usual succinimide anticonvulsant side and adverse effects. GI effects are the most common: nausea, vomiting, anorexia, cramps, weight loss, diarrhea. CNS effects are also common, esp. drowsiness, dizziness, headache, irritability, hyperactivity, lethargy, fatigue and ataxia. Sleep disturbances and night terrors have been reported in previously unaffected patients. **LEVELS**: Therapeutic: 40-100 µg/ml.
METHSUXIMIDE (Celontin)	**Seizure Disorders**: **PO**: 300 mg/d for 1 wk, each wk add 300 mg/d (maximum 1200 mg/d).	PO (Cap's): 150, 300 mg	Produrg; N-demethylmethsuximide is a CNS depressant. In general, drug of second choice in absence seizures. Methsuximide has less potential to precipitate tonic-clonic seizures than do ethosuximide or phensuximide; may be more useful in mixed forms of epilepsy. **SIDE EFFECTS**: Usual succinimide anticonvulsant side and adverse effects; GI effects prominent.

ANTICONVULSANTS: PETIT MAL SEIZURES - CLASSIC TYPE - SUCCINIMIDES *Continued*

DRUG	INDICATIONS & DOSAGE	DOSE FORMS	REMARKS
PHENSUXIMIDE (Milontin)	<u>**Seizure Disorders**</u>: **PO**: 500-1000 mg bid-tid (maximum 3 gm/d).	PO (Cap's): 500 mg	Least effective and least toxic of the succinimides. Tolerance often develops to the therapeutic effect. **SIDE EFFECTS**: Usual succinimide anticonvulsant side and adverse effects; GI effects prominent. CNS depression also prominent.
OXAZOLIDINEDIONES			
These more toxic drugs are used rarely in the treatment of absence seizures. **SIDE EFFECTS**: Potentially FATAL adverse effects: nephrosis, anemias (aplastic, hypoplastic), blood dyscrasias. Other serious reactions: myasthenia gravis, rash (progressive to erythema multiforme or exfoliative dermatitis; discontinue promptly upon evidence of any dermal reaction), SLE-like syndrome, lymphadenopathies, hepatitis. Major side effects are drowsiness and ataxia (tolerance may develop). **CAUTIONS**: Sudden discontinuation of therapy may precipitate absence seizures. **RECOMMENDATIONS**: Perform baseline and periodic urinalysis, CBC, LFTs.			
TRIMETHADIONE (Tridione)	<u>**Seizure Disorders**</u>: **PO**: 300 mg tid initially, each wk add 300 mg/d; maintenance 900-2400 mg/d. **Pediatric PO**: 300-900 mg/d in 3-4 doses.	PO (Tab's): 150 mg PO (Cap's): 300 mg Solution: 40 mg/ml	Oxazolidinedione and general anticonvulsant Group Remarks. Contains tartrazine dye.
PARAMETHADIONE (Paradione)	<u>**Seizure Disorders**</u>: **PO**: 300 mg tid initially, each wk add 300 mg/d; maintenance 900-2400 mg/d. **Pediatric PO**: 300-900 mg/d in 3-4 doses.	PO (Cap's): 150, 300 mg Solution: 300 mg/ml	Oxazolidinedione and general anticonvulsant Group Remarks. Solution contains approximately 65% alcohol.
VALPROIC ACID			
VALPROIC ACID (Depakene)	<u>**Seizure Disorders**</u>: **PO**: 15 mg/kg/d initially, each wk add 5-10 mg/kg/d; maintenance 30-60 mg/kg/d in 1-3 doses.	PO (Tab's): 125, 250, 500 mg PO (Cap's): 250 mg Syrup: 50 mg/ml	Used primarily for absence seizures, but may also be effective in psychomotor, temporal lobe, myoclonic, akinetic and photic-induced seizures. **SIDE EFFECTS**: GI effects most common: nausea, vomiting and diarrhea. CNS effects also common: sedation, drowsiness (heightened alertness has been reported) and headache. **LEVELS**: Therapeutic: approximately 50-100 μg/ml. **CAUTIONS**: Severe, FATAL hepatotoxicity has occurred (esp. during initial 6 months of therapy); may be preceded by loss of anticonvulsant efficacy, weakness or GI effects; perform baseline and periodic LFTs.

ANTICONVULSANTS: *Continued*

DRUG	INDICATIONS & DOSAGE	DOSE FORMS	REMARKS
MISCELLANEOUS AGENTS			
CLONAZEPAM (Klonopin)	<u>Seizure Disorders</u>: **PO**: 0.5 mg tid initially, increase by 0.5-1 mg q3d (maximum 20 mg/d). **Pediatric PO**: 0.01-0.03 mg/kg/d in 3 doses, increase by 0.5 mg/d q3d (maximum 0.2 mg/kg/d).	PO (Tab's): 0.5, 1, 2 mg	**SIDE EFFECTS**: See Benzodiazepine Sedative-Hypnotics. CNS effects are most prominent: sedation, drowsiness, ataxia, behavioral changes (occasionally in children). Minor cardiovascular, gastrointestinal and genitourinary effects. **NOTES**: Useful in petit mal variant, akinetic and myoclonic seizures; drug of second choice in absence seizures. **LEVELS**: Therapeutic: approximately 20-80 ng/ml.
PHENACEMIDE (Phenurone)	<u>Seizure Disorders</u>: **PO**: 500 mg tid initially, each wk add 500 mg/d; maintenance 2000-5000 mg/d. **Pediatric PO**: approximately 1/2 adult dose, given at the same intervals.	PO (Tab's): 500 mg	Should be used only as drug of last resort in the treatment of mixed epilepsy and psychomotor seizures; usefulness limited by toxicity. **SIDE EFFECTS**: Potentially FATAL adverse effects: hepatitis, jaundice, aplastic anemia, blood dyscrasias. Other serious side effects: personality changes (approximately 17% patients; may be severe/suicidal), nephritis (discontinue therapy at first abnormal urinalysis). Minor effects: GI disturbances, drowsiness. **CAUTIONS**: Concurrent ethotoin may precipitate paranoia.
ACETAZOLAMIDE (Diamox)	<u>Epilepsy</u>: **PO**: 8-30 mg/kg/d in 2-4 doses (start at 250 mg/d if adding to other seizure medication).	PO (Tab's): 125, 250 mg Injection: 500 mg/vial	Carbonic Anhydrase Inhibitor, see applicable Group Remarks (Ophthalmic Agents). Used as adjunctive medication in epilepsy (especially petit mal in children).

ANTIPSYCHOTIC TRANQUILIZERS

GROUP REMARKS: Antipsychotics suppress schizophrenic ideation and behavior; they reduce activity of grossly disturbed patients without inducing anesthesia. They are NOT effective against anxiety. **NOTES**: In general, clinical efficacy varies little between the various antipsychotics when equitherapeutic doses are administered. However, because of individual variation, lack of response to one drug doesn't preclude success of another. The various classes of antipsychotics differ mainly in the severity of characteristic side effects produced by each: anticholinergic effects, sedation and extrapyramidal effects. Optimal response occurs over a wide range of doses and therapy must be individualized. Initial doses may be gradually increased to control symptoms and then tapered to lowest effective maintenance dose. Therapeutic response may require weeks to months to fully develop. Debilitated, geriatric or adolescent patients may require lower doses; patients in an acute psychotic episode may require rapid increases in dose. Plasma levels are useful mainly for assessing patient compliance. No true withdrawal occurs, but abrupt cessation of therapy may precipitate mild withdrawal-like symptoms (nausea and vomiting). Acute overdosage toxicity is very low in adults. **SIDE EFFECTS**:

Nervous System Side Effects:

Antipsychotics, (also tricyclic antidepressants, antinauseants, antihypertensives, and antihistamines) induce an unpleasant sedation (unlike barbiturates and benzodiazepines). It is characterized by feelings of indifference or apathy, lassitude, tiredness and depression. Drowsiness is common (tolerance gradually develops). Decreased deep and increased REM sleep can induce nightmares. Occasional paradoxical excitement occurs with insomnia, agitation, euphoria, and exacerbation of psychotic symptoms. Cerebral edema, protein abnormalities in cerebral spinal fluid, hypothermia, respiratory distress occur rarely. Antipsychotics may lower the seizure threshold and precipitate seizures in patients with convulsive disorders.

Extrapyramidal Side Effects:

(1) Parkinson syndrome: Akinesia (slowing of voluntary movement), fine resting tremors, and muscular rigidity. Benztropine (Cogentin) may decrease rigidity but will also decrease chlorpromazine absorption/blood levels.

(2) Dystonias and dyskinesias: Most common in patients < 25 y.o. Jaw, neck, shoulder girdle usually involved in grimacing or torticollis; also athetoid and/or oculogyrate movements may occur. Diphenhydramine (Benadryl) is useful.

(3) Akathisia: Feeling of restlessness and/or need for constant movement of a leg or other part of the body, often very unpleasant.

Note: (1), (2), & (3) above are reversible when agents are discontinued or dosage is reduced.

Tardive dyskinesia: Face, jaws, lips and tongue are usually involved in stereotypical involuntary movements. Usually occurs late in therapy, is only slowly reversible (if at all) and is often intensified by phenothiazine withdrawal. At risk are patients > 40 y.o., women, and patients receiving large doses for 6 months to ≥ 2 years. Occurrence and severity of most extrapyramidal reactions are proportional to dose and drug class. Piperazinylpropyl agents (Compazine, Stelazine, Trilafon, Prolixin, etc.) cause the least sedation and most extrapyramidal symptoms.

Anticholinergic Effects (common with large doses): Dry mouth, dry skin, failure of visual accommodation, constipation (rarely, paralytic ileus) and urine retention.

Cardiovascular Effects: Vasodilation and orthostatic hypotension with dizziness & possible fainting (esp. with parenteral administration and early in treatment). Quinidine-like effects on heart: flattened T waves, prolonged P-R and QRS intervals (slowed conduction). May produce PVC's, ventricular fibrillation and sudden death (especially with high doses or pre-existing cardiac problems).

Endocrine Disorders: Amenorrhea, weight gain, decreased libido. Increased prolactin release (galactorrhea, gynecomastia). **Dermatologic Effects**: Photosensitivity and dermatoses (esp. early in treatment). Exposed skin can present mauve pigmentation (with long-term therapy). Ocular pigmentation/deposits (anterior lens capsule, posterior cornea; rarely, retina); can cause blurred vision (may reverse with cessation of therapy). **Other Side Effects**: Hematologic disorders (leukopenia or agranulocytosis) rare. Rarely, malignant neuroleptic syndrome (hyperthermia, muscular rigidity, sweating, salivation, dyspnea, tachycardia, leukocytosis) can develop over 1-3 d and persist 5-10 d after cessation of therapy. Oral syndrome with red oral mucosa, loosened dentition, vesicles, denture stomatitis, chelosis, black or beefy red tongue with thin, oral pseudomembrane. **CAUTIONS**: Antipsychotics decrease ability to do tasks needing mental alertness. Caution recommended in: severe cardiovascular disorders, seizure disorders (esp. if concurrent anticoagulant drugs), debilitated or geriatric patients, hepatic or renal disease, glaucoma, prostatic hypertrophy, chronic pulmonary disorders, and patients with

Continued, next page

ANTIPSYCHOTIC TRANQUILIZERS *Continued*

breast cancer. Use with caution in children when dehydrated, or if acutely ill. Neonates born of women on phenothiazines may have hyperreflexia, extrapyramidal signs, or jaundice. **RECOMMENDATIONS**: Reduce dose if other CNS depressants given concurrently. Perform periodic ophthalmologic examinations. To minimize orthostatic hypotension: decrease dose, switch to a different drug, or use several smaller doses throughout day. May have additive effects if administered with cardiac medications (e.g., quinidine); check EKG and serum drug levels. AVOID oral or parenteral solutions if discolored or precipitate is present. With parenteral use, patients should be supine for 30-60 min. AVOID concurrent epinephrine (hypotension). AVOID exposure to sun if photosensitivity develops. Periodically evaluate patient and attempt to lower dosage or discontinue drug. **CONTRAINDICATIONS**: Previous hypersensitivity reaction to an antipsychotic congener, comatose state, severe CNS depression, bone marrow depression, severe brain damage, and the first trimester of pregnancy.

AGENTS CAUSING PROMINENT EXTRAPYRAMIDAL SIDE EFFECTS

These agents are characterized by **weak-moderate anticholinergic** and **weak-moderate sedative** properties, **strong extrapyramidal** effects and **strong antiemetic** action. All may be used to treat intractable hiccups.

DRUG	INDICATIONS & DOSAGE	DOSE FORMS	REMARKS
PHENOTHIAZINES			
TRIFLUOPERAZINE (Stelazine)	<u>**Psychotic Disorders**</u>: **PO**: 2-5 mg bid; 2-40 mg/d maintenance in 2 doses. **IM**: 1-2 mg q4-6h (maximum 6-10 mg/d).	PO (Cap's): 1, 2, 5, 10 mg PO (Liquid): 10 mg/ml Injection: 2 mg/ml	**RECOMMEND**: Dilute oral concentrate (to 60 ml) prior to administration. Protect dosing preparations from light and heat.
PERPHENAZINE (Trilafon)	<u>**Psychotic Disorders**</u>: **PO**: 4-8 mg tid intially; 12-64 mg/d maintenance as 2-3 doses. **PO (Extended release)**: 8-32 mg bid. **IM**: 5 mg q6h (maximum 30 mg/d); then PO maintenance. <u>**Nausea & Vomiting**</u>: **PO**: 8-16 mg/d in 2-3 doses (maximum 24 mg/d). **IM**: 5 mg (maximum 10 mg). **IV**: 1 mg q1-2min until 5 mg total.	PO (Tab's): 2, 4, 8, 16 mg PO (Extended release): 8 mg PO (Liquid): 16 mg/ml Injection: 5 mg/ml	**RECOMMEND**: Dilute oral concentrate (to 60 ml) prior to administration.
FLUPHENAZINE (Prolixin) (Permitil)	<u>**Psychotic Disorders**</u>: **PO**: 0.5-10 mg/d in 3-4 doses (maximum 20 mg/d); usual maintenance = 1-5 mg/d. **Geriatric PO**: 1-2.5 mg/d initial dose. **IM**: 1.25 mg initially; 2.5-10 mg/d maintenance in 3-4 doses).	PO (Tab's): 0.25, 1, 2.5, 5, 10 mg PO (Liquid): 0.5, 5 mg/ml Injection: 2.5 mg/ml Injection (Extended release): 25 mg/ml	Enanthate or decanoate injection (ext'd release prep's): 12.5 mg initially, then 25-100 mg q2-6wks. Dose and interval must be individualized for each patient. Extrapyramidal effects occur 2-3 d after administration of ext'd release forms; persist for 5 d. Depression common with ext'd release prep's. **CAUTIONS**: Prolixin 2.5, 5, & 10 mg and Permitil 0.25 mg tablets contain tartrazine (possible allergic reaction, esp. if patient allergic to aspirin).

ANTIPSYCHOTIC TRANQUILIZERS: PHENOTHIAZINES WITH PROMINENT EXTRAPYRAMIDAL SIDE EFFECTS *Continued*

DRUG	INDICATIONS & DOSAGE	DOSE FORMS	REMARKS
PROCHLORPERAZINE (Compazine)	<u>**Psychotic Disorders**</u>: **PO**: 5-10 mg tid-qid initially; maintenance 50-150 mg/d. **Pediatric PO**: 2.5 mg bid-tid initially; maintenance 20-25 mg/d. **IM**: 10-20 mg q1-6h PRN; then PO maintenance. **Pediatric IM**: 0.13 mg/kg. <u>**Anxiety**</u>: **PO**: 5-10 mg tid-qid. **PO (extended release)**: 10 mg q12-24h (maximum 15 mg). **IM**: 5-10 mg q3-4h (maximum 40 mg/d).	PO (Tab's): 5, 10, 25 mg PO (Liquid): 1 mg/ml PO (extended release): 10, 15, 30, 75 mg Injection: 5 mg/ml	Typical antipsychotic side and adverse effects. High frequency of extrapyramidal reactions, especially in children. **CAUTIONS**: Extended release capsules contain tartrazine dye (potential for allergic reactions, especially in patients hypersensitive to aspirin). **CONTRAINDICATIONS**: Reye's syndrome, confirmed or suspected.
ACETOPHENAZINE (Tindal)	<u>**Psychotic Disorders**</u>: **PO**: 20 mg tid initially; maintenance 40-80 mg/d (maximum 400-600 mg/d, in hospitalized patients)	PO (Tab's): 20 mg	
MISCELLANEOUS			
HALOPERIDOL (Haldol)	<u>**Psychotic Disorders**</u>: **PO**: 0.5-2 mg bid-tid initially (3-5 mg if s/sx severe); maximum 100 mg/d. **Pediatric PO**: 0.5 mg/d initially, increase by 0.5 mg/d q1wk; maintenance 0.05-0.15 mg/kg/d in 2-3 doses(maximum 6 mg/d). **IM**: 2-5 mg q30min-8h, then PO maintenance dosing (maximum 10-30 mg/dose). <u>**Tourette's Syndrome/Non-Psychotic Disorders**</u>: **PO**: 0.5-2 mg bid-tid initially (3-5 mg if s/sx severe); maximum 100 mg/d. **Pediatric PO**: 0.05-0.075 mg/kg/d in 2-3 doses (maximum 6 mg/d).	PO (Tab's): 0.5, 1, 2, 5, 10, 20 mg PO (Liquid): 2 mg/ml Injection: 5 mg/ml	Haloperidol is a **Butyrophenone** antipsychotic. Typical antipsychotic side and adverse effects. Extrapyramidal effects and drowsiness common early in therapy. Autonomic effects are milder. Electrocardiographic changes, hepatic and hematologic effects are also uncommon. **CAUTIONS**: Haldol tab's 1, 5, 10 mg contain tartrazine dye (may precipitate allergic reactions). Avoid dermal contact with oral or injection solutions; contact dermatitis occurs rarely.
THIOTHIXENE (Navane)	<u>**Psychotic Disorders**</u>: **PO**: 2 mg bid-tid initially; maintenance 15-30 mg/d (maximum 60 mg/d). **IM**: 4 mg bid-qid initially; maintenance 15-30 mg/d.	PO (Cap's): 1, 2, 5, 10, 20 mg PO (Liquid): 5 mg/ml Injection: 2 mg/ml	Thiothixene is a **Thioxanthine** antipsychotic. Typical antipsychotic side and adverse effects. Drowsiness is most common but tolerance develops.

ANTIPSYCHOTIC TRANQUILIZERS: MISCELLANEOUS AGENTS WITH PROMINENT EXTRAPYRAMIDAL EFFECTS *Continued*

DRUG	INDICATIONS & DOSAGE	DOSE FORMS	REMARKS
LOXAPINE (Loxitane)	<u>**Psychotic Disorders**</u>: **PO**: 10 mg bid initially, increase rapidly; maintenance 20-100 mg/d in 2-4 doses (maximum 250 mg/d). **IM**: 12.5-50 mg q4-6h; then PO maintenance.	PO (Cap's): 5, 10, 25, 50 mg PO (Liquid): 25 mg/ml Injection: 50 mg/ml	Loxapine is a **Dibenzoxazepine** antipsychotic. Typical antipsychotic side and adverse effects.
MOLINDONE (Moban)	<u>**Psychotic Disorders**</u>: **PO**: 50-75 mg/d initially; maintenance 5-25 mg tid-qid (maximum 225 mg/d).	PO (Tab's): 5, 10, 25, 50, 100 mg PO (Liquid): 20 mg/ml	Molindone is an **Indole** antipsychotic. Occasional temporary changes in WBC counts and LFTs.

AGENTS CAUSING MODERATE EXTRAPYRAMIDAL SIDE EFFECTS

These agents have **strong anticholinergic** properties; **moderate to strong sedative** and **moderate to strong extrapyramidal** effects; **strong antiemetic** action.

PHENOTHIAZINES

DRUG	INDICATIONS & DOSAGE	DOSE FORMS	REMARKS
CHLORPROMAZINE (Thorazine) (CPZ)	<u>**Psychotic Disorders (Adults)**</u>: **PO**: 25 mg tid initially; 25-100 mg tid maintenance (maximum 400-500 mg/d). **IM**: 25 mg, can repeat in 1h; max. 400 mg q4-6h, then PO maintenance. <u>**Nausea & Vomiting**</u>: **PO**: 10-25 mg q4-6h PRN. **IM**: 25 mg initially; 25-50 mg q3-4h if no hypotension. <u>**Behavioral Disorders (Children)**</u>: **PO**: 0.5 mg/kg q4-6h. **IM**: 0.5 mg/kg q6-8h (maximum 40 mg/d if < 5 y.o.; 75 mg/d if 5-12 y.o.). **Rectal**: 1.1 mg/kg q6-8h. <u>**Intractable Hiccups**</u>: **PO**: 25-50 mg q6-8h.	PO (Tab's/Cap's): 10, 25, 30, 50, 75, 100, 150, 200 & 300 mg PO (liquid): 10 mg/5 ml, 30, 100 mg/ml Injection: 25 mg/m Suppositories: 25, 100 mg	Behavioral disorders treated = combativeness, hyperexcitability. Protect dosing preparations from light and heat. Sedation is prominent; extrapyramidal effects are moderate. **SIDE EFFECTS**: Gastrointestinal upset. Hyperthermic reactions, Candida infections, lowered seizure threshold. **NOTES**: Administer initial test dose of 25 mg tid, increase by 20-50 mg semi-weekly until acute psychotic state is controlled or 25-50 mg q3-4h as needed for sedation or nausea control, then decrease if possible. **RECOMMEND**: Discontinue therapy if WBC < 3500. **CONTRAINDICATIONS**: CNS depression, intoxication with alcohol or other sedative agents.

ANTIPSYCHOTIC TRANQUILIZERS: PHENOTHIAZINES WITH MODERATE EXTRAPYRAMIDAL EFFECTS *Continued*

DRUG	INDICATIONS & DOSAGE	DOSE FORMS	REMARKS
PROMAZINE (Sparine)	**Psychotic Disorders (Adults)**: **PO, IM**: 10-200 mg (usual 50-150 mg) q4-6h (maximum 1000 mg/d).	PO (Tab's): 10, 25, 50, 100 mg PO (Liquid): 10, 30 mg/ml Injection: 15, 50 mg	Sedation is prominent; extrapyramidal effects are moderate. Frequent drowsiness. Orthostatic hypotension marked. **CAUTIONS**: Tartrazine dye in preparations may cause allergic reactions. Contact dermatitis possible.
PIPERIDINES			
THIORIDAZINE (Mellaril)	**Psychotic Disorders**: **PO, IM**: 150-300 mg/d initially in 2-4 doses (maximum 800 mg/d). **Pediatric PO (2-12 y.o.)**: 0.5-3 mg/kg/d. **Behavioral Disorders (Children)**: **PO**: 10 mg q6-8h initially (maximum 3 mg/kg/d).	PO (Tab's): 10, 20, 15, 25, 50, 100, 150 & 200 mg. PO (Liquid): 30, 100 mg/ml; (Suspension): 5 & 20 mg/ml	Similar to Chlorpromazine. Sedation is prominent; extrapyramidal effects are weak-moderate; little antiemetic action. EKG changes, arrhythmias, and pigmentary retinopathy are more common with this agent.
MESORIDAZINE (Serentil)	**Psychotic Disorders**: **PO**: 50 mg tid initially; 100-400 mg/d maintenance in 3 doses. **IM**: 25 mg; can repeat at 0.5-1 h (maximum 200 mg/d). **Psychoneurotic Effects**: **PO**: 10 mg tid initially; 30-150 mg/d maintenance in 3 doses. **IM**: 25 mg; can repeat at 0.5-1 h (maximum 200 mg/d). **Alcohol Dependence**: **PO**: 25 mg bid initially (maximum 50-200 mg/d).	PO (Tab's): 10, 25, 50, 100 mg PO (Liquid): 25	Sedation is prominent; extrapyramidal properties are weak-moderate. Weak antiemetic action. **CAUTIONS**: Tablets contain tartrazine (possible allergic reaction, especially if patient is allergic to aspirin). Protect dosing preparations from light and heat.
MISCELLANEOUS			
TRIFLUPROMAZINE (Vesprin)	**Psychotic Disorders**: **IM**: 60 mg/d in 2-3 doses (maximum 150 mg/d). **Pediatric IM**: 0.2-0.25 mg/kg/d (maximum 10 mg/d). **Nausea & Vomiting**: **IM**: 5-15 mg q4h. **Pediatric IM**: 0.2-0.25 mg/kg q12-24h (maximum 10 mg/d). **Geriatric IM**: 2.5 mg q4h (maximum 15 mg/d). **IV**: 1 mg (max. 3 mg/d).	Injection: 10, 20 mg/ml	Triflupromazine is a **Piperizine** antipsychotic. Strong antiemetic action is present. **CAUTIONS**: Vesprin 25 and 50 mg tablets contain tartrazine dye (possibility of allergic reactions, esp. if patient allergic to aspirin). AVOID use in Reye's syndrome (may obscure symptoms). Protect dosing preparations from light and heat.

ANTIPSYCHOTIC TRANQUILIZERS: MISCELLANEOUS AGENTS WITH MODERATE EXTRAPYRAMIDAL EFFECTS *Continued*

DRUG	INDICATIONS & DOSAGE	DOSE FORMS	REMARKS
CHLORPROTHIXENE (Taractan)	<u>**Psychotic Disorders**</u>: **PO**: 25-50 mg tid-qid (maximum 600 mg/d). **Pediatric PO (> 6 y.o.)**: 10-25 mg tid-qid. **IM**: 25-50 mg tid-qid; PO maintenance.	PO (Tab's): 10, 25, 50, 100 mg PO (Liquid): 100 mg/5 ml Injection: 12.5 mg/ml	Chlorprothixene is a **Thioxanthene** antipsychotic. Sedation is prominent; extrapyramidal effects are moderate. Weak antiemetic action. Orthostatic hypotension more pronounced than with chlorpromazine. **RECOMMEND**: Increase dose cautiously in older/debilitated patients. **CAUTIONS**: Tablets contain tartrazine dye (possible allergic reaction; esp. if patient allergic to aspirin). Protect dosing preparations from light/heat. Contact dermatitis may occur.
PIMOZIDE (Orap)	<u>**Tourette's Syndrome**</u>: **PO**: 1-2 mg/d in 1-3 doses initially; increase dose q2d up to 2-20 mg/d maintenance.	PO (Tab's): 2 mg	Pimozide is a **Diphenylbutylpiperidine** agent. Major use = treatment of tics in Tourette's Syndrome. Shares most of the side effects of the antipsychotics; sedative and extrapyramidal effects less pronounced than with chlorpromazine. Rebound increased tic frequency occurs with decrease dosage or discontinuence of therapy (gradual dosage adjustment or withdrawal).

ANTI-MANIC AGENT

DRUG	INDICATIONS & DOSAGE	DOSE FORMS	REMARKS
LITHIUM (Lithium carbonate) (Lithium citrate)	<u>**Mania, Bipolar Disorders**</u>: **PO**: 1800 mg/d in 2-3 doses initially; maintenance 300 mg tid-qid. **PO (Ext'd release)**: same dose, bid-tid dosing. ***Note***: It is essential to monitor serum levels and adjust doses correspondingly.	PO (Tab's): 300 mg (8 mEq); carbonate PO (Cap's): 300 mg (8 mEq); carbonate PO (extended release): 300 (8 mEq), 450 (12 mEq) mg; carbonate PO (Liquid): 8 mEq/5ml; citrate	**NOTES**: **Very low therapeutic index.** 5 ml of citrate solution = 300 mg carbonate. **SIDE EFFECTS**: CNS and/or neuromuscular effects occur in 40-50% patients: headache, lethargy, confusion, mental dulling, weakness and tremor; GI effects also common (10-30% patients): nausea, vomiting, diarrhea, abdominal discomfort and anorexia; tolerance often develops. Polyuria, nephrogenic diabetes insipidus occur in 25-50% patients, due to decreased renal concentrating ability, and may persist; urinary tubular atrophy also occurs. Hypothyroidism and/or goiter develop in approximately 5% patients. T-wave depression on EKG occurs in 20-30% patients; EKG changes are asymptomatic and reversible. Reversible increased neutrophil, RBC and platelet counts may develop. **LEVELS**: Dosage must be controlled by reference to serum levels. **Therapeutic**: 0.6-1.2 mEq/l. **Mild intoxication**: 1.5-2.0 mEq/l; **significant intoxication**: 2-2.5 mEq/l; **potentially lethal intoxication**: > 2.5 mEq/l. If > 2 mEq/l, discontinue therapy for 24 h. **CAUTIONS**: Pregnancy should be avoided; major congenital defects occur in approximately 11% of first trimester exposures. Geriatric patients more susceptible to adverse (esp. CNS) effects. Acute encephalopathic syndromes have developed in some patients on concurrent antipsychotic medication. **RECOMMEND**: Monitor levels q3-4d until clinical status and serum Lithium levels are both stable; monitor levels q1-2months during maintenance. Draw blood for serum levels approximately 12 h after the last dose. Institute procedures to maintain normal fluid and sodium levels, avoid dehydration (especially if vomiting or diarrhea is present). Discontinue medication at first sign of intoxication. **CONTRAINDICATIONS**: Cardiovascular or renal disease; concurrent diuretic therapy.

TRICYCLIC ANTIDEPRESSANTS

GROUP REMARKS: Pharmacologic properties of the tricyclic antidepressants (TCAs) are the same as those of the phenothiazines and related antipsychotics. Primary actions, side effects and other properties are common to both classes. The major differences between the two "classes" are in the recommended dosages for their respective indications; antidepressant activity is achieved at lower relative doses than is antipsychotic activity. TCAs, when administered at their recommended doses, are effective in the treatment of endogenous depression, as distinct from the depression or fatigue of situational anxiety. In addition, imipramine and amitryptyline have demonstrated effectiveness for enuresis. **NOTES**: Therapeutic effect is delayed; following onset of therapy, a latent period of 2-3 weeks may occur prior to beneficial effect on depression. There is an increased risk of suicide during this period. Because of their long half-lives, most TCAs may be administered only once a day, usually at bedtime to minimize sedation. Plasma drug levels are useful only to monitor patient compliance. No one TCA is superior to the others; patient response is variable. **SIDE EFFECTS**: Postural hypotension occurs frequently and is the most common side effect limiting the use of the TCAs (tolerance may develop); weight gain is also common. **Anticholinergic Effects**: Dry mouth, dry skin, blurred vision (failure of accommodation), constipation (rarely, paralytic ileus) and urinary retention. Reduced tone of the esophageogastric sphincter may predispose to esophageal reflux. Some tolerance may develop to anticholinergic effects. **Nervous System Effects**: TCAs, like the antipsychotics, induce an unpleasant sedation characterized by feelings of indifference or apathy, lassitude, tiredness and depression. Drowsiness is common (tolerance gradually develops). Confusion, disorientation delusions, and hallucinations may occur, especially in geriatric patients. TCAs lower the seizure threshold; convulsions have been reported. Nightmares can result from a decreased depth of sleep and an increase in REM sleep. Occasional paradoxical excitement or worsening of psychosis or depression. Because of the relatively low doses employed, extrapyramidal effects are rare; tremor is the usual initial sign. Cerebral edema, protein abnormalities in cerebral spinal fluid and, hypothermia occur rarely. EEG alteration (occasionally seizures) reported. **Cardiovascular Effects**: Vasodilation (tolerance usually develops) and tachycardia occur (esp. with parenteral administration and early in treatment). Quinidine-like cardiotoxicity: flattened T waves; prolonged P-R and QRS intervals (slowed conduction); may produce PVC's, ventricular fibrillation (esp. with high doses or preexisting cardiac problems); sudden death may occur with therapeutic doses or as late effect of suicide attempts. Serious, rare side effects include: blood dyscrasias (agranulocytosis, thrombocytopenia, eosinophilia, leukopenia) and purpura; discontinue therapy at first sign. GI effects include elevated LFTs (asymptomatic), altered alkaline phosphatase levels, obstructive-type jaundice (reversible after cessation of therapy). Anorexia, nausea, vomiting, diarrhea, abdominal cramps may occur. Sudden discontinuance can precipitate: akathisia, anxiety, chills, muscle aches, headache, dizziness, nausea, vomiting. **CAUTIONS**: Toxicity of the TCAs is much greater in children than adults. Use cautiously in individuals with respiratory difficulties, pre-existing cardiovascular disease, predisposed to seizures or in whom excess anticholinergic activity would be potentially harmful (may precipitate acute angle-closure glaucoma or urinary retention in older males). Concurrent MAO inhibitor use has produced hyperpyrexia, hypertension and seizures. **RECOMMENDATIONS**: Minimize side effects by initiating therapy with low doses; increase gradually. Do NOT prescribe single large quantities to acutely depressed patients. Perform periodic EKG on ALL patients receiving higher than usual dosage, regardless of cardiac status. Discontinue medication upon first symptom of esophageal reflux; cautiously administer a concurrent cholinergic agent, such as bethanechol, if antidepressant therapy is essential. Discontinue medication several days prior to surgery (danger of hypertensive episodes). In suspected overdoses, monitor patient for ventricular arrhythmias (esp. during initial 24 h). **CONTRAINDICATIONS**: Contraindicated in the acute recovery phase after myocardial infarction.

TRICYCLIC ANTIDEPRESSANT DRUG INTERACTIONS:

Tricyclic Antidepressants: may inhibit action of ***Guanethidine*** and precipitate hypertensive crises; are additive with other ***CNS depressants***; may enhance cardiac stimulant and pressor activity of ***sympathomimetics*** to precipitate hypertensive crisis.

ANTIDEPRESSANTS: TRICYCLIC ANTIDEPRESSANTS *Continued*

DRUG	INDICATIONS & DOSAGE	DOSE FORMS	REMARKS
AMITRIPTYLINE (Elavil) (Amitril) (Emitrip) (Endep)	Endogenous Depression: **PO**: 75-100 mg/d initially in 3-4 doses; maintenance 25-150 mg/d. **Geriatric/adolescent PO**: 10 mg tid plus 20 mg at bedtime. **IM**: 20-30 mg qid.	PO (Tab's): 10, 25, 50, 75, 100, 150 mg Injection: 10 mg/ml	Start therapy with 50-100 mg at bedtime (maximum 150 mg). Higher doses possible in hospitalized patients (≤ 300 mg/d). **SIDE EFFECTS**: Typical TCA side and adverse effects, as in Group Remarks.
IMIPRAMINE (Tofranil) (Presamine) (Pramine) (Janimine)	Endogenous Depression: **PO**: 75 mg/d initially (single dose); maintenance 50-150 mg/d. **Geriatric/adolescent PO**: 30-40 mg/d initially; maintenance 30-100 mg/d. **IM**: 100 mg/d maximum. Enuresis: **PO**: 25 mg initially 1 h before bedtime; increase 10-25 mg q1-2wk PRN (maximum varies with age [see chart] but should NOT exceed 2.5 mg/kg/d).	PO (Tab's): 10, 25, 50 mg PO (Cap's): 75, 100, 125, 150 mg Injection: 12.5 mg/ml **Enuresis Maximum**: 5-6 y.o. 40 mg/d 6-8 y.o. 50 mg/d 8-10 y.o. 60 mg/d 10-12 y.o. 70 mg/d 12-14 y.o. 75 mg/d	Tofranil and janimine contain tartrazine dye (potential for respiratory symptoms, esp. in patients sensitive to aspirin). Higher doses possible in hospitalized patients (≤ 300 mg/d, divided). For enuresis: treat for 2-3 months, then slowly discontinue (taper). **SIDE EFFECTS**: Typical TCA side and adverse effects, as in Group Remarks.
AMOXAPINE (Asendin)	Endogenous Depression: **PO**: 150 mg/d initially in 2-3 doses; maintenance 200-400 mg/d. **Geriatric PO**: 25 mg bid-tid initially; maintenance100-300 mg/d.	PO (Tab's): 25, 50, 100, 150 mg	May have more rapid onset than amitriptyline or imipramine. Higher doses possible in hospitalized patients (≤ 600 mg/d). **SIDE EFFECTS**: Typical TCA side and adverse effects, as in Group Remarks.
DESIMIPRAMINE (Norpramin) (Pertofrane)	Endogenous Depression: **PO**: 75-200 mg/d initially in 1-3 doses; maintenance ≤ 300 mg/d. **Geriatric/adolescent PO**: 25-100 mg/d (maximum 150 mg/d).	PO (Tab's): 10, 25, 50, 75, 100, 150 mg PO (Cap's): 25, 50 mg	Norpramine tab's contain tartrazine dye (potential for respiratory symptoms, especially in patients sensitive to aspirin). **SIDE EFFECTS**: Typical TCA side and adverse effects, as in Group Remarks.
DOXEPIN (Adapin) (Sinequan)	Endogenous Depression: **PO**: 25-150 mg/d initially in 1-3 doses; maintenance 75-300 mg/d.	PO (Cap's): 10, 25, 50, 75, 100, 150 mg PO (Liquid): 10 mg/ml	Dilute oral solution with 120 ml of water, milk or juice. **SIDE EFFECTS**: Typical TCA side and adverse effects, as in Group Remarks.

ANTIDEPRESSANTS: TRICYCLIC ANTIDEPRESSANTS *Continued*

DRUG	INDICATIONS & DOSAGE	DOSE FORMS	REMARKS
NORTRIPTYLINE (Aventyl) (Pamelor)	<u>**Endogenous Depression**</u>: **PO**: 75-100 mg/d initially in 3-4 doses; maintenance 75-150 mg/d. **Geriatric PO**: 30-50 mg/d in 3-4 doses.	PO (Cap's): 10, 25, 75 mg PO (Liquid): 2mg/ml	Typical TCA side and adverse effects, as in Group Remarks.
PROTRIPTYLINE (Vivactil)	<u>**Endogenous Depression**</u>: **PO**: 15-40 mg/d initially in 3-4 doses; maintenance 15-60 mg/d. **Geriatric/adolescent PO**: 5 mg tid initially; maintenance 20 mg/d.	PO (Tab's): 5, 10 mg	Typical TCA side and adverse effects, as in Group Remarks.
TRIMIPRAMINE (Surmontil)	<u>**Endogenous Depression**</u>: **PO**: 75 mg/d initially in 2-4 doses; maintenance 50-200 mg/d. **Geriatric/adolescent PO**: 50 mg/d initially in 2-4 doses; maintenance 100 mg/d (may be single dose hs).	PO (Cap's): 25, 50, and 100 mg	Higher doses may be used in hospitalized patients (200-300 mg/d). **SIDE EFFECTS**: Typical TCA side and adverse effects, as in Group Remarks.
MAPROTILINE (Ludiomil)	<u>**Endogenous Depression**</u>: **PO**: 75-150 mg/d initially in 1-3 doses; maintenance 75-300 mg/d. **Geriatric PO**: 25 mg/d initially; maintenance 50-75 mg/d.	PO (Tab's): 25, 50, 75 mg	Typical TCA side and adverse effects, as in Group Remarks.
TRAZODONE (Desyrel)	<u>**Endogenous Depression**</u>: **PO**: 150 mg/d initially in 2-4 doses; maintenance 150-400 mg/d.	PO (Tab's): 50, 100 mg	Trazodone is slightly different chemically from the TCAs and antipsychotics, but shares many of the same pharmacological properties; it exhibits less anticholinergic activity and quinidine-like cardiotoxicity. Trazodone should be administered with food. Higher doses possible in hospitalized patients (≤ 600 mg/d). Follow all cautions and recommendations presented for the TCAs. **SIDE EFFECTS**: Sedation is prominent (20-50% patients); other CNS effect include dizziness, headache and insomnia. Dry mouth occurs in 15-30% patients; other "anticholinergic" effects are rare. Others include: orthostatic hypotension (5% patients), nausea, vomiting, priapism and muscle aches/pains. **CAUTIONS**: May be arrhythmogenic in patients with pre-existing cardiac disease. **CONTRAINDICATIONS**: Recovery phase of myocardial infarction.

MONOAMINE OXIDASE INHIBITORS

GROUP REMARKS: Monoamine oxidase inhibitors (MAO Inhibitors) are CNS stimulants generally similar to the sympathomimetics, such as amphetamine. They are NOT drugs of first choice and should be reserved for patients unresponsive or intolerant to other antidepressant medications. Patient response is quite variable. **NOTES**: MAO Inhibitor dosage should be adjusted for each patient to the lowest effective dose. Pharmacologic effects are rapidly apparent, but therapeutic action may be delayed. **SIDE EFFECTS**: Orthostatic hypotension is common and is dose related. CNS effects include: dizziness, headache, hallucinations, tremors or twitching, hyperreflexia, anxiety and hyperactivity. GI effects: constipation, nausea, diarrhea and abdominal pain. Other common effects include: edema, dry mouth, blurred vision and skin rashes. MAO Inhibitors may precipitate mania or hypomania. Hepatocellular jaundice occurs rarely. **Hypertensive crisis** is the most serious adverse reaction; it is characterized by occipital headaches, pupillary dilation with photophobia, palpitations, neck stiffness, sweating, nausea, vomiting, tachycardia/bradycardia and chest pain. A hypertensive crisis is usually due to ingestion of food containing tyramine or use of an OTC cold formulation containing a sympathomimetic amine and may occur up to 2 wks after last dose of MAO Inhibitor. Monitor blood pressure closely; discontinue medication upon palpitations or frequent, severe headaches. **RECOMMENDATIONS**: AVOID some foods with aged protein: aged cheeses (Camembert, cheddar, Stilton), sour cream, beer, red wines (esp. chianti), liver, pickled herring, raisins, chocolate, yeast extracts, fermented sausages (pepperoni, salami, summer sausage) and some meat tenderizers; all may have high tyramine content and can precipitate a hypertensive crisis. AVOID excessive caffeine intake. Perform periodic LFTs (discontinue at first sign of jaundice or hepatic dysfunction; NOT dose-related) and ophthalmalogic examinations (possible glaucoma). Discontinue 7-14d before elective surgery. Institute a 1-2wk drug-free interval when changing from another antidepressant to a MAO Inhibitor or from one MAO Inhibitor to another; initiate treatment at one-half the usual dosage. Institute a 4wk drug-free interval prior to starting levodopa therapy. **CAUTIONS**: MAO Inhibitors have variable effects on the seizure threshold; use cautiously in epileptics. Use cautiously/avoid in hyperexcitable patients. **CONTRAINDICATIONS**: MAO Inhibitors are contraindicated in pheochromocytoma, cerebrovascular disease, congestive heart failure or other states with altered cardiovascular responsiveness. Also contraindicated in elderly patients or those with serious hepatic or renal dysfunction.

MAO INHIBITOR DRUG INTERACTIONS:

MAO Inhibitors have numerous clinical actions and a high potential for serious interactions. **MAO Inhibitors** may potentiate the action of ***CNS depressants***. Concurrent ***methyldopa***, ***levodopa***, ***dopamine***, ***tryptophan***, or ***sympathomimetic agents*** (***phenylpropanolamine***, ***ephedrine***) present in cold, hay fever, or weight-reducing preparations have been associated with hypertension, headache and/or hyperexcitability. Interaction with ***meperidine*** can be severe or life threatening. Hypoglycemic episodes have occurred in patients on ***insulin*** or ***oral antidiabetic agents***. Possible precipitation of seizures with concurrent ***metrizamide***. Marked hypotension may occur with concurrent ***diuretics*** or ***antihypertensive agents***. Use of **MAO Inhibitors** and ***tricyclic antidepressants*** may produce hyperpyrexia, hypertension, tachycardia, confusion, and seizures (FATALITIES have occurred).

ANTIDEPRESSANTS: MONOAMINE OXIDASE INHIBITORS *Continued*

DRUG	INDICATIONS & DOSAGE	DOSE FORMS	REMARKS
ISOCARBOXAZID (Marplan)	<u>Endogenous Depression</u>: **PO**: 30 mg/d in 1-3 doses initially; maintenance 10-30 mg/d.	PO (Tab's): 10 mg	Typical MAO Inhibitor side and adverse effects.
PHENELZINE (Nardil)	<u>Endogenous Depression</u>: **PO**: 15 mg tid initially; increase rapidly to 60-90 mg/d; taper to 7.5-60 mg/d maintenance dose.	PO (Tab's):15 mg	Typical MAO Inhibitor side and adverse effects.
TRANYLCYPROMINE (Parnate)	<u>Endogenous Depression</u>: **PO**: 10 mg bid initially; maintenance 10-30 mg/d. <u>Adjunct to Electroconvulsive Therapy</u>: **PO**: 10 mg bid during ECT; maintenance 10 mg/d.	PO (Tab's): 10 mg	Typical MAO Inhibitor side and adverse effects. More hypertension and CNS stimulation than with other MAO Inhibitors. **RECOMMEND**: Use only in hospitalized or closely supervised patients and only if unresponsive to all other antidepressant therapy. Taper withdrawal. **CONTRAINDICATIONS**: AVOID in patients > 60 y.o. or those with history of hypertension, cerebrovascular disorders or headaches.
PARGYLINE (Eutonyl)		PO (Tab's): 10, 25 mg	Rarely used for antidepressant effect; some use as an antihypertensive. See Antihypertensive Adrenergic Inhibitors for more information. **SIDE EFFECTS**: GI disturbances, insomnia, urinary frequency, dry mouth, nightmares, impotence, edema. Congestive failure may occur in patients with reduced cardiac reserve. **CAUTIONS**: Eutonyl 25 mg contains tartrazine dye (potential for allergic reactions, especially in patients hypersensitive to aspirin).

SYMPATHOMIMETIC STIMULANTS

GROUP REMARKS: These CNS stimulants are ephredrine-type sympathomimetics exhibiting relatively greater CNS stimulation and relatively less cardiovascular effects. They are used to maintain wakefulness and suppress appetite (they have also been used to improve atheletic performance). Less potent members of this class (e.g. phenylisopropanolamine) are used in OTC "weight loss" preparations. The CNS stimulants are also used in treating attention deficit in "hyperkinetic" children; truly hyperkinetic or minimally brain damaged children respond with euphoria and improved psychomotor performance. Use in "hyperkinetic" children is NOT associated with long-term benefit and may interfere with normal growth. Amphetamine is also used treating narcolepsy. CNS effects include: increased mental alertness, diminished sense of fatigue, increased motor activity and mild euphoria. **NOTES**: Anxiety induced by these agents can interfere with performance. Euphoria induced by CNS stimulants is usually followed by mild depression and fatigue. Except with toxic doses, tolerance develops to the stimulant effect and the anorexic effect is lost in 2-3 wks (in controlled clinical trials). The doses given below are those permitted in labeling; most are excessive. Amphetamines are long-acting drugs; no benefit over a single morning dose is provided by sustained release preparations or by tid dosing. **SIDE EFFECTS**: **Acute side effects**: tremulousness, anxiety, cardiac awareness, dry mouth, irritability, altered sleep habits (e.g., insomnia), hypertension, tachycardia, dizziness, headaches, chilliness, flushing, blurred vision, mydriasis, constipation and hyperexcitability. Larger doses can induce fatigue, depression, disorientation, hallucinations, seizures, coma and respiratory failure. There is a large therapeutic index; death rarely occurs with overdosage. **Chronic toxicity** - long periods of wakefulness, marked weight loss, restlessness, intense anxiety (depression if deprived of the drug), feelings of depersonalization, altered perception and a state similar to paranoid schizophrenia (toxic psychosis) with auditory and visual hallucinations. **CAUTIONS**: Use cautiously in elderly or debilitated patients or those with psychiatric illness (e.g., psychopathic, suicidal, homicidal tendencies). Dependence or addiction can develop and abrupt withdrawal may precipitate lethargy and psychotic manifestations. **CONTRA-INDICATIONS**: Use is contraindicated in glaucoma, diabetes mellitus, nephritis, hyperthyroidism, hypertension, angina pectoris, or other cardiovascular diseases.

SCHEDULE II AGENTS

These first five agents are regarded as having greater abuse potential and therefore are classified as Schedule II drugs.

DRUG	INDICATIONS & DOSAGE	DOSE FORMS	REMARKS
AMPHETAMINE (d,l-amphetamine)			**NOTE**: This is the racemic mixture, formerly **Benzedrine**. It has been largely replaced by the dextro isomer which exhibits greater CNS activity; it remains in proprietary mixtures such as Biphetamine and Obetrol.
DEXTROAMPHETAMINE (Dexedrine) generic preparations	**Exogenous Obesity**: **PO**: 5-30 mg/d in 1-3 doses. **PO (Ext'd Release)**: 10-15 mg qAM. **Narcolepsy**: **PO**: 10 mg/d initially; increase 10 mg/d q1wk; maintenance 5-60 mg/d. **Attention Deficit**: **Pediatric PO**: **3-5 y.o.**: 2.5 mg/d initially; increase by 2.5 mg/d q1wk PRN; use lowest effective dose. **>6 y.o.**: 5 mg q12-24hinitially; increase by 5 mg/d q1wk; maintenance 10-40 mg/d.	PO (Tab's): 5, 10 mg PO (Cap's): 15 mg PO (Ext'd Release): 5, 10, 15 mg	Dextro isomer of amphetamine; exhibits greater CNS activity than racemic mixture. Once per day dosing preferred.

SYMPATHOMIMETIC STIMULANTS: SCHEDULE II AGENTS *Continued*

DRUG	INDICATIONS & DOSAGE	DOSE FORMS	REMARKS
METHAMPHETAMINE (Desoxyn)	<u>**Exogenous Obesity**</u>: **PO**: 2.5-5 mg bid-tid (30 min before meals). **PO (Ext'd Release)**: 10-15 mg qAM. <u>**Attention Deficit**</u>: **Pediatric PO**: 5 mg, q12-24h initially; increase 5 mg/d q1wk PRN; maintenance 20-25 mg/d.	PO (Tab's): 5, 10 mg PO (Ext'd Release): 5, 10, 15 mg	Generally equivalent to dextroamphetamine; slightly more potent. Simpler synthesis, therefore popular drug for abuse. Known as "speed" on the street.
METHYLPHENIDATE (Ritalin)	<u>**Narcolepsy**</u>: **PO**: 10-20 mg bid-tid. <u>**Attention Deficit**</u>: **PO**: 5 mg bid; increase 5-10 mg/d q1wk; maintenance 10-60 mg/d.	PO (Tab's): 5, 10, 20 mg PO (Ext'd Release): 20 mg	Prolonged use in children may interfere with normal growth. **SIDE EFFECTS**: May paradoxically aggravate behavioral disorder; reduce dosage or discontinue therapy. **CONTRA-INDICATIONS**: Motor tics or family history of Gilles de la Tourette's syndrome.
PHENMETRAZINE (Preludin)	<u>**Exogenous Obesity**</u>: **PO**: 25 mg bid-tid (1 h before meals). **PO (Ext'd Release)**: 75 mg qAM.	PO (Tab's): 25 mg PO (Ext'd Release): 50, 75 mg	Preludin 75 mg ext'd release tab's contain tartrazine dye (potential for allergic reactions, especially in patients hyper-sensitive to aspirin).
MISCELLANEOUS			
BENZPHETAMINE (Didrex)	<u>**Exogenous Obesity**</u>: **PO**: 25-50 mg/d initially; maintenance 25-150 mg/d in 1-3 doses.	PO (Tab's): 25, 50 mg	Didrex 25 mg tab's contain tartrazine dye (potential for aller-gic reactions, especially in patients hypersensitive to aspirin).
PHENDIMETRAZINE (Plegine) (Prelu-2)	<u>**Exogenous Obesity**</u>: **PO**: 35 mg bid-tid (1 h before meals). **PO (Ext'd Release)**: 105 mg qAM.	PO (Tab's): 35 mg PO (Cap's): 35 mg PO (Ext'd Release) 105 mg	

SYMPATHOMIMETIC STIMULANTS: MISCELLANEOUS AGENTS *Continued*

DRUG	INDICATIONS & DOSAGE	DOSE FORMS	REMARKS
PEMOLINE (Cylert)	Attention Deficit: **Pediatric PO**: 37.5 mg/d initially; increase 18.8 mg/d q1wk; maintenance 56-75 mg/d (maximum 112 mg/d).	PO (Tab's): 18.8, 37.5, 75 mg	**SIDE EFFECTS**: Elevations of LFTs may occur with chronic therapy; monitor periodically. **CAUTIONS**: Use cautiously in patients with hepatic dysfunction; discontinue if abnormal LFTs develop.
PHENTERMINE (Ionamin) (Phentrol) (Obermine)	Exogenous Obesity: **PO**: 8 mg tid (30 min before meals). **PO (Ext'd Release)**: 15-30 mg qAM.	PO (Tab's): 8, 37.5 mg PO (Cap's): 8, 15, 30 mg PO (Ext'd Release): 15, 30 mg	
FENFLURAMINE (Pondimin)	Exogenous Obesity: **PO**: 20 mg tid; increase 20 mg/d q1wk; maintenance 60-120 mg/d.	PO (Tab's): 20 mg	Fenfluramine usually produces CNS depression rather than stimulation and its pressor activity is much less than that of amphetamine. Anorexic potency similar to that of the amphetamines. **SIDE EFFECTS**: Drowsiness, diarrhea and dry mouth most common; others include: dizziness, headache, depression, anxiety, lack of coordination, nightmares, nausea, vomiting and constipation.

ANTIPARKINSONIAN AGENTS

GROUP REMARKS: Parkinsonism is due to a loss of dopaminergic input to the basal ganglia from degenerative changes in the substantia nigra or from the use of dopamine receptor blocking drugs. Distal to the dopamine system is a cholinergic system that becomes hyper-reactive subsequent to the loss of dopaminergic activity. Treatment depends then on restoring striatal dopamine activity or, much less effectively, blocking the cholinergic system.

DOPAMINE PRECURSORS, AGONISTS & RELATED AGENTS

These agents all act to augment DA action on the corpus striatum. They are generally more effective than anticholinergic agents in treating Parkinsonism.
Newer treatment approaches stress less drug use by:

1) Delaying treatment until disease impairs activities of daily living.
2) Low starting doses and slowly increasing q2-4wk until lost function returns (NOT until all symptoms eradicated); slow increase may allow lower final dose, fewer side effects.
3) Early use of a combination of agents; while still at submaximal doses of another agent.
4) Periodic drug holidays/dosage reductions (most effective in patients with less dyskinesia or on lower doses; side effects worse if patients have "on-off" phenomenon).

RECOMMENDATIONS: The response of different patients varies and dosage levels should be individualized by titration to the lowest effective dose.

DRUG	INDICATIONS & DOSAGE	REMARKS
LEVODOPA (L-Dopa) (Dopar) (Bendopa) (Larodopa)	**Parkinsonism**: **PO**: 250-500 mg bid initially; increase 100-750 mg/d q3-7d; maximum 8 gm/d. **DOSE FORMS**: PO (Tab's): 100, 250, 500 mg. PO (Cap's): 100, 250, 500 mg.	Levodopa enters the CNS (DA itself will not) and is decarboxylated to DA with a resultant increase in DA action in the basal ganglia. It is often administered with carbidopa, a peripheral decarboxylase inhibitor which allows more levodopa to enter the CNS; combination preparations are available. Effective in about 80% of patients; complete/partial relief of akinesia, rigidity and tremor; improved control of facial and pharyngeal muscles, speech, posture and locomotion; general well-being improved. Optimal response may require 3-6 months of therapy. Effectiveness decreases with prolonged use (esp. > 3 years); complete loss of efficacy usually at 6-7 years. Ineffective in drug-induced extrapyramidal symptoms. **SIDE EFFECTS**: Side effects are common, dose-related and usually reversible. Concurrent carbidopa decreases incidence of peripheral side effects. **CNS Side Effects**: Adventitous movements (choreiform, dystonic, dyskinetic) occur in 10-90% patients; "on-off" phenomenon (sudden return of Parkinsonian symptoms alternating with sudden reinstatement of therapeutic action) also occurs. With prolonged therapy: Parkinsonian symptoms may return between doses (minimize by increasing dosing frequency); "Start hesitation" may occur (patient "freezes" at the start of a purposeful movement, such as taking a step). Others: decreased attention and memory, agitation, indifference, nightmares, depression (may be suicidal), and dementia. **Peripheral Side Effects**: Also common. GI effects: loss of appetite, nausea and vomiting; may be relieved by decreasing dosage or administration with meals. Others: orthostatic hypotension, changes in breathing pattern, urinary frequency/retention, blurred vision, headache, weakness and elevated LFTs. Blood dyscrasias have occurred rarely. **CAUTIONS**: Allow for *beta*-adrenergic effects of DA. Phenothiazines/butyrophenones may interfere with therapeutic effect. Use with EXTREME caution in patients with recent myocardial infarction and evidence of continued arrhythmia, or in psychotic patients. Use cautiously in asthma or emphysema requiring use of sympathomimetics. **RECOMMEND**: Reduce dosage if given with concurrent anticholinergic. Discontinue MAO Inhibitors > 2 wk before levodopa therapy. Periodically evaluate liver and renal function and perform CBC; discontinue if leukopenia develops. **CONTRAINDICATIONS**: AVOID in patients with evidence of uncompensated endocrine, renal, hepatic, cardiovascular, pulmonary diseases or blood dyscrasias; also narrow-angle glaucoma, unless well controlled. AVOID also in patients with undiagnosed skin lesions or history of melanoma; may activate malignant melanoma. Do NOT administer concurrent with MAO inhibitors; may precipitate hypertensive crisis.

ANTIPARKINSONIAN AGENTS: DOPAMINE-RELATED AGENTS *Continued*

DRUG	INDICATIONS & DOSAGE	REMARKS
LEVODOPA:CARBIDOPA combination (Sinemet) **CARBIDOPA** (Lodosyn)	Determine optimal daily dosage by careful titration. Maximum daily dose: 200 mg. **Patients NOT currently receiving levodopa**: One tab of 100 mg/10 mg or 100 mg/25 mg (levodopa/carbidopa) tid initially; increase 1 tab qd or qod; maintenance 6 tab's/d. If additional levodopa required: substitute 250 mg/25 mg, 1 tab tid-qid; increase by 1 tab qd or qod; maximum: 8 tab/d. **Patients currently receiving levodopa**: Initiate ≥ 8 h since patient last received levodopa. Choose levodopa/carbidopa dose that will provide 25% of previous levodopa daily dosage. Suggested starting dosage: 1 tab of 250 mg/25 mg tid-qid; adjust by adding/omitting 1/2 to 1 tab qd. Some patients may need additional carbidopa (unresponsive nausea, vomiting when dosage is < 70 mg/d and levodopa < 700 mg/d); add 25 mg carbidopa to the first dose each day; 12.5-25 mg may be added to subsequent doses during the day. **Dosage adjustment**: Add or omit 1/2 to 1 tab per day.	Carbidopa is a peripheral decarboxylase inhibitor; it inhibits peripheral conversion of levodopa to DA, allowing greater fraction of the administered dose to escape destruction and enter the CNS. Concurrent carbidopa reduces levadopa requirements by 70-80%; side effects (esp. nausea, vomiting) also reduced. Use ONLY in combination with levodopa; NO therapeutic action when used alone. Peripheral dopa decarboxylase saturated by 70-100 mg/d carbidopa. Carbidopa does NOT interfere with CNS-related side effects of levodopa; it may actually promote them. **RECOMMEND**: Therapeutic/adverse effects occur more rapidly with combined therapy; closely monitor patients. Dyskinesia may require dosage reduction. Blepharospasm may be an early sign of excess dosage. **DOSE FORMS**: PO (Tab's), Lodosyn (carbidopa alone): 25 mg PO (Tab's), Sinemet (combination with levodopa): Levodopa 100 mg with carbidopa 10 mg Levodopa 100 mg with carbidopa 25 mg Levodopa 250 mg with carbidopa 25 mg
BROMOCRIPTINE (Parlodel)	**Parkinsonism**: **PO**: 1.25 mg bid initially; increase 2.5 mg/d q2-4wk; maximum 100 mg/d. Give with meals. **DOSE FORMS**: PO (Tab's): 2.5 mg. PO (Cap's): 5 mg.	A DA receptor agonist, it also lowers serum prolactin (inhibits release from anterior pituitary); may restore fertility in amenorrheic women and inhibit lactation. Allow 2 wk for establishment of therapeutic effect following dosage adjustment. **SIDE EFFECTS**: Incidence is higher (68% patients) than with levodopa, but most are mild-moderate. **Most common**: nausea, headache, dizziness, fatigue, abdominal cramps, lightheadedness, constipation, diarrhea, persistent mild hypotension. Others are common with doses > 100 mg/d: hallucinations, paranoid delusions, erythromelagia and nightmares,. Pulmonary infiltrates, effusion and pleural thickening have been reported with long-term, high-dose treatment. **RECOMMEND**: Monitor blood pressure periodically. **CONTRAINDICATIONS**: Patients with sensitivity to any ergot alkaloids.

ANTIPARKINSONIAN AGENTS: DOPAMINE-RELATED AGENTS *Continued*

DRUG	INDICATIONS & DOSAGE	REMARKS
AMANTIDINE (Symmetrel)	**Parkinsonism**: **PO**: 100 mg q12-24h; maximum 400 mg/d. **Drug-Induced Extrapyramidal Disorders**: **PO**: 100 mg bid; maximum 300 mg/d. **DOSE FORMS**: PO (Cap's): 100 mg PO (Liquid): 10 mg/ml	Amantadine is an anti-viral agent (see Antibiotics). It is less effective than levodopa, but some efficacy in approximately 50% patients. Allow 2-12 wks for optimal therapeutic effect; tolerance may develop at 1-3 months. Do NOT use in active cases of influenza or other respiratory disease or with CNS stimulants. **SIDE EFFECTS**: Most CNS effects are dose-related and reversible: nervousness, fatigue, insomnia, lack of concentration, psychoses. Dry mouth, GI upset and urinary disturbances also occur. Livedo reticularis (bluish skin mottling) occurs frequently on the legs. **CAUTIONS**: Probably embryotoxic and teratogentic. Abrupt withdrawal has precipitated Parkinsonian crises. Use cautiously in cases of hepatic disease, recurrent eczema, CHF, hypotension, psychiatric disorders, epilepsy or with concurrent CNS stimulants.

ANTICHOLINERGIC AGENTS AND RELATED

The agents in this second group all exert their pharmacologic effect through antagonism of ACh. They are less effective than augmentation of DA by levodopa and are used as adjunctive agents for their effect on rigidity and hypersalivation. They have little effect on tremor and tend to worsen dystonias associated with Parkinsonism. They are also used to treat the acute dystonias produced by antipsychotic drugs and , with a doubtful basis, to prevent the Parkinsonism also produced by those agents. These agents should NOT be used in tardive dyskinesias. **SIDE EFFECTS**: Typical atropine-like side effects: dry mouth, blurred vision, nausea, constipation and urinary retention. In addition they also produce an unpleasant sedation and some dizziness. With high doses, agitation, vertigo, confusion and hallucinations may occur. Psychotic reactions have been reported rarely for some of these agents. **RECOMMENDATIONS**: Treatment should be initiated with low doses and increased gradually until tolerance develops or the recommended maximum is achieved. Dosage adjustments should be made SLOWLY; abrupt changes may worsen symptoms. Administer these drugs with meals to diminish GI side effects, esp. nausea. **CAUTIONS**: These agents may be used (PO) in patients with glaucoma provided periodic ophthalmologic exams are performed.

PARASYMPATHOLYTIC AGENTS

BENZTROPINE (Cogentin)	**Parkinsonism**: **PO**: 0.5-1 mg/d initially; increase 0.5 mg/d q5-6d; maintenance 0.5-6 mg/d. **IM, IV**: 1-2 mg, then PO regimen. **Drug-Induced Extrapyramidal Disorders**: **PO**: 1-4 mg bid (re-evaluate need after 1-2 wk). **IM, IV**: 1-2 mg bid.	PO (Tab's): 0.5, 1, 2 mg Injection: 1 mg/ml	Produces less CNS stimulation than does trihexyphenidyl. IM = IV administration.

ANTIPARKINSONIAN AGENTS: ANTICHOLINERGIC AGENTS *Continued*

DRUG	INDICATIONS & DOSAGE	DOSE FORMS	REMARKS
TRIHEXYPHENIDYL (Artane) (Tremin)	<u>**Parkinsonism**</u>: **PO**: 1-2 mg/d initially; increase 2 mg/d q3-5d; maintenance 6-10 mg/d in 3-4 doses. <u>**Drug-Induced Extrapyramidal Disorders**</u>: **PO**: 1 mg initially, then 5-15 mg/d.	PO (Tab's): 2, 5 mg PO (Ext'd Release): 5 mg PO (Liquid): 2 mg/5 ml	CNS depression occurs at low doses, stimulation at high doses. **SIDE EFFECTS**: Typical anticholinergic side effects noted in 30-50% patients. High dose CNS effects include: agitation, delirium and hallucination.
PROCYCLIDINE (Kemidrin)	<u>**Parkinsonism**</u>: **PO**: 2.5 mg tid initially; maintenance 4-5 mg tid-qid. <u>**Drug-Induced Extrapyramidal Disorders**</u>: **PO**: 2.5 mg tid initially; increase 2.5 mg/d qd; maintenance 10-20 mg/d.	PO (Tab's): 5 mg	**RECOMMENDATION**: Administer after meals.
BIPERIDEN (Akineton)	<u>**Parkinsonism**</u>: **PO**: 2 mg tid-qid. <u>**Drug-Induced Extrapyramidal Disorders**</u>: **PO**: 2-6 mg/d in 1-3 doses **IM, IV**: 2 mg q30min; maximum 8 mg/d.	PO (Tab's): 2 mg Injection: 5 mg	**RECOMMENDATION**: Administer IV injections SLOWLY; increased risk of side effects.
MISCELLANEOUS AGENTS			
DIPHENHYDRAMINE (Benadryl) (Benylin) (Fenylhist) (Diphen)	<u>**Parkinsonism**</u>: **PO**: 25-50 mg tid-qid. **IM, IV**: 10-50 mg; maximum 400 mg/d. <u>**Drug-Induced Extrapyramidal Disorders**</u>: **PO**: 25-50 mg tid-qid. **IM, IV**: 10-50 mg; maximum 400 mg/d.	PO (Tab's): 25, 50 mg PO (Cap's): 25, 50 mg Injection: 10, 50 mg/ml Elixir/Syrup: 12.5 mg/5 ml	Most common use is treatment of acute dystonias produced by antipsychotic agents. **SIDE EFFECTS**: CNS side effects are prominent (especially sedation). **RECOMMENDATION**: Do NOT administer SC; highly irritating.
ETHOPROPAZINE (Parsidol)	<u>**Parkinsonism**</u>: **PO**: 50 mg q12-24h initially; maintenance 100-600 mg/d. <u>**Drug-Induced Extrapyramidal Disorders**</u>: **PO**: 50 mg q12-24h initially; maintenance 100-400 mg/d.	PO (Tab's): 10, 50 mg	A phenothiazine derivative suggested for treatment of tremor. **SIDE EFFECTS**: S.E.s in Group Remarks and typical phenothiazine S.E.s, including: EKG changes, endocrinologic effects and hyperpigmentation. **CAUTIONS**: See Group Remarks for the Phenothiazine Antipsychotics.

PARASYMPATHOLYTICS

GROUP REMARKS: These anticholinergic and related agents decrease tone and motility in the smooth muscle of the gastrointestinal (GI) and genitourinary (GU) tracts; they also decrease secretions in the GI and respiratory tracts. Their anti-spasmotic properties are the basis for their use in functional GI and GU distress. Inhibition of acid secretion is the basis for their adjunctive use in peptic ulcer therapy; their efficacy is questionable. Pre-operative use is to decrease laryngospasm; to inhibit oral, nasal and respiratory secretions; and to inhibit vagally-mediated bradycardia secondary to visceral stimulation. **NOTES**: Effects are dose-dependent: low doses inhibit saliva, sweat and bronchial secretion and slow the heart; moderate doses increase heart rate and pupillary diameter and inhibit accommodation; higher doses decrease tone and motility of the GI and GU tracts; very high doses inhibit gastric acid secretion. **SIDE EFFECTS**: Dry mouth, blurred near vision, urinary retention (esp. in older men), dizziness or lightheadedness and fatigue are all common side effects which limit chronic use. With overdosage, additional effects occur: constipation, tachycardia, hyperpyrexia, "atropine flush" (characteristic erythema of the blush area), sedation, delirium (phenothiazines should NOT be used), coma. Quaternary (4°) compounds manifest fewer CNS effects and should be used if CNS side effects limit therapy. **CONTRAINDICATIONS**: Anticholinergics should NOT be used in glaucoma, myasthenia gravis, known hypersensitivity to anticholinergics, prostatic hypertrophy.

DRUG	INDICATIONS & DOSAGE	DOSE FORMS	REMARKS
	TERTIARY (3°) PARASYMPATHOLYTICS		
These tertiary compounds readily cross biologic membranes including those of the blood-brain barrier, therefore CNS effects are prominent. For the same reason, they are also readily absorbed by the GI tract and are thus active orally.			
ATROPINE (in Lomotil) (in Donnatal)	**Hypermotility**: **PO**: 0.4-0.6 mg q4-6h. **Pre-Operative**: **IM, SC**: 0.5 mg prior to anesthesia; range 0.4-0.6 mg. **Cardiopulmonary Resuscitation**: **IV**: 0.5 mg q5min PRN. **Pediatric IV**: 0.02 mg/kg (maximum 1 mg, minimum 0.1 mg). **Organophosphate Poisoning**: **IV**: 1-3 mg q5-60min; then PO: 0.5-1 mg PRN.	Injection: 0.1, 0.3, 0.4, 0.5, 1, 1.2 mg/ml PO (Tab's): 0.3, 0.4, 0.6 mg Generic powder	Used to treat poisoning by organophosphates (cholinesterase inhibitors) and muscarinic effects of some mushrooms. Used during cardiopulmonary resusitation (ACLS) to treat bradycardia. Present in many "cold remedies." Lomotil = 2.5 mg diphenoxylate HCl, 0.025 mg atropine sulfate (per tablet or 5 ml liquid). Donnatal = 16.2 mg phenobarbital, 0.104 mg hyoscyamine sulfate, 0.0065 mg scopolamine hydrobromide, 0.019 mg atropine sulfate (per tablet, capsule or 5 ml liquid).
ATROPINE Aerosol (Dey-Dose)	**Bronchospasm**: **Via Nebulizer**: **Adult**: 0.025 mg/kg diluted in 3-5 ml saline, q6-8h; maximum 2.5 mg/dose. **Pediatric**: 0.05 mg/kg diluted in saline, q6-8h (maximum 1.5 mg for children 26-37 kg).	Nebulizer solution: 1, 2.5 mg/0.5 m	When administered by inhalation, atropine produces somewhat selective bronchodilation; large individual variation exists. The effect may be additive with *beta*-agonist bronchodilators, due to a different site of action. **SIDE EFFECTS**: Systemic atropinic effects may occur (large individual variation): dry mouth/nose, dry/flushed skin, headache, bradycardia, tachycardia/palpitations, mydriasis and blurred vision. **CONTRAINDICATIONS**: Glaucoma, iris-lens adhesions (synechia), prostatic hypertrophy.

PARASYMPATHOLYTICS *Continued*

DRUG	INDICATIONS & DOSAGE	DOSE FORMS	REMARKS
SCOPOLAMINE (Invenex) (Transderm-Scop)	<u>**Motion Sickness**</u>: **PO**: 025 mg 1 h before travel; repeat q4-6h PRN (maximum 1 mg/d). **Patch**: 0.5 mg/72 h. <u>**Pre-Operative**</u>: **IM, SC**: 0.3-0.65 mg q6-8h PRN.	PO (Cap's): 0.25, 0.4, 0.6 mg Injection: 0.3, 0.4, 0.5, 0.9, 1.0 mg/ml Transdermal Patch: 0.5 mg/72 h	Used mainly for motion sickness and adjunct to anesthesia. Drug of choice for motion sickness; transdermal patch may result in fewer side effects. Sedative and amnesic effects (prominent CNS depressive action) contribute to anesthesia. **SIDE EFFECTS**: CNS side effects include disorientation, memory disturbances, excitement. **RECOMMEND**: Wash hands after handling transdermal patch.
QUATERNARY (4°) PARASYMPATHOLYTICS			
Quaternary compounds penetrate membranes poorly and therefore produce only negligible CNS effects (they do NOT cross the blood-brain barrier) and are poorly absorbed following oral administration. Ocular effects (blurred vision, dilated pupils) are also less likely.			
DICYCLOMINE (Bentyl) (Dibent) (Byclomine) (A-Spaz) (Or-Tyl)	<u>**Hypermotility**</u>: **PO**: 20 mg q6-8h; maintenance 40 mg q6h. **IM**: 20 mg q6h; then PO maintenance.	PO (Tab's): 10, 20 mg Injection: 10 mg/ml Syrup: 2 mg/ml	Synthetic tertiary amine. Efficacy in combination with phenobarbital to treat irritable bowel syndrome is questionable, as is efficacy in infant colic syndrome.
CLIDINIUM BROMIDE (Quarzan) (in Librax)	<u>**Peptic Ulcer**</u>: **PO**: 2.5-5 mg q6-8h. <u>**Hypermotility**</u>: **PO**: 2.5-5 mg q6-8h.	PO (Cap's): 2.5, 5 mg	Used alone only as adjunct for peptic ulcer therapy; used in combination with chlordiazepoxide (Librax) for irritable bowel syndrome. Quaternary ammonium compound; poor absorption PO, little CNS action.
GLYCOPYRROLATE (Robinul)	<u>**Peptic Ulcer**</u>: **PO**: 1-2 mg q8-12h; maintenance 1 mg bid. **IM, IV**: 0.1-0.2 mg q6-8h PRN. <u>**Pre-Operative**</u>: **IM**: 0.004 mg/kg 30-60 min prior to anesthesia; then 0.1 mg IV q2-3min PRN. **Pediatric IM**: 0.004-0.008 mg/kg.	PO (Tab's): 1, 2 mg Injection: 0.2 mg/ml	**RECOMMENDATIONS**: NOT to be used in children < 12 y.o. for management of peptic ulcer.

beta-AGONISTS

GROUP REMARKS: *Beta*-adrenergic agonists are sympathomimetics that are devoid of *alpha* (vasoconstrictor) effects (EXCEPT for epinephrine). *Beta*-agonists relax vascular and non-vascular smooth muscle; they produce bronchiolar dilatation, uterine relaxation and vasodilatation. They stimulate the rate and force of contraction of the heart; they produce the same tremulousness and feeling of anxiety as epinephrine. **SIDE EFFECTS**: Most side effects are due to cardiac and CNS stimulation. CNS effects include: headache, restlessness, anxiety, tremor, weakness, dizziness and excitement. Cardiac effects include: flush, palpitations, tachycardia and variable changes in blood pressure (hypertension may result from overdose). Pharyngeal irritation may occur with prolonged use of powdered aerosols. **CAUTIONS/CONTRAINDICATIONS**: Use cautiously in patients with coronary disease, hypertension, stroke, arrhythmias, hyperthyroidism or diabetes. Paradoxical increases in airway resistance (asthmatic response) can develop from overuse of the inhalant forms of these drugs. Tolerance can develop to the actions of these drugs; reactivity is usually restored by temporary avoidance of the drug. With overuse, aerosol propellants from inhalation formulations may sensitize the myocardium to endogenous catecholamines; fatal arrhythmias can occur. The *beta*-stimulants should NOT be administered concurrently with other sympathomimetics (esp. epinephrine) due to the possibility of additive cardiac stimulation. **ABBREVIATIONS**: IPPB = intermittent positive pressure breathing, SL = sub-lingual, Sln = solution.

BRONCHODILATOR *beta*-AGONISTS

Some of the *beta*-agonists are somewhat selective for *beta*$_2$ effects; they act preferentially on vascular smooth muscle with minimal stimulation of the heart. This selectivity becomes less apparent as the dose is increased, but the *beta*$_2$ agonists are widely used to treat asthma (isoproterenol, the prototype "pure" *beta*-agonist, and epinephrine, a mixed *alpha/beta* agonist, are also used for asthma).

In asthma and in patients with obstructive pulmonary disease, these agents increase vital capacity, decrease residual volume and facilitate movement of pulmonary secretions. For bronchodilation, inhalation (mist or micronized powder) is the preferred route of administration; the therapeutic action is localized and systemic absorption (leading to side effects) is minimized.

DRUG	INDICATIONS & DOSAGE	DOSE FORMS	REMARKS
ISOPROTERENOL (Isuprel) (Norisodrine) *Continued, next page*	**Asthma. Bronchospasm**: **Metered Aerosol**: 1 inhalation, repeat (once only) at 2-5 min; maintenance 1-2 inhalations, 4-6 times/d (maximum 6 inhalations/h) [0.2%-0.25% sln of hydrochloride or sulfate]. **Nebulizer**: 5-15 inhalations, repeat (once only) in 5-10 min; maximum 5 times/d (0.5% (1:200) sln initially; 1% (1:100) sln if insufficient response). **IPPB**: 0.5 ml of 0.5% (in 2-2.5 ml of saline) over 15-20 min (maximum 5 times/d). **IV**: 0.01-0.02 mg, repeat PRN. **Sub-lingual**: 10-20 mg (maximum 60 mg/d in 3 doses); 5-10 mg (maximum 30 mg/d) in children. *Continued, next page*	Aerosol: 0.25% sln (0.12-0.13 mg/metered dose) of hydrochloride, 0.2% (0.08 mg/metered dose) of sulfate Nebulizer Solution: 0.25%, 0.5%, 1% sln of hydrochloride Injection: 0.2 mg/ml of hydrochloride SL Tablets: 10, 15 mg of hydrochloride	Mixed *beta*$_1$/*beta*$_2$-stimulant; prominent cardiac stimulation. Heart rate and force of contraction increase; myocardial O_2 need may outstrip increased coronary blood flow and myocardial hypoxia can result. Shortens conduction time and refractory period in AV block. Cardiac effects lessened, but NOT abolished, when administered by inhalation. May reduce arterial oxygen levels. With overuse, tolerance can develop to both bronchodilation and cardiac stimulation. Inhalation "dosage" for children is same as for adults; lower ventilation capacity provides lower drug intake. Pediatric status asthmaticus use is investigational. **SIDE EFFECTS**: Parotid gland swelling may occur with chronic use; discontinue drug. Powdered formulation may produce respiratory tract irritation. **RECOMMENDATIONS**: Have *Continued, next page*

beta-AGONISTS: BRONCHODILATORS *Continued*

DRUG	INDICATIONS & DOSAGE	DOSE FORMS	REMARKS
ISOPROTERENOL *Continued*	**Chronic Obstructive Pulmonary Disease**: **Metered Aerosol**: 1-2 inhalations q3-4h.	See previous page.	patient report any decrement of response to 3-5 inhalation treatments within 6-12 h; consider alternate therapy. Discontinue if: precordial distress, arrhythmias, angina. **CAUTIONS**: Arrhythmias (premature ventricular contractions, ventricular tachycardia, ectopic beats or fibrillation) may occur. May increase extent of ischemia in acute myocardial infarction. Rebound bronchospasm possible upon termination of action. **CONTRAINDICATIONS**: Tachycardia (especially from digitalis overdosage).
METAPROTERENOL (Alupent) (Metaprel)	**Asthma, Bronchospasm**: **Metered Inhaler**: 1-3 inhalations tid-qid (maximum 12 inhalations/d). **Nebulizer**: 10 inhalations undiluted (0.5%) sln q4h. **IPPB**: Dilute 0.2-0.3 ml in 2.5 ml 0.9% saline. **PO**: 20 mg tid-qid. **Pediatric PO (<6 y.o.)**: 1.3-2.6 mg/kg/d in 3-4 doses. **Pediatric PO (6-9 y.o.)**: 10 mg tid-qid.	Aerosol: 0.65 mg/inhalation Nebulizer solution: 5% strength Syrup: 10 mg/5 ml PO (Tab's): 10, 20 mg	Selective *beta*$_2$-stimulant, although less so than albuterol. Duration of action longer than isoproterenol and lower incidence of side effects; also, more effective following PO administration.
TERBUTALINE (Brethine) (Bricanyl)	**Asthma, Bronchospasm**: **PO**: 2.5-5 mg tid (maximum 15 mg/d in adults, 7.5 mg/d in children 12-15 y.o.). **SC**: 0.25 mg, repeat in 15-30 min once only (maximum 0.5 mg/4 h).	PO (Tab's): 2.5, 5 mg Injection: 1 mg/ml	Selective *beta*$_2$-stimulant. Administered PO, terbutaline has a longer duration of action and equal or greater efficacy than metaproterenol. Use to inhibit premature labor is investigational.
ALBUTEROL (Preventil) (Ventolin) (Salbutamol = sulfate)	**Bronchospasm**: **Metered Inhaler**: 1-2 inhalations q4-6h. **Exercise Asthma (Prevention)**: **Metered Inhaler**: 2 inhalations 15 min prior to exercise. **PO**: 2-4 mg tid-qid initially; gradually increase to maximum 32 mg/d. **Geriatric PO**: 2 mg tid-qid initially (maximum 32 mg/d).	PO (Tab's): 2, 4 mg (as sulfate) Aerosol: 0.09 mg/inhalation	Selecitve *beta*$_2$-stimulant. Wait 1-10 min between individual inhalations. Cautiously increase dose > 4 mg qid ONLY if no response to initial therapy. Reflex tachycardia may be more prominent with albuterol than some other *beta*$_2$-stimulants. Duration of action longer than isoproterol, possibly longer than metaproterenol. Oral administration as effective as inhalation, but with longer onset delay. May lower serum potassium levels in patients with familial hyperkalemic periodic paralysis; used investigationally to treat episodes of paralysis.

DRUG	INDICATIONS & DOSAGE	DOSE FORMS	REMARKS
ISOETHARINE (Bronkosol)	Asthma, Bronchospasm: **Oxygen Aerosolization**: 2-4 ml of 0.125% sln, 2.5 ml of 0.2% sln, 2 ml of 0.25% sln, 0.5 ml of 0.5% sln OR 0.25-0.5 ml of 1% sln diluted 1:3; q4h (maximum 5 times/d). **IPPB**: 2-8 ml of 0.125% sln, 2.5 ml of 0.2% sln, 2 ml of 0.25% sln, 0.5 ml of 0.5% sln OR 0.25-0.5 ml of 1% sln diluted 1:3; q4h (maximum 5 times/d). **Nebulizer**: 3-7 inhalations of 1% sln q4h (maximum 5 times/d). **Metered Aerosol**: 1-2 inhalations q3-4h PRN.	Aerosol: 0.34 mg/metered dose of the mesylate Solution: 0.125%, 0.2%, 0.25%, 0.5%, 1% of the hydrochloride	Selective *beta*$_2$-stimulant; longer duration of action than isoproterenol and less cardiac stimulation. Pediatric doses NOT established, but many believe inhalation "doses" are the same as for adults. **CAUTIONS**: Paradoxical bronchoconstriction from overuse may be severe.

beta-AGONISTS USED TO INHIBIT PREMATURE LABOR

These drugs are *beta*$_2$-stimulants which are orally and parenterally active with a longer duration of action than isoproterenol. They stimulate both the heart and the CNS; they also relax smooth muscle and act as vasodilators. All are used, at least investigationally, in deferring premature labor. IV infusion decreases the intensity and frequency of uterine contractions; it also produces dose-related increases in heart rate and contractility in both the mother and fetus. **SIDE EFFECTS**: Palpitations, tremor, GI upset (nausea, vomiting), headache, flush, nervousness and malaise may occur with IV treatment; likelihood of side effects is decreased with oral administration. Pulmonary edema, with FATAL outcome has occurred (may be associated with concurrent corticosteroid administration). **CONTRAINDICATIONS**: Do NOT use before the 20th week of pregnancy. Do NOT administer immediately postpartum. Others: eclampsia, hemorrhage, pulmonary hypertension, cardiac disease.

DRUG	INDICATIONS & DOSAGE	DOSE FORMS	REMARKS
RITODRINE (Yutopar)	Premature Labor: **PO**: 10 mg q2h for 24 h, then 10-20 mg q4-6h (maximum 120 mg/d). **IV**: 0.1 mg/min initially, increase by 0.05 mg/min q10 min; maintenance 0.15-0.35 mg/min.	PO (Tab's): 10 mg Injection: 10 mg/ml	Maintain infusion for 12 h following cessation of uterine contractions; switch to oral administration 30 min prior to halting infusion. Monitor amount and rate of IV fluid; maximum fluid = 850 ml/12 h. Observe for signs of pulmonary edema.
ISOXSUPRINE (Vasodilan) (Vasoprin) (Voxsuprine)	Vascular Disorders: **PO**: 10-20 mg q6-8h.	PO (Tab's): 10, 20 mg	Use in premature labor is investigational. Also used as adjunctive agent in peripheral or cerebral vascular diseases. Discontinue if rash occurs.

TREATMENT OF ANAPHYLAXIS

ANAPHYLACTIC SHOCK:
Anaphylactic shock is an immediate and potentially fatal immune reaction to foreign sera (esp. horse), drugs (esp. penicillin and other antibiotics) or insect stings. Anaphylaxis is due to the liberation of histamine from mast cells of sensitized individuals when they are re-exposed to the elicting antigen. Histamine constricts non-vascular smooth muscle, dilates blood vessels and causes localized edema. Anaphylaxis therefore manifests as hives, flushing, tachycardia, urge to defecate or urinate, fall in blood pressure (shock) and bronchospasm and laryngeal edema which may be rapidly FATAL. Epinephrine is especially well-suited for the treatment of anaphylaxis; it relaxes airway smooth muscle ($beta_2$-action) to reverse bronchoconstriction, it constricts blood vessels (*alpha* action) to inhibit edema formation and increase blood pressure, and it stimulates the heart ($beta_1$-action) to also increase blood pressure. Epinephrine is also used as a bronchodilator in asthma.

DRUG	INDICATIONS & DOSAGE	DOSE FORMS	REMARKS
EPINEPHRINE (Adrenalin) (Epipen) (Sus-Phrine)	**Anaphylactic Shock**: **IV**: 0.1-0.5 mg (0.1-0.5 ml of 1:1000 dilution) SLOWLY; repeat q5-15min PRN. **IM, SC**: 0.1-0.5 mg (0.1-0.5 ml of 1:1000 dilution). For SC: repeat q15-30min for 3-4 doses (maximum 1 mg/dose); or q4h PRN. **Pediatric IM, SC**: 0.01 ml/kg (0.1 ml/kg of 1:1000 dilution) or 0.3 mg/m^2 (0.3 mg/m^2 of 1:1000 dilution) to maximum of 0.5 ml; repeat q15-20min for 3-4 doses (maximum 0.5 mg/dose) or q4hPRN. **Bronchospasm**: **IM, SC**: 0.3-0.5 ml (1:1000 dilution) q20min-4h. **Pediatric IM, SC**: 0.01 ml/kg (1:1000 dilution) q20min-4h PRN (maximum 0.5 ml/dose). **Nebulizer**: 1-3 inhalations (1:100 dilution); repeat q5 min PRN (maximum 4-6 times/d). **Cardiac Arrest**: **IV**: 0.5-1 mg (5-10 ml of 1:10,000 dilution); repeat q5min PRN. **Pediatric IV, ET**: 0.01 mg/kg (0.1 ml/kg of 1:10,000 dilution).	Injection: 0.1 mg/ml (1:10,000), 1 mg/ml (1:1000) Aerosol: metered doses equivalent to 160, 200, 270 µg Suspension: 5 mg/ml (1:200) Nebulizer Solution: 1% (1:100), 2.25% (of racemic epinephrine)	**SIDE EFFECTS**: Anxiety, tension, headache, lightheadedness, nervousness, excitability, weakness. May precipitate or worsen psychogenic reactions. Nausea, weakness, pallor and sweating also occur. Tachycardia, palpitations, cardiac arrhythmias (esp. with large doses or if myocardium sensitized by halogenated anesthetics or digitalis) and hypertension may result from effect on the heart and vascular system. **NOTES**: Racemic mixture has approximately one-half the activity of epinephrine. **CAUTIONS**: Use cautiously in geriatric patients. **RECOMMEND**: AVOID use with concurrent cyclopropane or halogenated inhalation anesthetics. **CONTRAINDICATIONS**: Acute coronary disease, cardiac asthma, most arrhythmias, hyperthyroidism, cerebral arteriosclerosis, hypertension, diabetes. ET = via endotracheal tube

XANTHINES

GROUP REMARKS: The xanthines (or methyl xanthines) include theophylline used therapeutically; caffeine in coffee, tea and other beverages and theobromine in chocolate. Aminophylline is theophylline solubilized with ethylenediamine. Xanthines produce CNS and cardiac stimulation, blood vessel and smooth muscle relaxation, diuresis and secretion of gastric acid. Their use in asthma is based on relaxation of bronchiolar smooth muscle. **SIDE EFFECTS:** Xanthines cause GI irritation (nausea, vomiting, heartburn, abdominal discomfort), especially during chronic oral use. CNS stimulation causes headache, irritability, restlessness, nervousness and insomnia. Cardiac side effects: palpitations, tachycardia, rapid pulse. Other: fever, flush, rapid respiration, proteinuria, urine retention in males with prostatic enlargement. Pulmonary vasodilation may cause ventilation/flow mismatch with resultant hypoxemia. Severe toxic reactions: arrhythmias (esp. ventricular; treat with lidocaine), shock, hyperglycemia, convulsions.

Notes: In general, doses are expressed as anhydrous theophylline. Aminophylline is commonly used for IV administration, anhydrous theophylline for PO administration. The xanthines have a low therapeutic index (T.I.); care should be taken in setting dosage and the patient should be followed closely.

EQUIVALENT DOSAGES: Each of the following contains or is equivalent to 100 mg theophylline:

	Dosage	Multiplier
Theophylline anhydrous	100 mg	1.00
Theophylline monohydrate	110 mg	1.10
Theophylline sodium glycinate	217 mg	2.17
Theophylline calcium salicylate	208 mg	2.08
Aminophylline anhydrous	116 mg	1.16
Aminophylline dihydrate	127 mg	1.27

"Multiplier" is the factor by which the desired theophylline anhydrous dose is multiplied to yield the corresponding dose for an alternate formulation.

Bronchospasm:

IV: 5.5 mg/kg of aminophylline, loading dose given over 20 min for naive patients (4.7 mg/kg theophylline); then infusion of aminophylline (theophylline) as per:

	Initial 12 h (mg/kg/h)	Maintenance > 12 h (mg/kg/h)
Pediatric (6 mo-9 y.o.)	1.2 (0.95)	1.0 (0.79)
Pediatric (9-16 y.o.) and adult smokers	1.0 (0.79)	0.8 (0.63)
Adult (nonsmoking)	0.7 (0.55)	0.5 (0.39)
Geriatric (and cor pulmonale patients)	0.6 (0.47)	0.3 (0.24)
Congestive Heart Failure or liver decompensation	0.5 (0.39)	0.1-0.2 (0.08-0.16)

For patients already being treated with a xanthine, the IV loading dose should be reduced based on the patient's recent dosing history. As a rule of thumb, each 0.5 mg/kg (lean body weight) of anhydrous theophylline will increase serum theophylline levels by 1 µg/ml. If serum levels are not available and patient requires immediate therapy, a loading dose of approximately 2.5 mg/kg should be given and the chart above then followed.

PO: 6 mg/kg anhydrous theophylline, loading dose for naive patients, then:

	Initial 12 h	Maintenance
Pediatric (6 mo-9 y.o.)	4 mg/kg q4h (for 3 doses)	4 mg/kg q6h
Pediatric (9-16 y.o.) and adult smokers	3 mg/kg q4h (for 3 doses)	3 mg/kg q6h
Adult (nonsmoking)	3 mg/kg q6h (for 2 doses)	3 mg/kg q8h
Geriatric and corpulmonale patients	2 mg/kg q6h (for 2 doses)	2 mg/kg q8h
Congestive Heart Failure or liver decompensation	2 mg/kg q8h (for 2 doses)	1-2 mg/kg q12h

Chronic Bronchospasm:

PO: 16 mg/kg/d OR 400 mg/d (whichever is less) of anhydrous theophylline initially in 3-4 doses; increase by 25% q2-3d until therapeutic effect, toxicity or maximum dose (see below) is achieved.

Extended Release (PO): 12 mg/kg/d or 400 mg/d (whichever is less) initially in 2-3 doses; increase by 2-3 mg/kg/d q3d until therapeutic effect, toxicity or maximum dose (see below) is achieved.

Maximum oral doses (standard or extended release):

Children < 9 y.o.	24 mg/kg/d
Children 9-12 y.o.	20 mg/kg/d
Adolescents 12-16 y.o.	18 mg/kg/d
Adults >16 y.o.	13 mg/kg/d (or 900 mg/d, if lesser)

XANTHINES *Continued*

LEVELS: Serum levels expressed as anhydrous theophylline (peak levels):

< 20 μg/ml	Side effects uncommon
20-30 μg/ml	Mild-moderate side effects in 75% patients
> 30 μg/ml	Serious, possibly fatal toxicity (> 10 μg/ml in neonates)

Monitor serum levels; adjust dosage to acheive **therapeutic range** of 10-20 μg/ml. Doses should be determined on the basis of lean body weight (theophylline does not enter fat) and anhydrous theophylline content (see chart). Dosage within 48 h preceding a serum test should be typical of the prescribed regimen.

Dosage Adjustment Based on Serum Level:

5-7.5 μg/ml	(LOW)	Increase dose by 25%; recheck levels; increase further.
7.5-10 μg/ml	(LOW)	Increase dose by 25%; recheck at 3 days.
10-20 μg/ml	(NORMAL)	Maintain dosage; recheck at 6,12 months.
20-25 μg/ml	(HIGH)	Decrease dose by 10%; recheck at 3 days, 6,12 months.
25-30 μg/ml	(HIGH)	Eliminate the next dose; lower dosage by 25%.
> 30 μg/ml	(HIGH)	Eliminate the next 2 doses; lower dosage by 50%.

Peak serum levels after PO administration occur at 1-2 h with a standard preparation and 3-12 h with an extended release preparation.

CAUTIONS: May cause or aggravate cardiac arrhythmias. Children are very sensitive to CNS stimulation from xanthines. Use cautiously in: cardiovascular disease, hypertension, hyperthyroidism, hypoxemia, peptic ulcer, glaucoma and geriatrics (esp. males). Rectal suppositories cause a higher incidence of adverse effects (due to erratic absorption); use with caution. **CONTRAINDICATIONS:** Hypersensitivity to theophylline, caffeine or theobromine.

DRUG	DOSAGE	DOSE FORMS	REMARKS
AMINOPHYLLINE anhydrous (theophylline with ethylenediamine)	See GROUP REMARKS.	PO (Liquid): 21 mg/ml (18 mg/ml anhydrous theophylline) Generic powder	Aminophylline is theophylline (79%) plus ethylenediamine. **RECOMMENDATIONS:** IV administration by SLOW injection only (< 25 mg/min); rapid infusion can result in FATAL arrhythmias and/or convulsions, watch for signs of cardiovascular or central nervous system distress. Do NOT administer IM; severe tissue irritation may result. **CONTRAINDICATIONS:** Hypersensitivity to ethylenediamine.
AMINOPHYLLINE dihydrate (Aminodur) (Aminophyllin)	See GROUP REMARKS.	PO (Tab's): 100, 200 mg (79, 158 mg anhydrous theophylline) Ext'd Rel: 225, 300 mg (178, 237 mg anhydrous theophylline) PO (Liquid): 16.6 mg/ml (13.1 mg/ml anhydrous theophylline) Injection: 25 mg/ml (19.7 mg/ml anhydrous theophylline) Rectal: 250, 500 mg (197, 394 mg anhydrous theophylline)	

XANTHINES *Continued*

DRUG	DOSAGE	DOSE FORMS	REMARKS
THEOPHYLLINE Anhydrous (Theo-Dur) (Bronkodyl) (Aquaphyllin) (Slo-Phyllin) (Sprinkle) (Asmalix) (Elixophyllin) (Respbid) (Sustaire) (Accurbron)	See GROUP REMARKS.	PO (Tab's): 100, 125, 200, 225, 250, 300 mg Ext'd Rel Tab's: 100, 200, 250, 300, 500 mg PO (Cap's): 50, 100, 200, 250 mg Ext'd Rel Cap's: 50, 60, 75, 100, 125, 200, 250, 300 mg PO (Liquid): 5.4, 7.5, 10, 10.7 mg/ml (in 5 ml) Generic powder	See GROUP REMARKS.
THEOPHYLLINE Sodium Glycinate (Synophylate)	See GROUP REMARKS.	PO (Tab's): 330 mg (151.5 mg anhydrous theophylline) Injection: 22 mg/ml (10.1 mg/ml anhydrous theophylline)	
THEOPHYLLINE Monohydrate	See GROUP REMARKS.	Generic powder	
DYPHYLLINE (Lufyllin) (Dilor) (Neothyllin) (Dyflex) (Asminyl) (Dilin) (Droxine)	**Bronchodilation**: **PO**: 15 mg/kg q6h. **Acute Bronchospasm**: **IM**: 250-500 mg injected SLOWLY (maximum 15 mg/kg q6h).	PO (Tab's): 200, 400 mg PO (Liquid): 6.6, 10.6, 20 mg/ml Injection: 250 mg/ml	Dyphylline is a chemical derivative of theophylline with similar pharmacological profile; it is NOT metabolized to theophylline. Dosage NOT determined by theophylline "equivalent." Possibly less efficacious than theophylline and with fewer side effects. Can NOT monitor therapy by theophylline serum levels. Do NOT administer IV.

PARASYMPATHOMIMETICS

GROUP REMARKS: Drugs of this class are either 1) **Choline Esters** that act directly on effectors to mimic the effects of acetylcholine OR 2) **Cholinesterase Inhibitors** which allow the accumulation of acetylcholine at those sites where it is physiologically released. As a result, stimulation of non-vascular smooth muscle (increased propulsive activity of the GI tract, urinary bladder contraction, bronchiolar constriction, decreased pupillary size and accommodation of the eye for near vision) and exocrine glands (increased salivation, lacrimation, perspiration and respiratory tract secretion) occurs. Choline esters have mixed vasodilating (muscarinic) and vasoconstricting (nicotinic) effects. Cholinesterase inhibitors are vasoconstictors. Note: The organophosphate (OP) and carbamate types of insecticides are cholinesterase inhibitors.

INDICATIONS:

Choline Esters and Cholinesterase Inhibitors:

1) Stimulate redevelopment of normal tone and motility in the GI tract and urinary bladder following surgery.
2) Constrict the pupil to relieve intraocular pressure (see Ophthalmic Agents).
3) Facilitate the conversion of Paroxysmal Atrial Tachycardia by accentuating vagal effort.

Cholinesterase Inhibitors ONLY:

4) Reverse the non-depolarizing neuromuscular blockade produced by curariform agents (curare alkaloids) following surgery.
5) Treatment, and as a diagnostic test, for Myasthenia Gravis.

SIDE EFFECTS: Signs of cholinergic stimulation: vomiting, diarrhea, abdominal cramps, sweating, salivation, lacrimation, blurred distant vision, urinary urgency/incontinence. Cardiovascular effects: choline esters cause flushing and a mixed vasodilatation and vasoconstriction, cholinesterase inhibitors cause only vasoconstriction (nicotinic or ganglionic effect) and a rise in blood pressure; both slow the pulse. Cholinesterase inhibitor effects on voluntary muscle: fasciculations, cramping, weakness (including muscles of respiration). **RECOMMENDATIONS**: When cholinesterase inhibitors are used for treatment of Myasthenia Gravis, injectable atropine should be readily available during initial dosing of a new patient; some patients are over-reactive and may develop a cholinergic crisis. **CONTRAINDICATIONS**: Should NOT be used in the presence of mechanical obstruction of the GI or urinary tracts. AVOID use in abdominal/GI inflammatory diseases.

DRUG	INDICATIONS & DOSAGE	DOSE FORMS	REMARKS
CHOLINE ESTER			
BETHANECHOL (Urecholine) (Duvoid) (Vesicholine)	**Urine Retention (Post-operative)**: **PO**: 10-50 mg q6-12h. **SC**: 2.5-5 mg initially, repeat minimum effective dose tid-qid PRN. **Detrusor Hypotonia**: **PO**: 50 mg bid-qid.	PO (Tab's): 5, 10, 25, 50 mg Injection: 5 mg/ml	Bethanechol is the only direct-acting parasympathomimetic used systemically to any significant extent. **SIDE EFFECTS**: With PO administration, only minor effects occur on the cardiovascular system and negligible effects on voluntary muscle. **CONTRAINDICATIONS**: IV or IM use is contraindicated. Others: hyperthyroidism, peptic ulcer, asthma, coronary artery or cardiovascular disease.
CHOLINESTERASE INHIBITORS			
NEOSTIGMINE (Prostigmin) *Continued, next page*	**Urine Retention (Post-operative)**: **IM, SC**: 0.25 mg q4-6h for 2-3 d. **Acute Urine Retention**: **IM, SC**: 0.5 mg initially; repeat q3h for treatment. *Continued, next page*	PO (Tab's): 15 mg; generic powder (bromide) Injection: 0.25, 0.5, 1.0 mg/ml; generic powder (methylsulfate)	Neostigmine is a quaternary ammonium cholinesterase inhibitor. **SIDE EFFECTS**: Careful dosage adjustment can minimize side effects. Overdosage: CNS stimulation then depression, depolarization-type neuromuscular blockade producing respiratory depression/paralysis. **RECOMMEN-** *Continued, next page*

DRUG	INDICATIONS & DOSAGE	DOSE FORMS	REMARKS
NEOSTIGMINE *Continued*	**Reversal of Non-Depolarizing Neuromuscular Blockade**: **IV**: 0.5-2 mg SLOWLY (maximum 5 mg) + atropine; observe closely. **Myasthenia Gravis Symptoms**: **PO**: 15 mg q8h initially; increase gradually until maximal response, maintenance doses range 15-375 mg/d. **IM, IV, SC**: 0.5-2.5 mg PRN (+ atropine).	See previous page.	**DATIONS**: For existing post-operative urine retention, patient should be catheterized if no response within 1 h of initial dose. Atropine (IV: 0.6-1.2 mg) should be added when high parenteral doses of neostigmine are administered; muscarinic side effects are lessened, but transient arrhythmias may result. Injectable atropine should be readily available during initial dosing of a new patient; some patients are over-reactive and may develop a cholinergic crisis. **CAUTIONS**: Use cautiously in: epilepsy, asthma, arrhythmias, recent coronary occlusion, hyperthyroidism or peptic ulcer. Avoid large PO doses if megacolon, decreased GI motility; neostigmine may accumulate without being absorbed initially. **CONTRAINDICATIONS**: History of hypersensitivity to neostigmine or bromides (for bromide salt).
EDROPHONIUM (Tensilon)	**Reversal of Non-Depolarizing Neuromuscular Blockade**: **IV**: 10 mg given over 1 min, repeat q5-10min PRN (maximum 40 mg); + atropine, observe closely. **Myasthenia Gravis - Diagnosis**: **IV**: 2 mg initially; then 8 mg at 45 sec, if no response to initial dose (if a cholinergic reaction occurs to initial dose, discontinue test and administer atropine IV: 0.4-0.5 mg). Test may be repeated after 30 min if necessary. **Pediatric IV**: 1 mg initially if weight ≤ 34 kg, 2 mg if > 34 kg; then 1 mg q30-45sec (maximum 5 mg if ≤ 34 kg, 10 mg if > 34 kg). **IM**: 10 mg (if a cholinergic reaction occurs, 2 mg at 30 min to verify). **Pediatric IM**: 2 mg if weight ≤ 34 kg, 5 mg if > 34 kg. Other cholinesterase medications should be withdrawn 8h prior to the diagnostic test. **Myasthenia Gravis - Treatment Evaluation**: **IV**: 1-2 mg administered 1 h following last oral medication (if patient is apneic, establish controlled ventilation prior to test). Response assessment: — Myasthenic / Therapeutic / Cholinergic Crisis Muscle strength: increased / no change / decreased Fasciculations: none / occur/none / occur/none Side effects: none / minimal / severe	Injection: 10 mg/ml	Edrophonium is a rapidly reversible cholinesterase inhibitor with a significant direct cholinomimetic action on voluntary muscle. Onset and duration of action are much shorter than with Neostigmine: when administered IV, onset = 30-60 sec, duration = 5-10 min; when administered IM, onset = 2-10 min, duration = 5-30 min. **SIDE EFFECTS**: Side effects are uncommon and transient. Overdosage: CNS stimulation then depression, depolarization-type neuromuscular blockade producing respiratory depression/paralysis. **RECOMMENDATIONS**: Atropine (IV: 0.6-1.2 mg) should be added when high parenteral doses are administered.

INJECTABLE LOCAL ANESTHETICS

GROUP REMARKS: Local anesthetics (LAs) are applied topically or by injection to block nerve conduction from a painful area or one that will be subjected to a procedure. When a nerve or spinal root is anesthetized, conduction along all types of nerve fibers is blocked; pain perception and autonomic functions are blocked, and motor paralysis is produced. In general, nerve function is lost according to the order: pain, temperature, touch, vasomotor, proprioception and muscle tone. **SIDE EFFECTS**: **Dose-Related**: LAs can stimulate the CNS, producing: dizziness, excitement, respiratory stimulation, bradycardia, hypertension, anxiety, tremor, twitching, convulsions. CNS depression may supplant stimulation, resulting in: hypotension, respiratory depression and coma (unresponsive to treatment if due to hypoxic brain damage). All LAs can produce quinidine-like effects on the heart, resulting in arrhythmias. **Allergic reactions**: Frequent dermal use may produce topical sensitization. Other allergic reactions are very rare. **Common "faint"**: The intense anxiety often experienced during injection of LAs may occasionally be followed by a vasovagal syncope, which is harmless provided the patient is kept supine. **NOTES**: LAs are weak bases, that are usually dispensed and injected as acidic solutions of the water soluble hydrochloride (or other) salt. In the slightly alkaline environment after injection, more will exist as the uncharged free base which is lipid soluble and readily penetrates nerve membranes. LAs are rapidly absorbed from mucosal surfaces (toxic blood levels can be reached with relative ease); restrict total mucosal or injectable dose. Adjunctive epinephrine (1:250,000) produces local vasoconstriction which slows absorption, reduces toxicity and prolongs duration. Because the amount of epinephrine present is so small, LAs with 1:200,000 epinephrine may be used in angina patients for whom epinephrine is normally contraindicated, especially if the injection is slow. Topical LAs have no effectiveness on intact skin. Potency and potential for systemic toxicity vary together between different agents. Differences in "time to onset" are rarely important clinically; "duration" is roughly the same for all except dibucaine (which should be used only topically or under special conditions, because of toxicity). **RECOMMENDATIONS**: In a patient allergic to a LA of either chemical class (ester or amide), substitute an agent of the other class. Resuscitative equipment should be available whenever LAs are used. Administer oxygen between convulsions if accidental overdosage produces CNS stimulation; do NOT administer a CNS depressant. Use the lowest effective dose (concentration and volume). In general, decrease normal dose for children, the elderly or debilitated patients. Wait a few minutes between subsequent injections to markedly decrease the danger of adverse reactions. **CAUTIONS**: Avoid accidental (and potentially dangerous) IV injection by aspirating for blood each time the needle is moved during infiltrative anesthesia. **CONTRAINDICATIONS**: Do NOT inject into an infected area. Vasocontrictors should NOT be used in the fingers, toes, ears, nose or penis.

DRUG	ANESTHETIC CONCENTRATION	DOSE FORMS	REMARKS
	INJECTABLE AMIDES		
LIDOCAINE (Xylocaine)	**Infiltration**: 0.5-1% **Peripheral Nerve Block**: 1-2%	Injection: 0.5, 1, 2, 4% (with Epi): 1:100,000; 1:200,000	Most commonly used local anesthetic. High diffusability produces rapid onset and greater dependability when injected distant from the site. Maximal single dose = 4.5 mg/kg (300 mg in adults) lidocaine alone or 7 mg/kg (500 mg in adults) with Epi. For antiarrhythmic use see "Antiarrhythmics."
PRILOCAINE (Citanest)	**Infiltration**: 4% **Peripheral Nerve Block**: 4%	Injection: 1, 2, 3, 4%	Produces less vasodilation than lidocaine. May produce methemoglobinemia, especially at doses > 600 mg. Maximal single dose = 8 mg/kg (600 mg in adults); 400 mg in debilitated patients. Can repeat single dose only at ≥ 2 h. Approved for dental use. NOT to be used for spinal anesthesia.

INJECTABLE LOCAL ANESTHETICS: INJECTABLE AMIDES *Continued*

DRUG	ANESTHETIC CONCENTRATION	DOSE FORMS	REMARKS
MEPIVACAINE (Carbocaine)	Infiltration: 1% Peripheral Nerve Block: 1-2%	Injection: 1, 1.5, 2, 3%	Slightly less potent than procaine or lidocaine. Maximal single dose = 300 mg in adults; 5-6 mg/kg in children. Repeat interval ≥ 1.5 h. Total dose ≤ 1000 mg/d. Approved for dental use. NOT to be used for spinal anesthesia.
DIBUCAINE (Nupercaine)		Injection: 1:200**, 1:1500 Injection (Heavy): 2.5 mg/ml in 5% dextrose	Extended duration of action, but also much greater systemic toxicity than other LAs. Use in spinal anesthesia reserved only for special cases (mostly obstetric); see below for topical use. **1:200 preparation to be diluted with equal volume spinal fluid.
BUPIVACAINE (Marcaine)	Infiltration: 0.25% Peripheral Nerve Block: 0.25-0.5%	Injection: 0.25, 0.5, 0.75% (with Epi): 1:200,000	Lowest potential of all local anesthetics to cross placenta. Should NOT be used in children. Maximum dose: 400 mg/d.
ETIDIOCAINE (Duranest)	Infiltration: 0.5% Peripheral Nerve Block: 0.5-1%	Injection: 1, 1.5% (with Epi) 1:200,000	Efficacy similar to that of bupivacaine. Usual optimum dose = 225-300 mg; maximum dose 4 mg/kg (300 mg), 5.5 mg/kg (400 mg) with Epi.
INJECTABLE ESTERS			
PROCAINE (Novocaine)	Infiltration: 0.25-0.5% Peripheral Nerve Block: 0.5-2%	Injection: 1, 2, 10%	Once the prototype local anesthetic, now largely replaced by lidocaine.
CHLOROPROCAINE (Nesacaine)	Infiltration: 1-2% Peripheral Nerve Block: 1-2%	Injection: 1, 2, 3%	Maximum dose = 800 mg; 1000 mg with Epi.
TETRACAINE (Pontocaine)		Injection: 0.2, 0.3, 1% Injection: 20 mg	Long duration of action. More toxic than lidocaine. Used primarily for spinal anesthesia.
PROPOXYCAINE (Ravocaine)	Infiltration: 4% Peripheral Nerve Block: 4%	Injection: 0.4% (with procaine 2% and vasocontrictor)	Marketed in combination with 2% procaine and levonordefrin (1:20,000), a vasoconstrictor. Duration of action longer than with procaine. Primarily for dental use.

Section 4: ENDOCRINE AGENTS
Table of Contents

INSULINS

GROUP REMARKS: Injection of crystalline insulin protein (regular or "clean" insulin) produces an immediate (within 20min) hypoglycemic effect that is dissipated before the next meal (4 h). To eliminate the need for 3-4 injections/d, the solubility of insulin is reduced by combination with protamine or zinc, to extend its effect. Protamine zinc insulin [PZI] (and ultralente insulin) is absorbed over a period > 24 h. Isophane insulin (NPH) is equivalent to a 2:1 mixture of regular and PZI; it has a shorter period of absorption and acts less intensely during the overnight fast. Inuslin has, until recently, been extracted from porcine, bovine or mixed pancreas. Human insulin, synthesized by E. coli cells modified by recombinant DNA, is now also available. ("Genetically-engineered" insulin is indicated by "[prb]".) "Purified" insulins refer to insulins with proinsulin concentrations of < 10 ppm. **SIDE EFFECTS**: Insulin in excess of the amount dictated by the glucose level produces effects due to hypoglycemia and to the release of large amounts of epinephrine: fatigue, confusion, weakness, hungar, tremulousness, sweating, pallor, paresthesias, hypokalemia, agitation, convulsions, coma. Lipodystrophy (SC fibrosis and atrophy) may occur at injection site. Systemic allergic reactions (rarely urticaria) may occur. **RECOMMENDATIONS**: Rotate administration sites to prevent or diminish lipodystrophy. The distribution of calories among the meals and the time of injection must be held relatively constant. Use freehand mixtures of regular with PZI or lente insulins within 5 min.

DRUG INTERACTIONS:
Patients taking ***cardiac glycosides*** may experience LETHAL arrhythmias if **insulin** or diabetes causes potassium levels to drop significantly. ***Thiazide diuretics*** may elevate blood glucose levels. Exaggerated lowering of blood sugar may occur with concomitant administration of ***tetracycline, alcohol, sulfinpyrazone, MAO Inhibitors***, and ***phenylbutazone***. Some symptoms of hypoglycemia may be masked by ***beta-adrenergic blocking agents***. **Insulin** requirements may be increased by concomitant adminstration of ***oral contraceptives, thyroid hormone, corticosteroids, dobutamine***, and by smoking.

DOSES:
The dosage of insulin depends on the severity of diabetes. Insulin requirements may be increased by stress, illness, infections, trauma, exercise and pregnancy; may be decreased by hepatic or renal dysfunction. Usual route of administration is SC, but regular insulin is administered IV or IM in diabetic coma, hyperosmolar state, severe ketoacidosis and post-surgical or other states where diet is interrupted.

Notes to Tables:
The time periods listed here as duration of action and peak effect should be considered as guidelines only. rH = human, recombinant, sH = semisynthetic human, B = beef, pB = purified beef, P = pork, pP = purified pork.

PHARMACOKINETICS OF INSULIN PREPARATIONS:

	ONSET (hours)	PEAK (hours)	DURATION (hours)
Fast-Acting			
Insulin Injection	0.5-1	2-3	5-7
Insulin Zinc Suspension, Prompt	0.5-1.5	4-7	12-16
Intermediate-Acting			
Isophane (NPH)	1-1.5	4-12	18-24
Insulin Zinc Suspension	1-2.5	6-12	18-24
Long-Acting			
Protamine Insulin Zinc (PZI)	4-8	14-20	36
Insulin Zinc Suspension, Extended	4-8	12-25	>36

FAST-ACTING INSULINS

Regular insulin may be required for adequate control of some diabetics; the same dose is given 20 min before each meal and a fourth, smaller dose at bedtime. Calories are distributed 1/3, 1/3, 1/3 plus an hs snack. Regular insulin may also be used PRN post-operatively and in other situations where caloric intake may be irregular.

INDICATIONS AND DOSES:
Specific dosing information is presented for Regular Insulin.

Diabetic Ketoacidosis (Low-dose Method):
IV: 0.1 units/kg (regular insulin) IV push initially; then 0.1 units/kg/h continuous infusion. Decrease to 0.05-0.07 units/kg/h if rate of fall of serum glucose > 100 mg/dl/h. Increase to 0.14-0.20 units/kg/h if rate of fall of serum glucose < 50 mg/dl/h. Change to SC sliding scale regular insulin q4-6h when serum glucose falls to 250-300 mg/dl, blood pH is above 7.30, and ketosis has cleared. Continuous infusion at 0.02-0.06 units/kg/h may be continued along with 5% glucose infusion until the following morning, when oral feedings and SC insulin doses are initiated.

INDICATIONS AND DOSES *Continued*:

Diabetic Ketoacidosis (Conventional Method):

IV: 0.5-2 units/kg initially (1/2 may be given SC); then, 0.25-1 unit/kg q12h or 0.5-2 units/kg q4-6h until glucose < 300 mg/dl, acidosis is improving, and ketosis is clearing. Then use SC sliding scale regular insulin q4-6h for the next 12-36h before changing to intermediate-acting insulin preparation. During the acute phase, do NOT allow the serum glucose to fall > 100 mg/dl/h.

Hyperkalemia:

IV: Administer calcium gluconate and sodium bicarbonate initially; then 0.5-1 ml/kg of 50% dextrose and insulin at 1 unit/q4-5gm of glucose given (1 unit/q8-10 ml of D50W).

INSULIN INJECTION ("Regular", "Clear")

Trade Name	Type	Form (units/ml)
Humulin R	rH	100
Iletin II Regular Beef	pB	100
Iletin II Regular Pork	pP	100
Novolin R	sH	100
Regular Iletin I	B&P	40, 100
Regular Insulin	P	100
Velosulin Human	sH	100
Velosulin Porcine	pP	100

INSULIN ZINC SUSPENSION, PROMPT

Trade Name	Type	Form (units/ml)
Iletin I Semilente	B&P	40, 100
Semilente Insulin	B	100
Semilente Purified	pP	100

INTERMEDIATE-ACTING INSULINS

Control of the diabetic state with a single injection per day is often achieved in patients not controlled by diet or oral hypoglycemics and with an insulin requirement too great to allow the use of PZI or other long-acting insulins. Injection is given before breakfast and caloric intake is distributed 1/5, 2/5, 2/5 plus an hs snack.

ISOPHANE, Insulin Suspension (NPH, Neutral Protamine Hagedorn)

Trade Name	Type	Form (units/ml)
Beef NPH Iletin II	pB	100
Humulin N	rH	100
Insulatard NPH Human	sH	100
Insulatard NPH Porcine	pP	100
Mixtard	pP	100
Novolin 30/70	sH	100
Novolin N	sH	100
NPH Iletin I	B&P	40, 100
NPH Insulin	B	100
NPH Purified Pork	pP	100
Pork NPH Iletin II	pP	100

INSULIN ZINC SUSPENSION

Trade Name	Type	Form (units/ml)
Humulin L	rH	100
Lente Iletin I	B&P	40, 100
Lente Iletin II Beef	pB	100
Lente Iletin II Pork	pP	100
Lente Insulin	B	100
Lente Purified Pork Insulin	pP	100
Novolin L	sH	100

LONG-ACTING INSULINS

Depot insulins can be used in diabetics whose insulin requirement is minimal. Because of long, even effect, any reactions will tend to occur in early AM hours (before waking) and coma may be superimposed on sleep without warning. Diet as for NPH insulins.

PROTAMINE INSULIN ZINC SUSPENSION (PZI)

Trade Name	Type	Form (units/ml)
Protamine, Zinc & Iletin I	B&P	40, 100
Protamine, Zinc & Iletin II Beef	pB	100
Protamine, Zinc & Iletin II Pork	pP	100

INSULIN ZINC SUSPENSION, EXTENDED

Trade Name	Type	Form (units/ml)
Ultralente Iletin I	B&P	40, 100
Ultralente Insulin	B	100
Ultralente Purified Beef	pB	100

ORAL ANTIDIABETIC AGENTS

GROUP REMARKS: The sulfonylureas are orally-active agents that lower blood sugar by stimulating the release of insulin from pancreatic beta cells. They are effective in maturity-onset (usually > 40 y.o.) diabetes in patients still able to synthesize some insulin in the pancreas (insulin requirment < 40 units/d). Other features characteristic of an acceptable therapeutic response include: duration of diabetes < 5 years, normal or overweight physique, serum glucose ≤ 200 mg% (fasting) and lack of ketoacidosis or liver/kidney disease. **SIDE EFFECTS**: Hypoglycemia (may be exacerbated by renal or hepatic insufficiency [via decreased drug elimination], malnutrition, adrenal or pituitary insufficiency, exercise, alcohol ingestion or with agents having longer half-lives, such as chloropropamide). Other side effects: elevated LFTs, cholestatic jaundice, aggravation of hepatic porphyria, proctocolitis, weakness, dizziness, jaundice and malaise. Rarely: diarrhea, headache, elevation of BUN and creatinine, SIADH (associated with chloropropamide) is noted. Hypersensitivity reactions include urticaria, rash, bone marrow depression (leukopenia, thrombocytopenia, anemia), erythema multiforme, low-grade fever, eosinophilia. **RECOMMENDATIONS**: Insulin therapy is usually required when complications appear in diabetes initially controlled by sulfonylureas. Discontinue glipizide 1 month prior to delivery. Discontinue use of all others > 48h prior to delivery to avoid fetal hypoglycemia. **CAUTIONS**: In one study, patients on tolbutamide (1.5 gm/d) exhibited a relative risk of 2.5 for cardiovascular mortality; total mortality was NOT affected. Chlorpropamide and tolbutamide are excreted into breast milk. Safety of sulfonylureas in children has not been established. **CONTRAINDICATIONS**: Hypersensitivity to sulfonylureas (or other "sulfas"), complications of diabetes, thyroid disease, liver disease, renal impairment, uremia, glycosuria associated with renal disease, pregnancy (sulfonylureas are teratogenic in animal studies).

DRUG INTERACTIONS:
Sulfonylureas (induce liver enzymes; enhance metabolism of many other drugs); ***digitoxin*** half-life decreased. Drugs which may **enhance** the action of **sulfonylureas** (may cause hypoglycemia): ***insulin, dicumarol, NSAID agents, MAO inhibitors, chloremphenicol, sulfonamides, salicilates, sulfinpyrazone, probenecid, chlofibrate, fenfluramine, phenylbutazone***. Drugs which may **interfere** with **sulfonylureas** (may produce hyperglycemia and loss of diabetic control): ***birth control pills, estrogens, thyroid agents, phenytoin, calcium-channel blockers, isoniazid, sympathomimetics, thiazide diuretics***.

DRUG	DOSAGE	DOSE FORMS	REMARKS
TOLBUTAMIDE (Orinase) (Oramide)	**PO**: 1-2 gm/d in 1-2 doses (maximum 2 gm/d).	PO (Tab's): 250, 500 mg	Administer q12h to minimize gastric irritation. Generic preparations are available.
ACETOHEXAMIDE (Dymelor)	**PO**: 250-1500 mg/d in 1-2 doses (q12h dosing if > 1gm/d); maximum 1.5 gm/d.	PO (Tab's): 250, 500 mg	Generic preparations are available.
TOLAZAMIDE (Ronase) (Tolinase)	**PO**: Initial dose: 100 mg/d if fasting blood sugar < 200 mg%; 250 mg/d if fasting blood sugar > 200 mg% (maximum 1000 mg/d). Dose q12h if > 500 mg/d.	PO (Tab's): 100, 250, 500 mg	Generic preparations are available.
CHLORPROPAMIDE (Diabinese) (Glucamide)	**PO**: 250 mg/d initially; then 100-500 mg/d (maximum 750 mg/d).	PO (Tab's): 100, 250 mg	Generic preparations are available. Start with 250 mg/d in stable diabetics with mild to moderate disease and 100-125 mg/d in older patients.
GLYBURIDE (DiaBeta) (Micronase)	**PO**: 1.25-5 mg/d at breakfast initially, then 1.25-20 mg/d. Increase in increments of 2.5 mg/week while monitoring response (maximum 20 mg/d).	PO (Tab's): 1.25, 2.5, 5 mg	
GLIPIZIDE (Glucotrol)	**PO**: 2.5-5 mg before breakfast initially, then increase by 2.5-5 mg/d increments as determined by blood glucose response (maximum 15 mg/dose and 40 mg/d); dose q12h if > 15 mg/d.	PO (Tab's): 2.5, 5, 10 mg	Some patients will show better glucose control with bid dosing.

ANTI-INFLAMMATORY STEROIDS

GROUP REMARKS: The adrenal cortex normally secretes a number of steroids; the two major types are glucocorticoids, which regulate intermediary metabolism, and mineralocorticoids, which regulate salt retention by the kidney. Steroids with androgenic or estrogenic activity (depending on sex) are a third major class. Both natural and synthetic glucocorticoids are used to treat a number of inflammatory, allergic and some immunologic disorders. Adrenocortical deficiency states are also treated with these agents. Abrupt discontinuence following prolonged therapy may produce withdrawal: nausea, fatigue, cyspnea, hypotension, muscle/joint pain (taper discontinuance). **SIDE EFFECTS**: Adrenal suppression: degree of suppression is related to dose and length of steroid therapy; it is reversible, but may require months; ACTH does NOT suppress the adrenal cortex. Iatrogenic Cushing's syndrome: fat deposition at the trunk and face; growth of fine hair on trunk, thighs and face; weight gain; muscle wasting; thinning of the skin leading to bruising and striae; hyperglycemia; development of osteoporosis and diabetes with chronic therapy. Others: nausea; dizziness; peptic ulcer; cataracts; glaucoma; intracranial hypertension (benign); rare myopathy (more common with triamcinolone). Steroids with significant mineralocorticoid activity cause sodium and fluid retention and potassium loss; they may produce a hypokalemic/hypochloremic acidosis and hypertension; they rarely precipitate CHF. Large doses may induce psychosis. Growth retardation occurs in children receiving > 45 $mg/m^2/d$. Steroids may mask signs of other disorders, especially bacterial or mycotic infections.

DOSING: Use dose equivalents to guide relative dosing, depending on severity of condition. Example doses are given for prednisone:

Chronic PO Administration:
Prednisone: 10 mg q2d - 60 mg/d (q2d dosing minimizes adrenal atrophy).

Acute PO Therapy with Rapid Tapering:
Prednisone: 30-40 mg/d for 1d; then decrease 5-10 mg each day (i.e., 40 mg on day 1, 35 mg on day 2, 30 mg on day 3, etc.)

IV Use:
Prednisone: 0.5-1 mg/kg q6h.
Reserve for pre-/post- operative status, convulsive states, status asthmaticus.

Adrenal Replacement:
Use prednisone or similar steroid, add small doses of a mineralocorticoid for sodium retention.

Relative activities are given below for these agents' anti-inflammatory (systemic and topical) and salt-retaining potencies; equivalent doses are also given.

	Anti-Inflammatory Activity	Salt Retention	Topical Potency	Equivalent Oral Dose
SHORT-ACTING GLUCOCORTICOIDS: Biologic half-life = 8-12h.				
HYDROCORTISONE (Cortisol)	1	1	1	20 mg
PREDNISONE	4	0.3	none	5 mg
PREDNISOLONE	5	0.3	4	5 mg
METHYL-PREDNISOLONE	5	none	5	4 mg
MEPREDNISONE	5	none		4 mg
INTERMEDIATE-ACTING GLUCOCORTICOIDS: Biologic half-life = 18-36h.				
TRIAMCINOLONE	5	none	5	4 mg
PARAMETHASONE	10	none		2 mg
FLUPREDNISONE	15	none	7	1.5 mg
LONG-ACTING GLUCOCORTICOIDS: Biologic half-life = 36-54h.				
BETAMETHASONE	25-40	none	10	0.6 mg
DEXAMETHASONE	30	none	10	0.75 mg
MINERALOCORTICOIDS:				
FLUDROCORTISONE	10	250	10	2 mg
DESOXY-CORTICOSTERONE	none	20	none	

ESTROGENS

GROUP REMARKS: INDICATIONS: Estrogens are used: 1) as a component of **oral contraceptives**, 2) for treatment of **symptoms at menopause**, 3) during post-menopausal period to **prevent osteoporosis**, 4) for **atrophic vaginitis** and 5) to antagonize androgenic effects during **cancer of the prostate**. Equipotent doses: estradiol = 50 µg; diethylstilbesterol = 1 mg; mestranol = 80 µg; conjugated estrogens = 5 mg. **SIDE EFFECTS:** Nausea, vomiting ("morning sickness"), cramps. Sodium retention with elevated blood pressure, edema and headache. Endometrial hyperplasia, amenorrhea, irregular vaginal bleeding, endometrial carcinoma (absent progestin effect). Feminization (maturation), anabolic effects, but with epiphyseal closure. Abnormal LFTs, hepatic adenoma. Hypercalcemia in presense of bony metastases. Increased incidence of gall bladder disease. Breast tenderness and enlargement. Interferes with thyroid function tests. Altered glucose and insulin tolerance. See also adverse effects of Oral Contraceptives. **CAUTIONS:** Give cyclically (first 21 d of each month) or add progestin at intervals to produce withdrawal bleeding to reduce risk of endometrial cancer. Lower doses may be needed in presence of liver disease (inactivated primarily in the liver). **RECOMMENDATIONS:** Use the largest dose possible. In diabetics, monitor blood sugars and therapeutic needs closely when beginning estrogen therapy. Estrogen effectiveness for palliation of prostatic cancer can be evaluate by alkaline phosphatase determinations as well as by improvement in symptoms. **CONTRAINDICATIONS:** Active thrombophlebitis, thrombosis and thromboembolic disorders or history of same related to estrogen use. Pregnancy; limb defects and vaginal adenoma in daughters if given during first trimester. Hypersensitivity to estrogens, abnormal uterine bleeding (undiagnosed), breast cancer (except when used for treatment in selected patients) and estrogen-dependent neoplasia.

DRUG INTERACTIONS:
Drugs which may lower **estrogen** levels: ***barbiturates, primidone, phenytoin, carbamazepine*** and ***rifampin***. **Estrogens** may potentiate toxicity of ***tricyclic antidepressants***, reduce the effect of ***oral anticoagulants*** (monitor prothrombin times very closely when beginning estrogen therapy), and increase the need for ***insulin*** in diabetics. ***Antibiotics*** may inhibit gastrointestinal **estrogen** absorption.

DRUG	INDICATIONS & DOSAGE	DOSE FORMS	REMARKS
ESTRONE Various	**Menopausal Symptoms, Atrophic Vaginitis and Related Conditions**: **IM**: 0.1-0.5 mg 12-3 times/wk. **Post-Menopausal Estrogen Replacement**: **IM**: 0.1-1 mg/wk given as a single dose or divided (maximum 2 mg/wk). **Prostatic Cancer**: **IM**: 2-4 mg given 2-3 times/wk.	Injection: 2, 5 mg/ml (10, 30 ml)	Group Remarks.
ESTRADIOL (Estrace) Generics	**Menopausal Symptoms, Atrophic Vaginitis & Related Conditions, Post-Menopausal Estrogen Replacement**: **PO**: 1-2 mg/d initially. Cyclic therapy recommended: 3 wk of treatment, followed by 1 wk off. **Prostatic Cancer**: **PO**: 1-2 mg tid. **Breast Cancer (appropriately selected patients)**: **PO**: 10 mg tid for > 3 months.	PO (Tab's): 1, 2 mg	Group Remarks. Also available as a transdermal patch delivery system: 10 cm^2 delivers 0.05 mg/d (4 mg total), 20 cm^2 delivers 0.1 mg/d (8 mg total). Apply cyclically (3 wk on, 1 wk off). Do NOT apply to breasts. Start with smallest patch and adjust PRN.

ESTROGENS *Continued*

DRUG	INDICATIONS & DOSAGE	DOSE FORMS	REMARKS
ESTRADIOL CYPIONATE (DEPOT FORMS) Various	**Menopausal Symptoms**: **IM**: 1-5 mg q3-4wks. **Post-Menopausal Estrogen Replacement**: **IM**: 1.5-2 mg q4wks.	Injection: 1, 5 mg/ml (5 & 10 ml)	Group Remarks.
ESTRADIOL VALERATE (DEPOT FORMS) Various	**Menopausal Symptoms, Atrophic Vaginitis & Related Conditions, Post-Menopausal Estrogen Replacement**: **IM**: 10-20 mg q4wks. **Prevention of Postpartum Breast Enlargement**: **IM**: 10-25 mg in a single dose at the end of the first stage of labor. **Prostatic Cancer**: **IM**: 30 mg q1-2wks.	Injection: 10, 20, 40 mg/ml (5,10 ml)	Group Remarks.
CONJUGATED ESTROGENS (Conjugated Estrogens, primarily estrone sulfate) (Premarin) (Estrocon) (Progens) (Premarin Intravenous)	**Menopausal Symptoms**: **PO**: 1.25 mg/d initially. Start on day 5 of menstrual cycle. **Atrophic Vaginitis & Related Conditions**: **PO**: 0.3-1.25 mg/d; adjust PRN. **Female Hypogonadism**: **PO**: 2.5-7.5 mg/d in 3-4 doses for 20 d, followed by 10 d off drug at the end of which bleeding should occur. If bleeding does NOT occur, repeat cycle. If bleeding occurs prior to 10 d, initiate a 20 d combined estrogen-progestin cycle. **Post-Menopausal Estrogen Replacement**: **PO**: 1.25 mg/d initially. Cyclic therapy recommended: 3 wk of treatment, followed by 1 wk off drug. **Breast Cancer (appropriately selected patients)**: **PO**: 10 mg tid for > 3 months. **Prostatic Cancer**: **PO**: 1.25-2.5 mg tid. **Prevention of Postpartum Breast Enlargement**: **PO**: 3.75 mg q4h for 5 doses (alternate schedule: 1.25 mg q4h for 5 d). **Abnormal Uterine Bleeding**: **IM, IV**: 25 mg; repeat (once only) at 6-12 h PRN.	PO (Tab's): 0.3, 0.625, 0.9, 1.25, 2.5 mg. Injection: 5 mg/ml (in 5 ml vial for reconstitution)	Group Remarks.

ESTROGENS *Continued*

DRUG	INDICATIONS & DOSAGE	DOSE FORMS	REMARKS
ESTERIFIED ESTROGENS (Estratab) (Menest)	**Menopausal Symptoms, Atrophic Vaginitis & Related Conditions**: **PO**: 0.3-1.25 mg/d initially. Cyclic therapy recommended: 3 wk of treatment, followed by 1 wk off drug. **Female Hypogonadism**: **PO**: 2.5-7.5 mg/d in 3-4 doses for 20 d, followed by 10 d off drug at the end of which bleeding should occur. If bleeding does NOT occur, repeat cycle. If bleeding occurs prior to 10 d, initiate a 20 d combined estrogen-progestin cycle. **Post-Menopausal Estrogen Replacement**: **PO**: 2.5-7.5 mg/d in 3-4 doses for 20 d. During last 5 d, add an oral progestin. If bleeding occurs before schedule is complet-ed, discontinue therapy and restart on day 5 of bleeding.	PO (Tab's): 0.3, 0.625, 1.25, 2.5 mg. **Prostatic Cancer**: **PO**: 1.5-2.5 mg tid. **Breast Cancer (appropriately selected patients)**: **PO**: 10 mg tid for > 3 months.	Group Remarks.
ESTROPIPATE (PIPERAZINE ESTRONE SULFATE) (Ogen)	**Menopausal Symptoms, Atrophic Vaginitis & Related Conditions**: **PO**: 0.625-5 mg/d initially. Cyclic therapy recommended: 3 wk of treatment, followed by 1 wk off drug. **Post-Menopausal Estrogen Replacement**: **PO**: 1.25-7.5 mg/d for 3 wk, followed by 8-10 d off drug at the end of which bleeding may occur. If bleeding does not occur, repeat cycle. Give a progestin during the third week of the cycle if still unresponsive.	PO (Tab's): 0.625, 1.25, 2.5,5 mg	Group Remarks.
ETHINYL ESTRADIOL (Estinyl) (Feminone)	**Menopausal Symptoms**: **PO**: 0.02-0.05 mg/d cyclically. **Post-Menopausal Estrogen Replacement**: **PO**:0.02- 0.05 mg tid, taper upon clinical impreovement. Progestin may be added at mid-cycle. **Female Hypogonadism**: **PO**: 0.05 mg q8-24h during first 2wk of menstrual cycle, followed by progesterone during the last half of cycle. Continue 3-6 months, followed by 2 months without treat-ment, to see if cycle can be maintained without therapy.	PO (Tab's): 0.02, 0.05, 0.5 mg. **Female Breast Cancer (appropriately selected postmenopausal patients)**: **PO**: 1 mg tid. **Prostatic Cancer**: **PO**: 0.15-2 mg/d.	Group Remarks.

ESTROGENS *Continued*

DRUG	INDICATIONS & DOSAGE	DOSE FORMS	REMARKS
QUINESTROL (Estrovis)	<u>**Menopausal Symptoms, Atrophic Vaginitis & Related Conditions, Female Hypogonadism and Post-Menopausal Estrogen Replacement**</u>: **PO**: 100 µg/d for 7 d, followed by 100 µg/wk starting on day 14 of treatment (maximum maintenance dose: 200 µg/wk).	PO (Tab's): 100 µg	Group Remarks.
DIETHYLSTILBESTROL (DES)	<u>**Menopausal Symptoms**</u>: **PO**: 0.2-0.5 mg/d (cyclically). <u>**Atrophic Vaginitis & Related Conditions**</u>: **PO**: 0.2-2 mg/d (cyclically). Concomitant administration of DES in vaginal suppository form may hasten resolution of symptoms. Give 1 mg/d for 10-14 d at initiation of oral therapy. <u>**Prostatic Cancer**</u>: **PO**: 1-3 mg/d initially; tapered to 1 mg/d. <u>**Post-Coital Contraception (emergency treatment only)**</u>: **PO**: 25 mg bid for 5 d. Must initiate < 72 h after coitus.	Tablets: 0.25, 0.5, 1 & 5 mg	Group Remarks.
CHLOROTRIANISENE (Tace)	<u>**Menopausal Symptoms**</u>: **PO**: 12-25 mg/d (cyclically). <u>**Atrophic Vaginitis & Related Conditions**</u>: **PO**: 12-25 mg/d cyclically for 30-60 d. <u>**Female Hypogonadism**</u>: **PO**: 12-25 mg/d (cyclically). Progesterone IM 100 mg or an oral progestin may be given during last 5 d of therapy. Begin next cycle on day 5 of uterine bleeding. <u>**Prostatic Cancer**</u>: **PO**: 12-25 mg/d. <u>**Prevention of Postpartum Breast Enlargement**</u>: **PO**: 12 mg qid for 7 d (alternative schedule: 50 mg q6h for 6 doses or 75 mg bid for 2 d). For all schedules, give first dose within 8 h of delivery.	PO (Cap's): 12, 25, 72 mg	Combination forms with anti-anxiety agents in fixed proportions should NOT be used.

PROGESTINS

GROUP REMARKS: Progestins: act on the estrogen-primed uterus to lead to withdrawal bleeding; inhibit LH (luetinizing hormone) release which blocks follicle maturation and ovulation; inhibit uterin contraction; exhibit some androgenic and depressant activity. **SIDE EFFECTS**: Edema, hirsutism, masculinization of the female fetus, alopecia, depression, insomnia, hypersomnia, amenorrhea, withdrawal bleeding, cervical erosion, pyrexia, papilledema, retinal vascular lesions, decreased glucose tolerance in diabetic patients. **CAUTIONS**: Teratogenic (limb defects and others) during first 4 months of pregnancy. May precipitate acute intermittent porphyria or depression. Photosensitization may occur. **CONTRAINDICATIONS**: Active thromboembolic disorders, thrombophlebitis and cerebral hemorrhage or history of same. Vaginal bleeding (undiagnosed), breast or genital organ cancer, missed abortion and significant hepatic dysfunction.

DRUG	INDICATIONS & DOSAGE	DOSE FORMS	REMARKS
PROGESTERONE **Oil**: Generics (Bay Progest) (Femotrone in Oil) (Gesterol 50) **Powder**: Generics Progest-M	**Amenorrhea**: **IM**: 5-10 mg/d for 6-8 d. Withdrawal bleeding should occur 48-72 h after last injection. **Functional Uterine Bleeding**: IM: 5-10 mg/d for 6 doses. Bleeding should stop within 6 d. If used with estrogen, start progesterone 14 d after starting estrogen therapy. Stop injections when menses starts.	Injection: 25, 50, 100 mg/ml (10, 30 ml)	
MEDROXYPRO-GESTERONE (Provera) (Amen) (Curretab)	**Secondary Amenorrhea**: **PO**: 5-10 mg/d for 5-10 d. Withdrawal bleeding should occur 3-7 d after last dose. **Abnormal Uterine Bleeding**: **PO**: 5-10 mg/d for 5-10 d; start on day 16 or 21 of menstrual cycle. Withdrawal bleeding should occur 3-7 d after last dose. Continue therapy for 2 cycles after bleeding is controlled.	PO (Tab's): 2.5, 10 mg	
HYDROXYPRO-GESTERONE Generics (Hyroxon) (Duralutin) (Gesterol L.A. 250) (Hy-Gestrone) (Hylutin) (Hyprogest 250) (Hyproval P.A.) (Pro-Depo)	**Primary/Secondary Amenorrhea, Abnormal Uterine Bleeding**: **IM**: 375 mg (single dose); if no bleeding after 21 d, begin cyclic estrogen-progestin therapy for 4 cycles; observe patient for 2-3 cycles after cessation of therapy. **Stage 3 or 4 Uterine Adenocarcinoma**: **IM**: 1-7 gm/wk (single dose). Continue until relapse occurs or 12 wk total therapy. **Test for Endogenous Estrogen Production**: **IM**: 250 mg (single dose). To confirm, repeat after 4 weeks. Normal nonpregnant patients should develop bleeding in 7-14 d.	Injection: 125, 250 mg/ml (5, 10 ml)	Depot form in oil; for IM use only.

PROGESTINS *Continued*

DRUG	INDICATIONS & DOSAGE	DOSE FORMS	REMARKS
NORETHINDRONE (Norlutin)	**Amenorrhea and Abnormal Uterine Bleeding**: **PO**: 5-20 mg/d; begin on day 5, end on day 25 of menstrual cycle. **Endometriosis**: **PO**: 10 mg/d for 2 wk; increase by 5 mg q2wk until 30 mg/d is reached (10 wk); continue at 30 mg/d for 6-9 months. If break-through bleeding occurs, discontinue therapy temporarily.	PO (Tab's): 5 mg	
NORETHINDRONE ACETATE (Norlutate) (Aygestin)	**Amenorrhea and Abnormal Uterine Bleeding**: **PO**: 2.5-10 mg/d; begin on day 5, end on day 25 of menstrual cycle. **Endometriosis**: **PO**: 5 mg/d for 2 wk; increase by 2.5 mg q2wk until 15 mg/d is reached (10 wk), continue at 15 mg/d for 6-9 months. If break-through bleeding occurs, discontinue therapy temporarily.	PO (Tab's): 5 mg	

ORAL CONTRACEPTIVES

GROUP REMARKS: Oral contraceptives (OCs) differ in the strength of their estrogenic and progestational components. There are three types of oral contraceptives: monophasic, biphasic and triphasic. Monophasic types deliver a constant progestin:estrogen ratio throughout the cycle. Biphasic types maintain a constant estrogen level throughout, but have a lower progestin:estrogen ratio during the first half of the cycle. Triphasic types vary estrogen and/or progestin levels throughout the entire cycle. The contraceptive action of these agents is mainly due to suppression of ovulation or implantation. **SIDE EFFECTS**: Thromboembolic disorders are 2-11 times more likely in OC users than in controls. Risk of myocardial infarction is increased, particularly: when use > 10 years, in smokers or in patients > 40 y.o. Other increased risks: development of ocular lesions and, possibly, carcinoma. Hepatic lesions noted particularly in patients > 30 y.o. or when OC use > 4 years. Risk of gallbladder disease risk may double after 5 years of use. Blood sugar and lipid metabolism alterations and menstrual irregularities are all seen. OCs may cause congenital abnormalities. OCs may precipitate acute intermittent porphyria, jaundice, depressed serum folate levels, fluid retention, hypertension, depression (5-30% patients), or enlargement of uterine fibroids. All risks are lower with current "low estrogen potency" preparations than with the earlier "strong" pill. **CAUTIONS**: Cigarette smoking markedly increases the risk of cardiovascular problems in women taking OCs, especially after age 35. **RECOMMENDATIONS**: Use an additional method of birth control during the first week of therapy. Rule out pregnancy before initiating OC use and before continuing therapy if two consecutive menstrual periods are missed. Discontinue OC use in nursing mothers. **CONTRAINDICATIONS**: Pregnancy, abnormal vaginal bleeding, benign or malignant liver tumors, estrogen-dependent tumors, breast cancer, thrombophlebitis, history of deep venous thrombophlebitis, cerebral vascular disease, myocardial infarction, coronary artery disease.

DRUG INTERACTIONS:
Many drugs (***antibiotics, analgesics, phenytoin, etc.***) inhibit **Oral Contraceptive** function in the laboratory; clinical efficacy is NOT affected.

INDICATIONS AND DOSES:
Prevention of pregnancy is the major use of these agents; 1 pill/d taken at intervals not to exceed 24 h. Some are also used in estrogen replacement therapy.

MONOPHASIC ORAL CONTRACEPTIVES

The FDA has recently advised that oral contraceptive formulations containing > 50 µg of estrogen no longer be marketed. Since 1970, the FDA has advised physicians to prescribe the lowest effective dose oral contraceptive.

In March 1988, a number of pharmaceutical firms advised physicians they would discontinue formulations containing 75-100 µg estrogen.

ESTROGEN = 50 µg Mestranol

	PROGESTIN
Norinyl 1+50 21-Day Norinyl 1+50 28-Day Ortho-Novum 1/50 21 Ortho-Novum 1/50 28	1 mg norethindrone

ESTROGEN = 50 µg Ethinyl estradiol

	PROGESTIN
Ovcon-50	1 mg norethindrone
Norlestrin 21 1/50 Norlestrin Fe 1/50	1 mg norethindrone acetate
Demulen 1/50-21 Demulen 1/50-28	1 mg ethynodiol diacetate
Norlestrin 21 2.5/50 Norlestrin Fe 2.5/50	2.5 mg norethindrone acetate
Ovral Ovral-28	0.5 mg norgestrel

ESTROGEN = 35 µg Ethinyl estradiol

	PROGESTIN
Norinyl 1+35 21-Day Norinyl 1+35 28-Day Ortho-Novum 1/35 21 Ortho-Novum 1/35 28 Brevicon 21-Day Modicon Modicon 28	1 mg norethindrone

ESTROGEN = 35 μg Ethinyl estradiol *Continued*

	PROGESTIN
Ovcon-35	0.4 mgnorethindrone
Demulen 1/35-21 Demulen 1/35-28	1 mg ethynodiol diacetate

ESTROGEN = 30 μg Ethinyl estradiol

	PROGESTIN
Loestrin 21 1.5/30 Liestrin Fe 1.5/30	1.5 mg norethindrone acetate
Lo/Ovral-21 Lo/Ovral-28	0.3 mg norgestrel
Nordette-21 Nordette-28	0.15 mg levonorgestrel

ESTROGEN = 20 μg Ethinyl estradiol

	PROGESTIN
Loestrin 21 1/20 Loestrin Fe 1/20	1 mg norethindrone

BIPHASIC ORAL CONTRACEPTIVES

	ESTROGEN	PROGESTIN	Duration
Ortho-Novum 10/11-21, Ortho-Novum 10/11-28:			
Phase 1:	35 μg ethinyl estradiol	0.5 mg norethindrone	10 d
Phase 2:	35 μg ethinyl estradiol	1 mg norethindrone	11 d

TRIPHASIC ORAL CONTRACEPTIVES

	ESTROGEN	PROGESTIN	Duration
Tri-Norinyl:			
Phase 1:	35 μg ethinyl estradiol	0.5 mg norethindrone	7 d
Phase 2:	35 μg ethinyl estradiol	1 mg norethindrone	9 d
Phase 3:	35 μg ethinyl estradiol	0.5 mg norethindrone	5 d
Followed by an inert tablet for 7 d.			
Ortho-Novum 7/7/7:			
Phase 1:	35 μg ethinyl estradiol	0.5 mg norethindrone	7 d
Phase 2:	35 μg ethinyl estradiol	0.75 mg norethindrone	7 d
Phase 3:	35 μg ethinyl estradiol	1 mg norethindrone	7 d
Followed by an inert tablet for 7 d.			
Triphasil-21, Tri-Levlen:			
Phase 1:	30 μg ethinyl estradiol	0.005 mg levonorgestrel	6 d
Phase 2:	40 μg ethinyl estradiol	0.75 mg levonorgestrel	5 d
Phase 3:	30 μg ethinyl estradiol	0.125 mg levonorgestrel	10 d
Followed by an inert tablet for 7 d.			

PROGESTIN-ONLY CONTRACEPTIVES

	PROGESTIN
Micronor Nor-Q.D.	0.35 mg norethindrone
Ovrette	0.075 mg norgestrel

THYROID REPLACEMENTS

GROUP REMARKS: T_4 is treatment of choice for hypothyroidism. T_3 has more rapid onset and decay of effects. **SIDE EFFECTS**: Palpitations, tachycardia, chest pain, widened pulse pressure, weight loss, heat intolerance, sweating, nausea, diarrhea, insomnia, headache, anxiety, tremulousness; rash occurs rarely. **CAUTIONS**: In hypothyroidism, initial thyroid replacement therapy may accelerate metabolism and precipitate adrenocortical insufficiency. In this situation lower initial doses of thyroid hormone or supplemental glucocorticoids may be needed. In hypothyroidism caused by hypopituitarism, adrenocortical insufficiency with thyroid administration is very likely. T_3 produces wider swings in thryoid effects than does T_4. **RECOMMENDATIONS**: In the treatment of adult hypothyroidism without myxedema, perform clinical re-evaluation q30d and laboratory re-evaluation q90d. In children use the pulse rate while asleep and morning temperatures as guidelines to effectiveness of treatment. **CONTRAINDICATIONS**: Thyrotoxicosis, acute myocardial infarction (provided no hypothyroidism exists), uncorrected adrenal insufficiency, hypersensitivity to preparation constituents.

DRUG INTERACTIONS:
Thyroid hormones may enhance the effects of the ***tricyclic antidepressants***, such as ***imipramine***. The effect of ***digitalis*** may be inhibited. Concomitant administration of ***ketamine*** may precipitate high blood pressure and tachycardia. ***Estrogen*** use may increase requirement for thyroid replacement. ***Cholestyramine*** may inhibit intestinal absorption of thyroid hormone.

DRUG	INDICATIONS & DOSAGE	DOSE FORMS	REMARKS
	CRUDE THYROID HORMONE EXTRACTS		
THYROID DESICCATED (USP) (Armour Thyroid) (Thyro-Teric) (Thyrar (Bovine)) (S-P-T (Porcine)) (Thyroid USP Enseals) (Thyroid Strong)	**Hypothyroidism (without myxedema)**: **PO**: 65 mg/d initially, increase by 65 mg q30d PRN. **Pediatric PO**: 16 mg/d for 2 wk, then 32 mg/d for 2 wk; increase q2wk as needed. Thyroid hormone requirements for children may be > adults (metabolic requirements for growth may be greater). **Hypothyroidism with Myxedema**: **PO**: 16 mg/d for 2 wk, then 32 mg/d for 2 wk, then 65 mg/d for 2 wk, maintenance: 65-195 mg/d.	PO (Tab's): 16, 32, 65, 98, 130, 195, 260, 325 mg PO (Tab's, enteric): 32, 65, 130 mg PO (Cap's): 65, 130, 195, 325 mg Thyroid Strong (Tab's sugar coated): 32, 65, 130, 195 mg (50% more potent than Thyroid USP tab's)	Group Remarks. Perform clinical evaluation every month, laboratory exam every 3 months.
THYROGLOBULIN (Proloid)	**Hypothyroidism**: **PO**: 32 mg/d initially, increase q2-3wk PRN; maintenance 65-200 mg/d.	PO (Tab's): 32, 65, 100, 130, 200 mg	Group Remarks.

THYROID REPLACEMENTS *Continued*

DRUG	INDICATIONS & DOSAGE	DOSE FORMS	REMARKS
CRYSTALLINE THYROID HORMONES			
LEVOTHYROXINE (T_4) (Levothroid) (Synthroid) (Syroxine) (Synthrox)	**Hypothyroidism**: **PO**: 0.1-0.2 mg/d maintenance (maximum 0.4 mg/d). In healthy adults with recent hypothyroidism, institute full dosage immediately; in debilitated, aged or long-standing hypothyroid conditions: 0.025 mg/d initially, increase by 0.025 mg/d q3-4wks PRN. **Pediatric PO**: 0-6 months: 8-10 µg/kg/d. 6-12 months: 6-8 µg/kg/d. 1-5 years: 5-6 µg/kg/d. 6-12 years: 4-5 µg/kg/d. > 12 years: 2-3 µg/kg/d. **Severe Hypothyroidism or Cretinism**: **Pediatric PO**: 0.025-0.5 mg/d initially, increase by 0.05-0.1 mg/d q7d PRN (maximum 0.3-0.4 mg/d).	PO (Tab's): 0.025, 0.05, 0.75, 0.1, 0.125, 0.15, 0.175, 0.2, 0.3 mg Injection: 200, 500 µg/vial (6 & 10 ml vials) Injection, reconstituted: 100 µg/ml (6 & 10 ml)	Group Remarks. **Hypothyroidism with Myxedema, Coma or Obtundation**: **IM, IV**: 0.2-0.5 mg (solution ≤0.1 mg/ml); 0.1-0.3 mg or more on day 2 if no improvement. Maintain daily injections until oral dosing is tolerated. Do NOT administer parenteral thyroxine if patient has heart disease unless all risks associated with therapy are considered.
LIOTHYRONINE (T_3) (Cytomel) (Cyronine)	**Hypothyroidism**: **PO**: 25 µg/d initially, increase by 12.5-25 µg/d q1-2wks; maintenance 25-75 µg/d. **Myxedema**: **PO**: 5 µg/d initially, increase by 5-10 µg/d q1-2wk until 25 µg/d, then increase by 12.5-25 µg/d q1-2wk; maintenance 50-100 µg/d. *Note*: In elderly,use 5 µg/d initially, increase 5 µg q1-2wks PRN.	PO (Tab's): 5, 25, 50 µg	Group Remarks. **Severe Hypothyroidism or Cretinism**: **Pediatric PO**: 5 µg/d initially, increase by 5 µg/d q3-4d PRN: 6-12 months: maintenance 20 µg/d. 1-3 years: maintenance 50 µg/d.
LIOTRIX **4:1 mixture of T_4 & T_3** (Euthroid) (Thyrolar)	**Untreated Hypothyroidism**: **PO**: 15-30 mg/d initially, increase by 15 mg q1-2wks.	Tablet strength (thyroid equivalent in mg's): 1/4 (15), 1/2 (30), 1 (60), 2 (120), 3 (180)	60 mg liotrix = 65 mg desiccated thyroid or 0.1 mg levothyroxine or 25 µg liothyronine.

ANTITHYROID AGENTS

DRUG	INDICATIONS & DOSAGE	DOSE FORMS	REMARKS
IODINE PREPARATIONS (Strong Iodine Solution) (Lugol's Solution)	**Preparation of Hyperthyroid Patients for Thyroidectomy**: **PO**: 2-6 qtt tid for 10 d prior to surgery. **Thyroid Crisis Adjunct**: **IV**: 2 gm/d. **Block Thyroid Uptake of Isotopes**: **PO**: 6 qtt/d or 130 mg/d for10 d. **Pediatric PO (< 1 y.o.)**: 3 qtt/d or 65 mg/d for 10 d.	Lugol's sln: 5% iodine + 10% potassium iodide (KI) PO (Tab's): 130 mg KI Injection: 10% NaI Sol'n, KI: 21 mg/drop (30 ml dropper bottles)	
PROPYLTHIOURACIL & METHIMAZOLE			
GROUP NOTES: These agents inhibit the synthesis of thyroid hormones. **SIDE EFFECTS**: Agranulocytosis is the most significant side effect; have patient report any fever or sore throat. Vascular, hyperplastic thyroid (TSH not inhibited); treat with iodine 10-21 days before surgery. Drug fever, jaundice. Methimazole somewhat more allergenic than propylthiouracil.			
PROPYLTHIOURACIL (PTU)	**Hyperthyroidism**: **PO**: 300-400 mg/d initially (rarely 600-900 mg/d); maintenance 100-150 mg/d. **Pediatric PO**: 6-10 years: 50-150 mg/d. >10 years: 150-300 mg/d	PO (Tab's): 50 mg	
METHIMAZOLE (Tapazole)	**Mild Hyperthyroidism**: **PO**: 15 mg/d initially; maintenance 5-15 mg/d in 3 doses. **Pediatric PO**: 0.4 mg/kg/d initially; maintenance 0.2 mg/kg/d in 3 doses. **Moderate Hyperthyroidism**: **PO**: 30-40 mg/d initially; maintenance 5-15 mg/d in 3 doses. **Severe Hyperthyroidism**: **PO**: 60 mg/d initially; maintenance 5-15 mg/d in 3 doses.	PO (Tab's): 5 mg	

POSTERIOR PITUITARY HORMONES

DRUG	INDICATIONS & DOSAGE	DOSE FORMS	REMARKS
GROUP REMARKS: The posterior pituitary secretes two major hormones with characteristically different actions, vasopressin and oxytocin. Vasopressin (a.k.a. antidiuretic hormone, ADH) stimulates resorption of water from the renal tubules; it also stimulates vascular constriction, mainly of the portal and splanchnic beds, resulting in increased GI motility and tone. Diabetes insipidus results from a deficiency of vasopressin and is its main therapeutic indication. Oxytocin and its analogs are discussed elsewhere.			
VASOPRESSIN (8-Arginine Vasopressin) (Pitressin, synthetic)	**Diabetes Insipidus**: **IM, SC**: 5-10 units q8-12h PRN. **Post-Operative Ileus and Distention**: **IM**: 5-10 units initially, repeat q3-4h PRN.	Injection: 20 pressor units/ml (0.5, 1 ml ampules)	Duration of action = 2-8 h.
VASOPRESSIN Tannate (Pitressin Tannate)	**Diabetes Insipidus**: **IM**: 0.3-1 ml PRN.	Injection: 5 pressor units/ml (1 ml) in oil	Depot form of vasopressin; duration of action = 24-96 h.
LYPRESSIN (8-Lysine Vasopressin) (Diapid)	**Diabetes Insipidus**: **Nasal spray**: 1-2 sprays q4-6h (maximum 10 sprays/nostril q3-4h).	Nasal spray = 50 USP posterior pituitary pressor units/ml: 0.185 mg (8 ml bottles)	1 spray = 2 posterior pituitary pressor units. Quick onset (30-60 min) with duration of action = 3-8 h. May produce nasal irritation.
DESMOPRESSIN (DDAVP) (Stimate)	**Diabetes Insipidus**: **IV, SC**: 2-4 μg/d (0.5-1 ml/d) in 2 doses. **Nasal**: 0.1-0.4 ml/d in 1-2 doses. **Pediatric Nasal (3 mo.-12 y.o.)**: 0.05-0.3 ml/d in 1-2 doses. **Type I von Willebrand's Disease, Hemophilia A**: **IV**: 0.3 μg/kg (SLOWLY, over 15-30 min); dilute in 50 ml normal saline. **Pediatric IV (< 10 kg)**: 0.3 μg/kg SLOWLY (over 15-30 min); dilute in 10 ml normal saline.	Nasal spray: 0.1 mg = 400 IU arginine vasopressin: 0.1 mg/ml (2.5 ml) Injection: 4 μg/ml (10 ml)	Synthetic analog of arginine-vasopressin with duration of action = 8-20 h. Antidiuretic effect more specific than with natural vassopressin; vasopressor effects not normally seen at therapeutic doses. Monitor blood pressure and pulse during IV infusion.
POSTERIOR PITUITARY PREPARATIONS (Posterior Pituitary) (Pituitrin)	**Diabetes Insipidus**: **IM, SC**: 5-20 units PRN. **Nasal spray**: 1-2 sprays q6-8hPRN.	Nasal spray cap's: 40 mg (= 45 IU ADH activity + 45 U oxytocin activity). Injection: 20 units/ml 1 ml)	Both of these are preparations of animal posterior pituitary gland. Pituitrin is for IM injection, Posterior Pituitary is for intranasal installation. Both are used to control symptoms of diabetes insipidus. Hypersensitivity reactions may occur because of the animal nature of these products.

MISCELLANEOUS HORMONES

DRUG	INDICATIONS & DOSAGE	DOSE FORMS	REMARKS
ADRENOCORTICO-TROPHIC HORMONE (ACTH) (Corticotropin) (Acthar)	<u>**Various**</u>: **IM, SC**: 20 units q6h. <u>**Multiple Sclerosis, Exacerbations**</u>: **IM, SC**: 80-120 units/d for 2-3 wks.	Injection: 25 & 40 units/vial.	ACTH may be effective in a wide variety of miscellaneous disorders. However, it is generally of limited utility in conditions responsive to corticosteroids.
(DEPOT FORMS) (Corticotropin Gel) (Cortige) (Cotropic-Gel) (Cortrophin Gel) (H.P. Acthar Gel)	<u>**ACTH-Responsive Conditions**</u>: **IM, SC**: 40-80 units q24-78h.	Injection: 40 & 80 units/ml (1, 5 ml vials)	
(Cortrophin-Zinc)	<u>**ACTH-Responsive Conditions**</u>: **IM**: 40-80 units q24-72h deeply into gluteal muscle.	Injection: 40 units/ml (5 ml vials)	
COSYNTROPIN (Cortrosyn)	<u>**Test of Adrenal Function**</u>: **IM, IV**: 0.25-0.75 mg (single dose).	Injection: 0.25 mg/vial	Synthetic ACTH. Can be given as an IV infusion over 4-8 h for greater adrenal gland stimulation.
HUMAN GROWTH HORMONE (SOMATREM) (Protropin) (Humatrope)	<u>**Growth Failure**</u>: **IM**: 0.16 IU/kg 3 times/wk (Protropin maximum 0.2 IU/kg).	Injection: 10 IU/vial	Recombinant DNA product.
CALCITONIN-SALMON (Calcimar)	<u>**Hypercalcemia**</u>: **IM, SC**: 4 IU/kg q12h initially; after 2-4 doses, increase to 8 IU/kg q12h if needed; after next 4 doses, increase to a maximum of 8 IU/kg q6h if needed. <u>**Osteoporosis (postmenopausal)**</u>: **IM, SC**: 100 IU/d; patient should be concurrently taking a minimum calcium supplement of 1.5 gm/d and 400 units/d vitamin D.	Injection: 200 IU/ml (2 ml vials)	

Section 5: GASTROINTESTINAL SYSTEM AGENTS
Table of Contents

Antidiarrheal Agents

ANTACIDS

GROUP REMARKS: Antacids in common use are all non-systemic (i.e., non-absorbed). Some may be systemic (i.e., absorbed), such as sodium bicarbonate. All of the others listed below react to neutralize HCl in the stomach but are regenerated to their original form in the alkaline intestinal contents. Antacids chelate or complex with many drugs (most notably tetracycline, cimetidine, phenytoin) and thus interfere with their absorption; do not administer within 2h before or after such agents. Aluminum hydroxide is also used to reduce absorption of phosphate in chronic renal insufficiency.

DRUG	INDICATIONS & DOSAGE	DOSE FORMS	REMARKS
SUCRALFATE (Carafate)	**Gastric Acidity:** **PO**: 1 gm qid 1h before meals and hs; continue 4-8w ks.	PO (Tab's)1 gm	Inhibits pepsin activity in gastric juice, negligible acid-neutralizing ability. **SIDE EFFECTS**: Constipation, nausea, indigestion, diarrhea, rash, pruritis, vertigo, drowsiness, dry mouth and back pain. **RECOMMENDATIONS**: Antacids should NOT be taken within 1/2 h before or after sucralfate. Take on empty stomach 1 h before or 2 h after eating.
ALUMINUM HYDROXIDE GEL (Amphojel) (Gelumina) (Alternagel) (AluCaps)	**Gastric Acidity:** **PO**: 500-1800 mg 3-6 times/d (between meals and at bedtime). **PO**: 1-2 tsp in water (1/2 glass). **PO**: 1-2 tab's chewed; follow by 1/2 glass water.	PO (Cap's): 475, 500 mg PO (Tab's): 300, 600 mg Gel Suspension: 320 mg/5 ml (360 ml) Gel Liquid: 600 mg/5 ml (150, 360 ml)	Constipation, phosphorus depletion, excessive mobilization of bone salts.
MILK of MAGNESIA (magnesium hydroxide)	**Gastric Acidity:** **PO**: 5-15 ml (650-1300 mg) qid. **PO**: 2 tab's chewed qid.	PO (Tab's): 325 mg Liquid: 390 mg/5 ml	Soluble, but not absorbed. Magnesium ion exerts laxative effect.
ALUMINUM HYDROXIDE with MAGNESIUM HYDROXIDE (Maalox) (Mylanta) Various others	**Gastric Acidity:** **PO**: 5-10 ml qid. **PO**: 1-2 tab's qid.		Laxative and constipating effects more or less balanced. Much variation in patient preference.

ANTACIDS *Continued*

DRUG	INDICATIONS & DOSAGE	DOSE FORMS	REMARKS
ALUMINUM HYDROXIDE with MAGNESIUM TRISILICATE (Gelusil)	**Gastric Acidity**: **PO**: 1-2 tsp's. **PO**: 2 tab's.		Same as for aluminum hydroxide with magnesium hydroxide.
CALCIUM CARBONATE (Tums) Various others	**Gastric Acidity**: **PO**: 500-1500 ng q2-4h.	PO (Tab's): 350, 420, 500, 650, 750, 850 mg	Constipating. Some excess calcium absorption.
BISMUTH SUBGALLATE	**Gastric Acidity**: **PO**: 500-1000 mg qid.		
SODIUM BICARBONATE (SODA)	**Gastric Acidity**: **PO**: 300-2000 mg q6-24h.	PO (Tab's): 350, 520, 650,	Systemic effects to rebound hypersecretion. Used by patients, but not prescribed.

H_2 ANTAGONISTS

DRUG	INDICATIONS & DOSAGE	DOSE FORMS	REMARKS
CIMETIDINE (Tagamet)	**Duodenal/Gastric Ulcer, Acid Hypersecretion**: **PO**: 300 mg qid (with meals and at bedtime), or 400 mg bid; maximum 2400 mg/d. Continue 4-6 wks for ulcer. **Ulcer (Prophylaxis/Maintenance)**: **PO**: 400 mg qhs. **IM, IV**: 300 mg q6-8h; maximum 2400 mg/d. ***Note***: For IV use, infuse sln over 15-20 min. **Above with Impaired Renal Function**: **PO, IM, IV**: 300 mg q8-12h; may accumulate.	PO (Tab's): 200, 300, 400 mg Ampules: 150 mg/ml (2, 8 ml) PO (Liquid): 300 mg/5 ml (240 ml)	**SIDE EFFECTS**: Diarrhea, dizziness, myalgia, rash, gynecomastia, confusion or psychosis (reversible), elevated creatinine, elevated SGOT and SGPT, possibly neutropenia, cutaneous vasculitis, thrombocytopenia, somnolence. **CAUTIONS**: Rare cardiac arrhythmias and hypotension have occurred with rapid IV administration. Risk factors for reversible confusional state include renal impairment, liver disease, age > 50, serum [cimetidine] > 125 µg/ml. **RECOMMENDATIONS**: Give antacids and cimetidine at different times. Take with meals. **CONTRAINDICATIONS**: History of hypersensitivity. **DRUG INTERACTIONS**: **Cimetidine** use increases blood levels of ***procainamide, benzodiazepines, theophylline, lidocaine, caffeine, quinidine, beta-adrenergic blocking agents, phenytoin, warfarin-type anticoagulants***. Concurrent administration with ***antacids*** or ***metoclopramide*** may impair **cimetidine** absorption. ***Digoxin*** level may decrease with coadministration of **cimetidine**. Incompatible in solution with ***aminophylline*** and ***barbiturates***.
RANITIDINE (Zantac)	**Duodenal Ulcer and Hypersecretory Conditions**: **PO**: 100-150 mg bid. **IM, IV**: 50 mg q6-8h. IV: Infuse sln over 15-20 min. **Above with Impaired Renal Function**: **PO**: 150 mg/d if creat. clearance < 50 cc/min. **IM, IV**: 50 mg q18-24h if creat. clearance < 50 cc/min. (Administer after end of hemodialysis sessions.)	PO (Tab's): 150 mg Injection: 25 mg/ml (2, 10 ml)	**SIDE EFFECTS**: Rash, headache, diarrhea, dyspepsia, impotence, decreased sexual drive, dizziness, confusion, increased serum prolactin, gynecomastia, bradycardia, transient increase in serum creatinine, rare malaise, agitation, depression, hallucination. Rare depression of blood-forming elements, rare hypersensitivity. **CAUTIONS**: Potential problems in pregnancy and with children not known. **CONTRAINDICATIONS**: Hypersensitivity to ranitidine.
FAMOTIDINE (Pepcid)	**Duodenal/Gastric Ulcer, Acid Hypersecretion**: **PO**: 20-40 mg/d at bedtime. **IV**: 20 mg SLOWLY (infuse over ≥ 2 min) q12h.	PO (Tab's): 20, 40 mg Suspension: 40 mg/5 ml Injection: 10 mg/ml (2, 4 ml)	**SIDE EFFECTS**: Headache, dizziness, constipation or diarrhea, fatigue. No significant interactions with drugs metabolized by liver microsomal enzymes (as occur with above 2 agents).

EMETICS AND ANTIEMETICS

DRUG	INDICATIONS & DOSAGE	DOSE FORMS	REMARKS
EMETICS			
APOMORPHINE	<u>Emesis Induction</u>: **SC**: 5 mg (range 2-10 mg); once only. **Pediatric SC**: 0.1 mg/kg; once only.	Soluble Tablets: 6 mg (with lactose)	**SIDE EFFECTS**: CNS or respiratory depression; violent vomiting. **CONTRAINDICATIONS**: Ingestion of acid, alkali or petroleum distillates; absent gag reflex; coma, seizures; opiate, alcohol or barbiturate narcosis.
IPECAC	<u>Emesis Induction</u>: **PO**: 15 ml followed by 1-2 glasses water. **Pediatric PO (< 1 y.o.)**: 5-10 ml followed by 0.5-1 glass water. May repeat in 20 minutes if ineffective; ONCE only.	Syrup: 15, 30 ml	**SIDE EFFECTS**: GI irritation, diarrhea common. Cardiotoxicity remotely possible. **RECOMMENDATIONS**: If emesis does NOT occur within 30 min, remove ipecac from the stomach by gastric lavage. **CONTRAINDICATIONS**: Ingestion of acid, alkali, strychnine or petroleum distillates; absent gag reflex; convulsions; coma.
ANTIEMETICS FOR MOTION SICKNESS			
CYCLIZINE (Marezine)	<u>Motion Sickness</u>: **PO**: 50 mg 1/2 h before departure; repeat q4-6h; maximum 200 mg/d. **Pediatric PO**: 25 mg; tid maximum. **IM**: 50 mg q4-6h when needed.	PO (Tab's): 50 mg Injection: 50 mg/ml	**SIDE EFFECTS**: CNS: Drowsiness, excitation, blurred vision at normal doses; hallucinations and convulsions with overdosage. Others: rash, dry nose/mouth/throat, urinary frequency.
MECLIZINE (Antivert) (Antivert-25) (Bonine)	<u>Motion Sickness</u>: **PO**: 25-50 mg 1 h before departure; repeat q24h as needed. <u>Vertigo</u>: **PO**: 25-100 mg/d bid-tid.	PO (Tab's): 2.5, 25, 50 mg	**SIDE EFFECTS**: Same as for cyclizine (above).
DIMENHYDRINATE (Dramamine) (Dramocen) (Reioamine)	<u>Motion Sickness</u>: **PO**: 50-100 mg q4-6h; maximum 400 mg/d. **Pediatric PO**:25-50 mgq6-8h; maximum 150 mg/d. **IM**: 50 mg q4-6h PRN; maximum 300 mg/d. **IV**: 50 mg in 10 ml saline over 2 min.	PO (Tab's): 50 mg PO (Liquid): 3.1 mg/ml Injection: 50 mg/ml	Dimenhydrinate is the chlortheophyllineate salt of diphenhydramine. **SIDE EFFECTS**: See cyclizine (above). Substantially unpleasant sedation is prominent.

DRUG	INDICATIONS & DOSAGE	DOSE FORMS	REMARKS
GENERAL ANTIEMETICS			
BENZQUINAMIDE (Emete-con)	**Nausea, Vomiting**: **IM**: 50 mg (0.5-1 mg/kg), repeat at 1 h, then q3-4h PRN. Administer ≥ 15min prior to emergence from anesthesia. **IV**: 25 mg (0.2-0.4 mg/kg) slowly (0.5-1 ml/min); follow with IM maintenance.	Injection: 50 mg/vial	**NOTES**: IM route preferable. **SIDE EFFECTS**: Common: Dry mouth, blurred vision, chills, sweating. **CAUTIONS**: Sudden increased blood pressure, transient arrhythmias may follow IV administration. **RECOMMEND**: AVOID IV use in patients with CV disease, and possibly elderly or debilitated patients.
DIPHENIDOL (Vontrol)	**Nausea, Vomiting**: **PO**: 25-50 mg q4h. **Pediatric PO**: 0.88 mg/kg q4h; maximum 5.5 mg/kg/d. **Vertigo**: **PO**: 25-50 mg q4h.	PO (Tab's): 25 mg	**SIDE EFFECTS**: Dry mouth, drowsiness, hallucinations, disorientation, confusion. **RECOMMEND**: Use ONLY in hospitalized or closely supervised patients
THIETHYLPERAZINE (Torecan)	**Nausea, Vomiting**: **IM**: 10-30 mg/d bid-qid.	PO (Tab's): 10 mg. Suppositories: 10 mg IM Injection: 5/ml	**NOTES**: A phenothiazine, see Antipsychotics for a more complete discussion. **SIDE EFFECTS**: Drowsiness, dry mouth, orthostatic hypotension. **CONTRAINDICATIONS**: Contraindicated in pregnancy, severe CNS depression, coma.
TRIMETHOBENZAMIDE (Tigan)	**Nausea, Vomiting**: **PO**: 250 mg q6-8h. **Rectal**: 200 mg q6-8h. **IM**: 200 mg q6-8h. **Pediatric PO**: 100-200 mg q6-8h. **Pediatric Rectal**: 100-200 mg q6-8h.	PO (Cap's): 100, 250 mg Suppositories: 200 mg Pediatric Suppositories: 100 mg Injection: 100 mg/ml	**SIDE EFFECTS**: Drowsiness claimed to be rare. Pain at IM injection site.
METOCLOPRAMIDE (Reglan)	**Diabetic Gastroparesis**: **PO**: 10 mg 30 min before meals and at bedtime, for 2-8 wk. **Gastroesophageal Reflux**: **PO**: 10-15 mg 30 min before measl and at bedtime; maximum 45 mg/d.	PO (Tab's): 10 mg Syrup: 1 mg/ml Injection: 5 mg/ml **Chemotherapy-Induced Emesis**: **IV Infusion**: 1-2 mg/kg over 15 min. Administer 30 min prior to chemotherapy, repeat q2-3h. **IV Injection**: 10 mg as a single dose over 1-2 min. If extrapyramidal symptoms occur, add 50 mg diphenhydramine IM.	**SIDE EFFECTS**: Drowsiness and dizziness in 10% of patients. May produce or worsen extrapyramidal symptoms; usually reversible in 24 h.

DRUGS USED IN HEPATIC FAILURE

DRUG	INDICATIONS & DOSAGE	DOSE FORMS	REMARKS
NEOMYCIN (Mycifradin) (Neobiotic)	Hepatic Coma: **PO**: 4-12 gm/d, divided q6h. **Pediatric PO**: 50-100 mg/kg/d, divided q6h. Chronic Hepatic Insufficiency: **PO**: 4 gm/d, divided q6h.	PO (Tab's): 500 mg PO (Liquid): 125 mg/5 ml (60 ml, pints)	**SIDE EFFECTS**: Laxative effect, rare renal and 8th nerve toxicity with oral use. **CAUTIONS**: Some preparations contain tartrazine; possible allergic reactions. **CONTRAINDICATIONS**: Hypersensitivity to neomycin or tartrazine. See Antibiotics for additional information.
PAROMOMYCIN SULFATE (Humatin)	Hepatic Coma: **PO**: 4 gm/d, divided q8h for 5-6 d. Intestinal Ameblasis: **PO**: 25-35 mg/kg/d, divided q8h for 5-10 d.	PO (Cap's): 250 mg	NOT effective in extraintestinal amebic infections. **SIDE EFFECTS**: Nausea, abdominal cramps, diarrhea (esp. with doses > 3 gm/d). **CAUTIONS**: May cause bacterial overgrowth of nonsusceptible organisms (e.g., fungi). In situations of increased GI absorption, ulcerative lesions of the bowel may occur with resultant aminoglycoside toxicity. **RECOMMENDATIONS**: Give with meals. Observe closely for overgrowth of intestinal microorganisms. **CONTRAINDICATIONS**: Hypersensitivity to paromomycin, intestinal obstruction.
KANAMYCIN SULFATE (Kantrex)	Suppression of Intestinal Bacteria: **PO**: 1 gm q1h for 4h, then 1 gm q6h for 36-72 h. Hepatic Coma: **PO**: 8-12 gm/d in divided doses.	PO (Cap's): 500 mg	Approximately 1% of a PO dose is absorbed through normal GI tract. **SIDE EFFECTS**: Nausea, vomiting, diarrhea, malabsorption syndrome may occur with prolonged use. **CAUTIONS**: Concurrent use of nephrotoxic, ototoxic and/or potent diuretic agents may increase toxicity of oral neomycin. **RECOMMENDATIONS**: Reduce dose in renal insufficiency. Perform baseline and periodic audiometric testing, urinalysis and hematologic evaluations during prolonged therapy (especially in patients with renal failure). **CONTRAINDICATIONS**: Hypersensitivity to kanamycin, intestinal obstruction.

LAXATIVES

DRUG	DOSAGE	ONSET	REMARKS
	IRRITANT OR STIMULANT LAXATIVES		
CASTOR OIL	**Adult:** 15-60 ml (mild laxative) preparatory for abdominal X-ray.	3 h	Administer chilled or with juice; flavored preparations available.
CASCARA	**Fluid Extract:** 5 ml. **Tablets:** 1 (often with 30 ml milk of magnesia).	6-10 h	Administer at bedtime. May discolor urine.
BISACODYL (Dulcolax)	**Adult:** 10-15 mg (maximum 30 mg). **Rectal:** 10 mg. **Child:** 5-10 mg.	PO: 6-10 h Rectal: 15-60 min	Administer tablets at bedtime, do not chew.
	BULK LAXATIVES		
MAGNESIA (MILK of) (magnesia magma) (magnesium hydroxide)	**Adult:** 5-30 ml. **Child:** 0.25-0.5 of Adult dose.	0.5-3 h	Use may affect fluid and electrolyte status. Administer with a glass of water.
SODIUM PHOSPHATE	**Adult:** 4-8 gm with water before break-fast.	15-30 min	Probably less effective than milk of magnesia. Administer with a glass of water.
METHYLCELLULOSE (Citrucel) (Cologel) (Maltsuprex)	**Adult:** 1-2 Tbsp 1-3 times/d.	12-24 h	Administer with a glass of water.
PYSILLIUM (Serutan) (Metamucil) (Naturacil)	**Adult:** 3.5-7.5 gm 1-3 times/d.	12-24 h	Very safe. Administer with a glass of water.

LAXATIVES *Continued*

DRUG	DOSAGE	ONSET	REMARKS
FECAL SOFTENER LAXATIVES			
GROUP REMARKS: The fecal softener laxatives are detergents or emulsifiers. They are especially useful if the feces are dry and hard or in cases where passage causes pain or should not require extreme effort.			
DOCUSATE (Colace) (Doxinate)	**Adult:** 50-240 mg. **Child:** 40-120 mg. **3-6 y.o.:** 20-60 mg.	24-48 h	
MINERAL OIL	**Adult:** 15-30 ml. **Child:** 5-20 ml.	6-18 h	Available neat or as flavored emulsifiers.

ANTISPASMODICS

GROUP REMARKS: Although technically not a separate class, these anticholinergic agents are presented as one because they are used primarily to inhibit smooth muscle tone and secretion in the gastrointestinal, biliary and urinary tracts. The effects of these anticholinergics are dose-related: inhibition of salivary and bronchial secretions (along with sweating) occurs at low doses; effects on the eye (pupillary dilatation, inhibition of accommodation) and the heart (increased rate) occur at higher doses; inhibition of GI and urinary tract motility occur at even higher doses; inhibition of gastric acid secretion occurs at very high doses. Those anticholinergics that are tertiary amines are rapidly absorbed after PO administration and readily cross the blood-brain barrier to produce CNS effects; subjectively unpleasant sedation or lassitude or, in toxic doses, excitement and disorientation. Those anticholinergics that are quaternary amines do not sufficiently cross the blood-brain barrier to cause these CNS effects. Therefore, when used to decrease GI motility or acid secretion, significant side effects will occur. See Parasympatholytics for a more complete discussion of these agents.

DRUG	INDICATIONS & DOSAGE	DOSE FORMS	REMARKS
BELLADONNA (Bellafoline) (in Donnatal)	Peptic Ulcer, Hypermotility: **Extract**: 15 mg tid-qid. **Tincture**: 0.6-1 ml tid-qid.	Extract (Tab's): 15 mg Tincture (Liquid): 0.3 mg/ml	Contains the alkaloids hyoscyamine (forms atropine upon extraction) and scopolamine. Both are tertiary anticholinergics and produce CNS effects at therapeutic doses.
PROPANTHELINE (Pro-Banthene)	Peptic Ulcer, Hypermotility: **PO**: 15 mg 30 min prior to meals, 30 mg prior to bedtime. **Geriatric PO**: 7.5 mg tid.	PO (Tab's): 7.5, 15 mg	Quaternary anticholinergic agent, negligible CNS side effects.

ANTIDIARRHEAL AGENTS

DRUG	INDICATIONS & DOSAGE	DOSE FORMS	REMARKS
KAOLIN + PECTIN (Kaopectate) (K-Pek) (Pektamalt)	**Adults**: 60-120 ml. **Child**: 30-60 ml. **3-6 y.o.**: 15-30 ml.	Suspension: **Regular**: Kaolin 200 mg + Pectin 4.3 mg per ml **Concentrate**: Kaolin 290 mg + Pectin 6.5 mg per ml	Decrease dose with concentrated product. Other proprietary adsorbents are available by prescription or over the counter (Pepto-Bismol).
DIPHENOXYLATE (Lomotil) Generic forms	**Adult**: 5 mg q6h. **8-12 y.o.**: 2 mg 5 times/d. **5-8 y.o.**: 2 mg 4 times/d. **2-5 y.o.**: 2 mg 3 times/d.	PO (Tab's): 2.5 mg diphenoxylate + 0.025 mg atropine PO (Liquid): 0.5 mg/ml diphenoxylate + 0.005 mg/ml atropine	A weak narcotic and atropine. May cause drowsiness, dizziness, dry mouth. **CONTRAINDICATIONS**: Liver disease, concurrent MAO Inhibitors.
LOPERAMIDE (Imodium)	**Adult**: 4 mg initially, then 2 mg PRN (maximum 16 mg/d). **8-12 y.o.**: 2 mg q8h initially, then 0.1 mg/ kg PRN (maximum 6 mg/d). **5-8 y.o.**: 2 mg q12h initially, then 0.1 mg/ kg PRN (maximum 4 mg/d). **2-5 y.o.**: 1 mg q8h initially, then 0.1 mg/ kg PRN (maximum 3 mg/d).	PO (Cap's): 2 mg PO (Liquid): 1 mg/5 ml	A weak narcotic. May cause drowsiness, dizziness, dry mouth, abdominal discomfort. **CONTRAINDICATIONS**: Severe infectious diarrhea. See other narcotics for further discussion.
PAREGORIC (opium camphorated tincture)	**Adult**: 5-10 ml q6-24h. **Child**: 0.25-0.5 ml/kgq6-24h.	Liquid: contains 2 mg morphine per 5 ml	Side effects primarily constipation and lethargy. See other narcotics for further discussion.

Section 6: DERMATOLOGIC AGENTS
Table of Contents

TOPICAL STEROIDS

GROUP REMARKS: In the chart, preparations with the same active ingredient but with different concentrations have been repeated in separate classes. Even with the same concentration of active ingredient, different preparations may have differing potencies (e.g., betamethasone dipropionate 0.05%). This multiple listing, though somewhat repetitious, facilitates the identification of the relevant functional class for a given concentration of a specific agent. **CAUTIONS**: Systemic effects can occur from the transcutaneous absorption of steroids. This is of especial concern with: (1) more potent steroid preparations, (2) occlusive dressings, (3) prolonged use, (4) use over large body surface areas, (5) use > 50 gm/week in adults or > 15 gm/week in children. Because of this absorption and because steroids have been shown to be teratogenic in animals at relatively low doses, use during pregnancy is potentially dangerous. **SIDE EFFECTS**: See also: Anti-Inflammatory Steroids. All of the known side effects of systemic steroids can occur upon systemic absorption of topical steroids, including suppression of the pituitary adrenal axis. Other side effects include: local irritation, secondary infection, striae (especially when high potency agents are used on face or genitalia), glaucoma and cataracts (especially when high potency agents are used for prolonged periods around the eyes), skin atrophy (the authors have reported observation of total fingerprint eradication after 20 years of continuous use). **CONTRAINDICATIONS**: Hypersensitivity to any component of the different preparations, fungal infection, tuberculosis of the skin, varicella, vaccinia, herpes simplex infection. **RECOMMENDATIONS**: Discontinue if secondary infection occurs. AVOID prolonged use around eyes, genitalia or rectum. Apply sparingly in a thin film.

DRUG	INDICATIONS & DOSAGE	REMARKS
VERY HIGH POTENCY		
CLOBETASOL (0.05%)	**Topical**: Apply bid for ≤ 14d; maximum 50 gm/wk.	Available as ointment and cream.
BETAMETHASONE DIPROPIONATE (0.05%) (special base)	**Topical**: Apply 1-4 times/d for ≤ 14d; maximum 45 gm/wk. Do NOT use with occlusion. **Spray**: Spray for ≤ 3sec, 3-4 times/d, from a distance of 10-15cm.	Available as cream, lotion and ointment. **Propylene glycol base** gives this preparation optimal potency. Recent studies show clobetasol more effective for treatment of psoriasis.
HIGH POTENCY		
FLUOCINONIDE ACETONIDE (0.05%)	**Topical**: Apply 2-4 times/d.	Available as ointment, cream, gel and solution.
TRIAMCINOLONE (0.5%)	**Topical**: Apply 2-4 times/d. **Spray**: Spray for ≤ 3sec, 3-4 times/d, from a distance of 10-15cm.	Availabel as ointment, lotion, cream, spray, foam and dental paste.
DESOXIMETASONE (0.25%)	**Topical**: Apply 2-3 times/d.	Available as ointment and cream.
FLUOCINOLONE (0.2%)	**Topical**: Apply 3-4 times/d.	Available as cream.
DIFLORASONE (0.05%)	**Topical**: Apply cream 2-4 times/d. Apply ointment 1-3 times/d.	Available as ointment and cream.
HALCINONIDE (0.1%)	**Topical**: Apply 2-3 times/d.	Available as ointment, cream and solution.

TOPICAL STEROIDS: HIGH POTENCY *Continued*

DRUG	INDICATIONS & DOSAGE	REMARKS
BETAMETHASONE DIPROPIONATE (0.05%)	**Topical**: Apply 1-4 times/d; maximum 45 gm/wk. Do NOT use with occlusion. **Spray**: Spray for ≤ 3sec, 3-4 times/d, from a distance of 10-15 cm.	Available as ointment, cream, lotion, aerosol spray, gel, ear/eye/nose drops, enema and suppositories.
AMCINONIDE (0.1%)	**Topical**: Apply 2-3 times/d.	Available as ointment and cream.
	MEDIUM POTENCY	
TRIAMCINOLONE (0.1%)	**Topical**: Apply 2-4 times/d.	Available as ointment, cream, lotion and spray.
BETAMETHASONE VALERATE (0.1%)	**Topical**: Apply 1-4 times/d.	Available as ointment, cream and lotion.
BETAMETHASONE BENZOATE (0.025%)	**Topical**: Apply 1-4 times/d.	Available as ointment, cream, lotion and gel.
HALCINONIDE (0.025%)	**Topical**: Apply 2-3 times/d.	Available as cream.
DESOXIMETASONE (0.05%)	**Topical**: Apply 2-3 times/d.	Available as ointment and gel.
FLUOCINOLONE (0.025%)	**Topical**: Apply 3-4 times/d.	Available as ointment and cream.
FLURANDRENOLIDE (0.05%)	**Topical**: Apply 2-3 times/d. **Topical (tape)**: Apply as occlusive dressing q12h on clean dry skin.	Available as ointment, cream, lotion and tape.
	LOW POTENCY	
TRIAMCINOLONE (0.025%)	**Topical**: Apply 2-4 times/d.	Available as ointment, cream and lotion.
BETAMETHASONE VALERATE (0.01%)	**Topical**: Apply 1-4 times/d.	Available as ointment, cream, lotion, aerosol spray, gel, ear/eye/nose drops, enema and suppositories.
FLUOCINOLONE (0.01%)	**Topical**: Apply 3-4 times/d.	Available as cream and lotion.

TOPICAL STEROIDS: LOW POTENCY *Continued*

DRUG	INDICATIONS & DOSAGE	REMARKS
FLURANDRENOLIDE (0.025%)	**Topical**: Apply 2-3 times/d.	Available as ointment and cream.
HYDROCORTISONE VALERATE (0.2%)	**Topical**: Apply 2-3 times/d.	Available as ointment and cream.
CLOCORTOLONE (0.1%)	**Topical**: Apply 1-4 times/d.	Available as cream.
DESONIDE (0.05%)	**Topical**: Apply 2-4 times/d.	Available as ointment and cream.
LOWEST POTENCY		
HYDROCORTISONE (0.25% to 2.5%)	**Topical**: Apply 2-4 times/d.	Available as ointment, cream, lotion, talc, aerosol spray, rectal foam, retention enema, otic solution/suspension, scalp lotion, scalp aerosol spray and urethral insert.
METHYLPREDNISO-LONE (0.25%, 1.0%)	**Topical**: Apply 1-4 times/d.	Available as ointment.
DEXAMETHASONE (0.1%)	**Topical**: Apply 3-4 times/d. **Spray**: Spray for 1-2 sec 2-4 times/d from a distance of 15 cm.	Available as cream, gel, ear ointment, ear solution and aerosol spray.
ALCLOMETASONE (0.05%)	**Topical**: Apply 2-3 times/d.	Available as ointment, cream, ear ointment, ear solution and aerosol spray.

TOPICAL ANTIBIOTIC AND ANTIFUNGAL AGENTS

DRUG	INDICATIONS & DOSAGE	DOSE FORMS & REMARKS
TOPICAL ANTIBIOTICS		
TRIPLE SULFA (Trisulfapyramidines) (Koro-sulf) (Sultrin) (Trysul)	**Vaginal**: 2.5-5 gm (1 applicator) bid for 4-6 d initially, then 1/2-1/4 applicator bid for a total of 7-14 d OR 1 tab bid for 10 d.	Vaginal creams: 3.42 & 10% sulfthiazole component (in 78, 82.5, 85 gm applicator) Vaginal tablets: 172.5 mg (of sulfthiazole component) **NOTES**: Contains sulfthiazole, sulfacetamide, sulfabenzamide and urea.
TRIPLE ANTIBIOTIC OINTMENT (Neosporin; OTC)	**Topical**: Apply 1-5 times/d.	Powder: 5,000 units polymyxin B sulfate, 3.5 mg neomycin base, 400 units bacitracin and 10 mg diperodon HCL/gm. Cream: 10,000 units polymyxin B sulfate & 3.5 mg neomycin base/gm.
TOPICAL ANTIFUNGAL AGENTS		
UNDECYLENIC ACID (Desenex; OTC) (Pedi-Dri; OTC)	**Topical**: Apply 1-5 times/d.	Available as powder (with zinc undecylenate, aluminum chlorhydroxide, menthol, formaldehyde), ointment, cream, liquid, foam and soap.
MICONAZOLE (Micatin; OTC) (Monistat)	**Topical**: Apply bid for 2-4 weeks. **Vaginal**: One applicator (Monostat-3) qhs for 3 d OR one applicator (Monostat-7) qhs for 7 d OR 1 suppository qhs for 7 d.	Available as cream (2%), lotion (2%), vaginal cream (2%) or vaginal suppositories.
ECONAZOLE NITRATE (Spectazole)	**Tinea Versicolor**: **Topical**: apply qd for 2 wk. **Tinea (corporis, pedis, cruis)**: **Topical**: apply bid for 2-4 wk. (Tenia pedis may take longer to resolve.)	Available as cream (1%).
CICLOPIROX OLAMINE (Loprox)	**Topical**: Apply bid; rethink diagnosis if no improvement after 4 wk.	Available as cream (1%).
CLOTRIMAZOLE (Gyne-Lotrimin) (Mycelex)	**Topical**: Apply bid; rethink diagnosis if no improvement after 4 wk. **Vaginal**: 1 applicator (5 gm) qd for 14 d OR one 100 mg tablet qhs for 7 d OR one 500 mg tablet at bedtime (once only).	Available as cream (1%), lotion (1%), solution (1%), vaginal cream (1%) or vaginal tablets.

DRUG	INDICATIONS & DOSAGE	DOSE FORMS & REMARKS
TRIACETIN (Fungoid) (Glyceryl Triacetate)	**Topical**: Apply bid for up to 1 week after lesions resolve.	Available as liquid (triacetin, cetylpyridinium chloride & chloroxylenol), solution (triacetin, cetylpyridinium chloride, chloroxylenol & benzalkonium chloride in a nonaqueous vehicle) and cream (triacetin, cetylpyridinium chloride & chloroxylenol in a vanishing cream base).
ACRISORCIN (Akrinol)	**Topical**: Apply bid after scrubbing lesions with soap and brush.	
HALOPROGIN (Halotex)	**Topical**: Apply bid for 2-4 weeks.	Available as cream (1%) and solution (1%).
TOLNAFTATE (Aftate) (Tinactin)	**Topical**: Apply bid for 2-4 wk (may extend up to 4-6 wk). (Use powders only as adjunctive therapy.)	Available as cream (1%), powder (1%), liquid aerosol (1% with 36% alcohol) and solution (1%).
NYSTATIN (Mycostatin) (Nilstat) (Candex)	**Topical**: Apply 2-3 times/d for 1 wk after lesions are gone. **Vaginal**: 1 tablet qd for 14 d.	Available as: Cream: 100,000 units/gm Ointment: 100,000 units/gm Lotion: 100,000 units/gm Powder: 100,000 units/gm Vaginal tablets: 100,000 & 500,000 units
AMPHOTERICIN B (Fungizone)	**Topical**: Apply to lesions 2-4 times/d for 1-3 weeks.	Available as cream (3%), lotion (3%) and ointment (3%).

TOPICAL LOCAL ANESTHETICS

GROUP REMARKS: Local anesthetics (LAs) are effective on mucosal surfaces, but have no effect on intact skin. They are used topically for the temporary relief of pain and itching due to minor burns (including sunburn), minor cuts and abrasions, insect bites or other minor skin irritation. Some preparations are used for the temporary relief of pain and itching associated with hemorrhoids. Some are also used to anesthetize sensitive mucosal surfaces prior to minor surgery or other procedures, especially bronchoscopy, gastroscopy and urethral catheterization. **NOTES**: See Group Remarks for Injectable Local Anesthetics. **RECOMMENDATIONS**: When used for hemorrhoids with rectal bleeding, examine for colon disease. **CAUTIONS**: Oral use may interfere with swallowing (pharyngeal stage), restrict food intake for 1h following use. Use of large doses, especially in highly vascular areas, can result in absorption of enough LA to produce systemic toxicity, including convulsions and death (see Injectable Local Anesthetics).

DRUG	ANESTHETIC CONCENTRATION	DOSE FORMS	REMARKS
TOPICAL AMIDES			
DIBUCAINE (Nupercaine)	<u>Topical</u>: 0.5-1%	Ointment: 1% Cream: 0.5% (water soluble) Suppositories	Primarily for dermal use; may be used rectally (with applicator) for hemorrhoids. Do NOT use in or near eyes. Slow onset (≤ 15 min) and long duration (2-4 h) relative to other LAs; also more toxic. Maximum use (of 1% preparation): 30 gm/d (adults), 7.5 gm/d (children) of the ointment. Available OTC.
LIDOCAINE (Xylocaine)	<u>Topical</u>: 2.5-5%	Ointment: 2.5 (water soluble), 5% Cream: 3% Jelly: 2% Solution: 2, 4, 10%	
TOPICAL ESTERS			
TETRACAINE (Pontocaine)	<u>Topical</u>: 0.5-2%	Ointment: 0.5% Cream: 1% Solution: 0.5, 2%	Ophthalmic use: tonometry, gonioscopy, removal of foreign bodies or sutures and short procedures; use 0.5% ointment or solution; onset at 30 sec, duration 15 min. Does not usually affect pupillary reactions, accommodation or intraocular pressure. Prolonged ophthalmic use NOT recommended.
BENZOCAINE (Ethyl aminobenzoate)	<u>Topical</u>: 0.5-20%	Ointment: 2% Cream: 1, 5, 6% Gel: 6.3, 7.5, 10, 20% Lotion: 0.5, 2% Solution: 2, 3, 5, 9.5, 20% Lozenges: 3, 5, 6.25, 10 mg	Available OTC. Used in minor sore throat pain, dental conditions, local pruritis and hemorrhoids. Do NOT use in or near the eyes. Repeated use may produce sensitization.

TOPICAL LOCAL ANESTHETICS: TOPICAL ESTERS *Continued*

DRUG	ANESTHETIC CONCENTRATION	DOSE FORMS	REMARKS
COCAINE	<u>**Topical**</u>: 1-4%	Solution: 40, 100 mg/ml Soluble Tab's: 135 mg	Local anesthetic and vasoconstrictor (sympathomimetic) properties. Produces euphoria and stimulation of the CNS similar to amphetamine. Use cautiously in patients with hypertension, CV disease, thyrotoxicosis, or on other medications potentiating catecholamine action. Do NOT add Epi. Maximum single dose = 1 mg/kg.
HEXYLCAINE (Cyclaine)	<u>**Topical**</u>: 5%	Solution: 5%	Local tissue irritation and sloughing may occur. Urethritis may occur after urethral use for catheterization. NOT for ophthalmic use. Maximum single dose = 500 mg.
MISCELLANEOUS			
CYCLOMETHYCAINE (Surfacaine)	<u>**Topical**</u>: 0.5-1%	Ointment: 1% Cream: 0.5% Jelly: 0.75%	Used mainly for mucosal anesthesia of the urethra, vagina or rectum prior to minor procedures; should NOT be used as the sole anesthetic in bronchoscopy. May produce initial irritation. Maximum dose = 30 ml/d.
DYCLONINE (Dyclone) (OTC: Sucrets)	<u>**Topical**</u>: 0.5-1%	Solution: 0.5, 1% Gel: 1%	Possesses some bacteriocidal and fungicidal activity. Used for pain of cold sores in addition to usual indications for mucosal local anesthetics. Maximum dose = 300 mg.
PRAMOXINE (Tronothane) (Proxine) (OTC: Tronolane)	<u>**Topical**</u>: 1%	Cream: 1% Foam: 1% Jelly: 1%	Apply cream to skin 5 times/d, foam to hemorrhoids 2-3 times/d. Will NOT abolish the gag reflex. NOT for use in or near eyes or nose.

ACNE AGENTS

DRUG	INDICATIONS & DOSAGE	DOSE FORMS	REMARKS
ISOTRETINOIN (Accutane)	<u>**Severe Cystic Acne**</u>: **PO**: 0.5-1 mg/kg/d (maximum 2 mg/kg/d) divided q12h for 15-20 wks. For persistent acne: repeat after 2 month intermission. See Newer Agents/Newer Uses for information on use on weather-damaged skin.	PO (Cap's): 10, 20, 40 mg	Recent studies claim that isotretinoin applied topically can aid weather-damaged skin. Investigational use in psoriasis. **SIDE EFFECTS**: Corneal opacities, pseudotumor cerebri, hypertriglyceridemia, inflammatory bowel disease, cheilitis, conjunctivitis, eye irritation, pruritis, epistaxis, dry mouth, dry skin, nausea, vomiting, abdominal pain, anorexia, lethargy, headache, pyuria, proteinuria, hematuria, abnormal menses, muscle pain, joint stiffness, disseminated herpes simplex, LFT elevations, increased serum glucose, hyperuricemia. **CAUTIONS**: Highly photosensitive. Alcohol consumption may potentiate hypertriglyceridemia. Known human teratogen. May interact with antidepressants. **RECOMMENDATIONS**: Take with meals. Women of child bearing age should ENSURE proper CONTRACEPTION during and for one month following therapy. Avoid prolonged exposure to sunlight. **CONTRAINDICATIONS**: Pregnancy, sensitivity to parabens.
BENZOYL PEROXIDE (PanOxyl) (Xerac B.P.) (Desquam-X) (Benzac) Generics	<u>**Mild-Moderate Acne**</u>: **Topical**: Massage into skin once/d for 3 d; then increase to bid application PRN.	Gel: 2.5, 5, 10% Lotion: 5, 5.5, 10% Bar: 5, 10% Liquid: 5, 10%	For external use only. **SIDE EFFECTS**: Allergic contact sensitization potential, excessive drying of skin. **RECOMMENDATIONS**: Discontinue use if skin irritation develops. **CONTRAINDICATIONS**: Hypersensitivity.

Section 7: OPHTHALMOLOGIC AGENTS
Table of Contents

Ophthalmic Antiviral Agents

Ophthalmic Antifungal Agents

AGENTS USED FOR THE TREATMENT OF GLAUCOMA

GROUP REMARKS: Increased pressure of the aqueous humor can develop acutely (narrow-angle, angle-closure glaucoma) or chronically (open-angle glaucoma). Aqueous humor is formed at the ciliary processes, enters the posterior chamber, passes through the pupil into the anterior chamber and is resorbed through the trabecular meshwork. The drugs listed below reduce intraocular pressure by one of two mechanisms, either they 1) decrease the formation of aqueous or 2) increase outflow, possibly by pulling open the drainage channels in the trabecular meshwork via stimulating constriction of the ciliary muscle.

RECOMMENDATIONS: Instruct patient as follows:

1) Drops should be applied into the "cup" formed when the lower lid is gently pulled away from the surface of the eye (NOT directly onto the surface) while the head is tilted back.

2) For 1 min following instillation, pressure should be applied with the thumb and fingers to the bridge of the nose (at the inner canthus of the eye). This prevents drainage of the drug into the naso-lacrimal duct, which can produce systemic effects.

3) Solutions should be protected from the possibility of contamination and NOT used if their color has changed. Droppers should NOT touch any surface and should be recapped immediately.

Adjust concentration and frequency to achieve maximal individual response. **ABBREVIATIONS**: IOP = intraocular pressure, sln = solution.

DRUG	DOSAGE	DOSE FORMS	REMARKS
SYMPATHOLYTICS			
TIMOLOL (Blokadren) (Timoptic)	Instill 1 drop bid (0.25% sln initially, 0.5% sln if inadequate response); decrase to 1 drop/d when possible.	Solution: 0.25, 0.5%	Timolol is a *beta*$_1$/*beta*$_2$-blocker. Decreased IOP occurs within 15-30 min and persists for 24 h. Adjust concentration to achieve maximal individual response. Effect may be additive with concurrent epinephrine or a carbonic anhydrase inhibitor. **SIDE EFFECTS**: Ocular irritation: conjunctivitis, blepharitis, keratitis, blepharoptosis; refractive changes. Systemic sympatholytic effects if absorbed via naso-lacrimal duct.
BETAXOLOL (Betopic)	Instill 1 drop bid.	Solution: 0.5% (5.6 [5 mg base] mg/ml)	Betaxolol exhibits some selectivity for *beta*$_1$-blockade; potentially fewer systemic side effects if absorbed via naso-lacrimal duct. Decreased IOP occurs within 30 min and persists for 12 h. Efficacy equivalent to timolol.
LEVOBUNOLOL (Betagan)	Instill 1 drop 1-2 times/d.	Solution: 0.5%	Levobunolol is a *beta*$_1$/*beta*$_2$-blocker. Decreased IOP occurs within 60 min and persists for 24 h.
SYMPATHOMIMETIC			
EPINEPHRINE (Epitrate) (Glaucon) (Epinal) (Eppy)	Instill 1-2 drops, 1-2 times/d; decrease frequency to q2d-q3d when possible, based on IOP measurement.	Solution: 0.1, 0.25, 0.5, 1, 2%	Use ONLY in open-angle glaucoma. Decreases aqueous production and increases outflow; also produces mydriasis without cycloplegia. Used mainly as an adjunct to miotics (may reduce spasm) or carbonic anhydrase inhibitors. Add a CA inhibitor when used as a mydriatic. **SIDE EFFECTS**: Frequent: ocular irritation/inflammation, headache. Rare, transient: INCREASED IOP when used without a concurrent miotic. Corneal edema, pigment deposits after prolonged use. Systemic sympathomimetic effects.

AGENTS USED FOR THE TREATMENT OF GLAUCOMA *Continued*

DRUG	DOSAGE	DOSE FORMS	REMARKS
PARASYMPATHOMIMETIC			
PILOCARPINE (Isopto) (Pilocar) (Ocusert)	**Solution**: Instill 1-2 drops q4h. Adjuxt concentration (usually = 0.5-4%) and frequency based on optimal response. **Ocusert**: 1 unit/wk (preferable to install at bedtime).	Solution: 0.25, 0.5, 1, 2, 3, 4, 5, 8, 10% Depot (Ocusert): 20, 40 µg/h	Pilocarpine is the drug of choice for glaucoma. Decreased IOP occurs within 15-30 min and persists for 4-6 h, miosis persists ≤24 h. Also used to reverse effects of cycloplegic or mydriatic agents. Ocusert is a drug delivery unit placed in the eye which continuously releases pilocarpine for 1 wk/unit; 20 µg/h is similar to 1% drops, 40 µg/h to 2%. Myopia of variable persistence may occur following instillation of drops or the delivery unit.
CHOLINESTERASE INHIBITORS			
GROUP NOTES: The cholinesterase inhibitor miotics may produce cataracts and may activate latent iritis or uveitis; iridial cysts or posterior synchies may occur. Perform periodic ophthamologic examinations, including pupillary dilation.			
ISOFLUROPHATE (DFP) (Floropryl)	Apply 0.5 cm q8-72h. Adjust to lowest effective frequency.	Ointment: 0.025%	Irreversible cholinesterase inhibitor. Miosis occurs within 5-10 min and persists for 1 week; IOP decreases within 24 h and persists for 1 week. Hydrolysis yields hydrogen fluoride, which is very irritating to the eye. Rarely used.
ECHOTHIOPHATE (Phospholine Iodide)	Instill 1 drop, 2 times/wk-1-2 times/d. Adjust to lowest effective concentration and frequency.	Powder for solution: 0.03, 0.06, 0.125, 0.25%	Irreversible cholinesterase inhibitor. Miosis occurs within 10-30 min and persists for days-4 weeks; IOP decreases within 24 h and persists for days-weeks.
DEMECARIUM (Humorsol)	Instill 1-2 drops, qod-2 times/d. Adjust to lowest effective concentration and frequency.	Solution: 0.12, 0.25%.	Irreversible cholinesterase inhibitor. If no response within 24 h of initial dose, switch to alternate therapy.
PHYSOSTIGMINE (Eserine)	**Solution**: Instill 1-2 drops, 3-4 times/d. **Ointment**: Apply small amount 1-3 times/d.	Solution: 0.25, 0.5% (+/- Pilocarpine) Ointment: 0.25% Generic powder	Reversible cholinesterase inhibitor. Miosis occurs within 10-30 min and persists for 12-48 h. Frequent conjunctivitis with chronic use. High potential to produce allergic reactions.
CARBONIC ANHYDRASE INHIBITORS			
GROUP NOTES: Carbonic anhydrase (CA) inhibitors may be used chronically in open-angle glaucoma, but ONLY ACUTELY in acute, angle-closure glaucoma; they decrease IOP by inhibiting formation of aqueous humor. CA inhibitors also act briefly as sodium diuretics. In addition, they akalinize the urine and produce respiratory and metabolic acidosis with high dose, long-term therapy. **SIDE EFFECTS**: Most are dose-related: paresthesias, nausea, vomiting, diarrhea, sedation, nervousness, seizures, renal calculi, hyper-			

Continued, next page

AGENTS USED FOR THE TREATMENT OF GLAUCOMA: CARBONIC ANHYDRASE INHIBITORS *Continued*

DRUG	DOSAGE	DOSE FORMS	REMARKS
uricemia, hyperchloremia. Rarely: Thrombocytopenia, aplastic anemia, hypokalemia, hyperglycemia. May precipitate hepatic coma in liver disease. **RECOMMENDATIONS:** If patient is intolerant to one CA inhibitor, another may be effective. **CAUTION**: CA inhibitors increase tissue CO_2 retention; may worsen pulmonary disease. **CONTRAINDICATIONS**: Hyperchloremic acidosis. Hepatic, adrenal or renal insufficiency. NOT for use in chronic closed-angle glaucoma.			
ACETAZOLAMIDE (Diamox)	<u>Chronic Glaucoma</u>: **PO**: 250-1000 mg/d in 3-4 doses. <u>Acute Glaucoma</u>: **PO**: 500 mg initially, then 125-250 q4h. **IV, IM**: 500 mg bolus, then 125-250 mg q2-4h.	PO (Tab's): 25, 250 mg PO (extended release): 500 mg	For decreased IOP: Onset: PO = 1 h; ext'd release = 2 h; IV = 2 min. Peak: PO = 2-4 h; extended release = 8-18 h; IV = 15 min. Duration: PO = 8-12 h; extended release = 18-24 h; IV = 4-5 h. IM, IV use only when rapid decrease in IOP required.
DICHLORPHENAMIDE (Daranide)	**PO**: 100-200 mg initially, then 100 mg q12h; maintenance 25-50 mg q8-12h.	PO (Tab's): 50 mg	Decreased IOP: Onset = 0.5-1 h; Peak = 2-4 h; Duration = 6-12 h.
METHAZOLAMIDE (Neptazane)	**PO**: 50-100 mg 2 or 3 times/d.	PO (Tab's): 50 mg.	Decreased IOP: Onset = 2-4 h; Peak = 6-8 h; Duration = 10-18 h.

OSMOTIC AGENTS

GROUP NOTES: Osmotic agents do not enter the aqueous humor. Therefore, they extract water from aqueous into extra-ocular fluid by osmotic forces. These agents are useful in acute angle-closure glaucoma and in preparation for intraocular surgery.			
UREA (Ureaphil)	**IV**: 500-1500 mg/kg (30% sln; rate < 4 ml/min); maximum 120 gm/d.	IV: 40 gm	See discussion under Osmotic Diuretics. Possible rebound increase in IOP.
MANNITOL (Osmitrol)	**IV**: 1.5-2 gm/kg (15-20% sln) over 30-60 min.	Solution: 5, 10, 15, 20, 25%	See discussion under Osmotic Diuretics. Possible rebound increase in IOP. Less toxic and more stable in solution than urea.
GLYCERIN (Glyrol) (Osmoglyn) (Ophthalgan)	**PO**: 1-1.5 gm/kg.	PO: 50, 65% solution	Density: 1 ml weighs 1.25 gm. Fewer side effects than mannitol. Used to reduce IOP in angle-closure glaucoma prior to iridectomy. Topical glycerin (anhydrous) relieves corneal edema. Lesser diuretic effect than urea, mannitol. **SIDE EFFECTS**: Occasional nausea, vomiting, and headache.

MYDRIATICS

GROUP REMARKS: Mydriatics dilate the pupil and are used mainly to aid the ophthalmolscopic examination. Cycloplegic mydriatics also interfere with accommodation for near vision and are used to facilitate refraction and prevent formation of synechia in uveitis. Mydriatics (whether cycloplegic or not) should NOT be used in eyes with narrow angles in the anterior chamber; can precipitate angle-closure glaucoma; their use is contraindicated in angle-closure glaucoma. **SIDE EFFECTS**: May elevate IOP. Blurred vision and photophobia from cycloplegia. **RECOMMENDATIONS**: As for all ocular drugs, the following procedures should be employed:

1) Drops should be applied into the "cup" formed when the lower lid is gently pulled away from the surface of the eye (NOT directly onto the surface) while the head is tilted back.
2) For 1 min following instillation, pressure should be applied with the thumb and fingers to the bridge of the nose (at the inner canthus of the eye). This prevents drainage of the drug into the naso-lacrimal duct, which can produce systemic effects.
3) Solutions should be protected from the possibility of contamination and NOT used if their color has changed. Droppers should NOT touch any surface and should be recapped immediately.

DRUG	INDICATIONS & DOSAGE	DOSE FORMS	REMARKS
NON-CYCLOPLEGIC MYDRIATIC			
PHENYLEPHRINE (Neo-Synephrine)	Instill 1-2 drops (2.5-10% sln); repeat in 60 min if needed. Precede by local anesthetic.	Solution: 0.12, 2.5, 10%.	NOT a cycloplegic; may be applied with concurrent cycloplegic mydriatic. Mydriasis onset = 30 min; duration = 2-3 h. Hydroxyamphetamine or eucatropine may be substituted in patients allergic to phenylpherine.
CYCLOPLEGIC MYDRIATICS			
ATROPINE	**Uveitis**: **Adults**: Instill 1-2 drops q6h. **Children**: Instill 1-2 drops q8h. **Refraction**: **Adults**: Instill 1 drop (1% sln) 1 h before the refraction. **Children**: Instill 1-2 drops (0.25-0.5% sln) 2 times/d for 1-2 d before examination, then 1-2 drops 1 h before the refraction.	Solution: 0.5, 1, 2, 3% Ointment: 0.5, 1%.	An effective, long-acting cycloplegic; drug of choice for refraction in children. Onset = 30-40 min; duration ≤ 2 weeks in a normal eye; duration shortened greatly in an inflamed eye (administer several times/d). **SIDE EFFECTS**: May elevate IOP; ocular irritation and inflammation may occur with prolonged use. Restlessness and excitement, flush, dry mouth and fever are prominent systemic side effects, particularly in young children. Block naso-lacrimal duct following instillation.
SCOPOLAMINE	**Refraction**: **Adults**: Instill 1-2 drops 1 h before procedure. **Uveitis**: **Adults**: Instill 1-2 drops q8-12h.	Solution: 0.25%.	Cycloplegia occurs in 15-30 min; duration ≤ 1 week in normal eyes (shorter than atropine); shorter duration in inflamed eyes. **SIDE EFFECTS**: May elevate IOP; ocular irritation and inflammation may occur with prolonged use. Potential systemic side effects: restlessness and behavioral disorders, vomiting and urinary incontinence.

MYDRIATICS: CYCLOPLEGIC MYDRIATICS *Continued*

DRUG	INDICATIONS & DOSAGE	DOSE FORMS	REMARKS
HOMATROPINE	**Refraction**: Instill 1-2 drops immediately before procedure, repeat q5-10min PRN. **Uveitis**: Instill 1-2 drops q3-4h.	Solution: 1, 2, 5%.	Short-acting mydriatic and cycloplegic: onset = 10-30 min; duration approximately 3 h (complete recovery within 36 h). **SIDE EFFECTS**: May increase IOP (esp. in glaucoma patients); ocular irritation and inflammation may occur with prolonged use.
CYCLOPENTOLATE (Cyclogyl)	**Refraction**: Instill 1 drop (1-2% sln) 40-50 min before procedure, repeat after 5-10 min.	Solution: 0.5, 1%.	Rapid onset and shorter duration of action than atropine or scopolamine: onset within 30-60 min; duration $\leq$ 24 h. **SIDE EFFECTS**: May increase IOP. Transient irritation upon instillation (less pronounced with 0.5% sln). Allergic ocular irritation may develop with prolonged use. Potential pyschotic reactions and behavioral disorders in children.
TROPICAMIDE (Mydriacyl)	**Mydriasis**: Instill 1-2 drops (0.5-1% sln) 15-20 min before procedure, repeat q30min PRN. **Cycloplegia**: Instill 1-2 drops (1% sln), repeat at 5 min.	Solution: 0.5, 1%	Onset = 20-25 min; duration = 5-6 h. Mydriatic effect greater than cycloplegic effect. **SIDE EFFECTS**: May increase IOP. Produces transient irritation upon instillation. Systemic effects include: dry mouth, headache and tachycardia.

OPHTHALMIC STEROIDS

GROUP REMARKS: Topical corticosteroids are used in the eye to reduce pain, photophobia and scarring associated with inflammatory conditions. The anti-inflammatory effect of topical steroids is especially useful in the eye because of the destructive effect of scarring on vision. These topical steroids should be used in conjunction with appropriate specific treatment such as antimicrobial or antiviral agents.

INDICATIONS:

Topical corticosteroid therapy is indicated for inflammation of the anterior structures of the eye, whether due to allergic, autoimmune, infectious or traumatic causes:

- anterior uveitis
- blepharitis
- conjunctivitis
- episcleritis
- scleritis
- phlyctenulosis
- superficial/interstitial keratitis

Systemic corticosteroid therapy is indicated for inflammation of the more posterior structures of the eye and optic nerve:

- posterior uveitis
- endophthalmitis
- optic neuritis
- sympathetic ophthalmia

Administration and Dosage:

Solutions/Drops:
Instill 1-2 drops into conjunctival sac q1h a during daytime, q2h at night; reduce to 1 drop q4h, then q6-8h as response develops.

Ointments:
Apply a thin coat to the conjunctival sac q6-8h; reduce to q12h, then q24h as response develops.

SIDE EFFECTS:

Glaucoma and photophobia occur commonly, cataract formation is rare; glaucoma is less likely with systemic steroid therapy. Side effects are NOT less common with low dosage steroids.

CONTRAINDICATIONS:

Herpes simplex keratitis; spreading ulceration or perforation of the cornea can occur from enhanced viral activity. Fungal diseases; steroids may cause overgrowth.

For a complete discussion on steroids see: Endocrine Agents; Steroid Hormones & Related Agents.

TOPICAL CORTICOSTEROIDS FOR OPHTHALMIC USE:

Solutions/Drops:

Preparation	Strength
Prednisolone acetate suspension	0.125,1%
Prednisolone sodium phosphate solution	0.125, 0.5, 1%
Dexamethasone suspension	0.1%
Dexamethasone phosphate solution	0.1%
Medrysone suspension	1%
Fluorometholone suspension	0.1%

Ointments:

Preparation	Strength
Dexamethasone phosphate	0.05%
Fluorometholone	0.1%

OPHTHALMIC LOCAL ANESTHETICS

GROUP REMARKS: Local anesthetics are used topically in the eye during tonometry, removal of foreign bodies and other short corneal or conjunctival procedures. They are NOT for prolonged use, as they may retard corneal healing or cause erosion, scarring or opacification.

DOSAGE:

Solutions/Drops:

Instill 1-2 drops into the conjunctival sac a few minutes prior to the procedure.

Ointments:

Apply a thin coat to the conjunctival sac a few minutes prior to the procedure.

SIDE EFFECTS:

May cause irritation, tearing or photophobia.

CONTRAINDICATIONS:

Hypersensitivity to local anesthetics.

See Local Anesthetics for a more complete discussion.

LOCAL ANESTHETICS FOR OPHTHALMIC USE:

TETRACAINE
(Pontocaine)

DOSE FORMS:
Solution: 0.5%
Ointment: 0.5%

PROPARACAINE
(AK-Taine)
(Alcaine)
(Ophthaine)
(Opthetic)

DOSE FORMS:
Solution: 0.5%

OPHTHALMIC ANTIBIOTICS

GROUP REMARKS: Only ocular doses and pertinent information regarding uses in the eyes are presented here. See discussion in Antibiotics section for further information. Infections that are only superficial may be treated by topical application alone, others may require concurrent systemic therapy. Adherence and viscosity of ointments provide a longer duration of action and protection in cases of eyelid and corneal infections. It is often prudent to continue treatment ≥ 48 h after infection clears.

DRUG	DOSAGE	DOSE FORMS	SPECTRUM OF ACTION	REMARKS
GENTAMICIN (Garamycin)	**Solution**: Instill 1-2 drops q4h (maximum 2 drops/h). **Ointment**: Apply small amount 2-3 times/d.	Solution: 0.3% Ointment: 0.3%	**Gram negative**: most. **Gram positive**: most.	Low toxicity potential with topical use; transient irritation may occur.
CHLORAMPHENICOL (Chloromycetin) (Chloroptic) (Econochlor)	**Solution**: Instill 1-2 drops q3-6h. **Ointment**: Apply small amount q3-6h.	Solution: 0.5% Powder for solution Ointment: 1%	**Gram negative**: most. **Gram positive**: most.	Hypersensitivity reactions (ocular irritation) occur rarely. Adjust concentration and frequency for optimal response.
BACITRACIN (Baciguent)	Apply small amount of ointment ≥ once/d.	Ointment: 500 units/gm	**Gram negative**: Gonococci, Meningococci. **Gram positive**: most. **Anerobes**: Fusobacterium species, Treponema pallidum. **Misc**.: Actinomyces israeli, T. vincenti.	Low toxicity potential; rash and allergic reactions may occur.
SULFACETAMIDE (Sulamyd)	**Ointment**: Apply 1.25-2.5 cm q6h. **Solution**: Instill 1-2 drops q1-3h.	Ointment: 10%. Solution: 10, 15, 30%	**Gram negative**: most. **Gram positive**: most.	Alter concentration of solution and frequency of instillation for maximal individual response. Transient ocular irritation may occur. Should NOT be used with silver nitrate or gentamicin.
SULFISOXAZOLE (Gantrisin)	**Ointment**: Apply small amount 1-3 times/d & hs. **Solution**: Instill 2-3 drops ≥ 3 times/d.	Solution: 4% Ointment: 4%.	**Gram negative**: most. **Gram positive**: most.	Should NOT be used with silver nitrate or gentamicin.
ERYTHROMYCIN (Ilotycin)	Apply small amount of ointment ≥ once/d.	Ointment: 0.5%	**Gram positive**: bacilli, cocci. **Gram negative**: H. influenza, Neisseria, Moraxella lacunata. **Anerobes**: Chlamydia, Treponema.	More effective than topical tetracycline.

OPHTHALMIC ANTIBIOTICS *Continued*

DRUG	DOSAGE	DOSE FORMS	SPECTRUM OF ACTION	REMARKS
TETRACYCLINE (Achromycin) **CHLORTETRACYCLINE** (Aureomycin)	**Ointment**: Apply small amount q2-12h. **Suspension**: Instill 1-2 drops q6-12h.	Ointment: 0.5,1% Suspension: 1%	**Gram negative**: most. **Gram positive**: most. **Misc.**: Rickettsia, Chlamydia, Mycoplasma, spirochetes.	Topical use alone effective for: blepharitits, conjunctivitis and keratitis. Toxicity and sensitization potentials are low; dermatitis and ocular irritation occur rarely.
NEOMYCIN (Myciguent)	**Ointment**: Apply small amount q3-4h. **Solution**: Instill 1-2 drops q6-12h PRN.		**Gram negative**: most aerobic species. **Gram positive**: some aerobic species.	Neomycin available in many combinations, especially with polymyxin B, bacitracin and hydrocortisone (must consider reduced host resistance to infection produced by the latter). **SIDE EFFECTS**: Prevalent contact sensitization (5-15% patients).
POLYMYXIN B	**Solution**: Instill 1-3 drops (10,000-25,000 units/ml) q1h. Decrase frequency as response develops. **Ointment**: Apply small amount q3-4h.	Powder	**Gram negative**: many (esp. Pseudomonas aeruginosa; most Proteus and Neisseria are resistant).	Polymyxin B available in many combinations, especially with neomycin and bacitracin. **SIDE EFFECTS**: Mild ocular irritation.
TOBRAMYCIN (Tobrex)	**Ointment**: Apply 1 cm 2-3 times/d. **Solution**: Instill 1-2 drops q4h (q30-60 min for severe infections).	Ointment: 0.3% Solution: 0.3% Powder for Injection	**Gram negative**: most aerobic. **Gram positive**: various.	Drug of choice in ocular Pseudomonas aeruginosa infections; sub-conjunctival injection may be necessary in corneal and anterior chamber infections. Ophthalmic solution is NOT for injection.

OPHTHALMIC ANTIVIRAL AGENTS

DRUG	DOSAGE	DOSE FORMS	SPECTRUM OF ACTION	REMARKS
IDOXURIDINE (Dendrid) (Herplex) (Stoxil)	**Solution**: Instill 1-2 drops q1h (daytime) and q2h (nighttime) initially. **Ointment**: Apply small amount 4-6 times/d.	Solution: 0.1% Ointment: 0.5%	Herpes simplex (types I and II), Varicella-zoster, Vaccinia, Cytomegalovirus, some DNA viruses.	Used in the treatment of herpes simplex keratitis. Decrease frequency of administration after healing appears complete and continue therapy for 5-7 d. May produce ocular irritation.
VIDARABINE (Vira-A)	Apply 1 cm q3h.	Ointment: 3%	Herpes simplex (types I and II), Varicella-zoster, Vaccinia, Cytomegalovirus, Hepatitis B virus.	May produce ocular irritation. Consider alternate therapy if no response within 7 d or if re-epithelialization is not complete after 21 d. Decrease frequency of administration after healing appears complete and continue therapy for 5-7 d.

OPHTHALMIC ANTIFUNGAL AGENTS

DRUG	DOSAGE	DOSE FORMS	SPECTRUM OF ACTION	REMARKS
NATAMYCIN (Natacyn)	Instill 1 drop q1-6h. Decrease frequency q3-4d.	Suspension: 5%	Aspergillus, Candida, Cephalosporium, Fusarium, Penicillium, Microsporum, Epidermophyton, Blastomyces dermatitidis, Coccidioides immitis, Cryptococcus neoformans, Histoplasma capsulatum, Sporothrix schenkii. Some activity against Trichomonas vaginalis.	Administer more frequently in keratitis, less frequently in conjunctivitis and blepharitis.
NYSTATIN (Mycostatin)	NOT approved for ophthalmologic use, and NOT available in ophthalmic dosage form. However, topical and injectable forms have been used in the treatment of fungal infection of the eye.			

Section 8: CANCER CHEMOTHERAPEUTIC AGENTS
Table of Contents

ALKYLATING AGENTS

GROUP REMARKS: Bone marrow depression (esp. granulocytes, platelets and megakaryocytes; RBC count usually only mildly reduced) occurs with most agents and may be SEVERE with excessive doses. Some agents produce cell-line specific depression. WBC nadir usually at 10-12 d, with recovery at 21-42 d. Ovarian or testicular failure a common late sequela. Tumor resistance normally class specific, with some exceptions. Hyperuricemia (esp. with large tumor burden). **MANUFACTURERS' RECOMMENDATIONS**: Monitor CBC weekly, discontinue treatment if WBC < 3,000 or platelets < 100,000.

DRUG	ACUTE TOXICITY	SIDE EFFECTS & REMARKS
BUSULFAN (Myleran)	Diarrhea.	Frequent hyperpigmentation, hyperuricemia. Possibly leukemogenic. Others: pulmonary fibrosis, adrenal insufficiency, alopecia, gynecomastia, amenorrhea, menopausal symptoms, chromosome aberrations, skin reactions, cataracts (rare). **RECOMMENDATIONS**: Perform monthly DL_{CO} (discontinue if decreases > 30%).
CHLORAMBUCIL (Leukeran)	None.	Pulmonary fibrosis, leukemia, hepatic toxicity, chromosomal damage. Q2wk dosing may decrease bone marrow depression. Seizures occur with overdose. Hysteria occurs rarely. **RECOMMENDATIONS**: Perform weekly CBC.
CYCLOPHOSPHAMIDE (Cytoxan) (Endoxan)	Nausea & vomiting (delayed 6-18 h).	Platelet toxicity less severe, alopecia (33%), SIADH. Hemorrhagic cystitis (< 20% patients)-may decrease with hydration. Occasional hemorrhagic colitis and diarrhea. Rare hemolytic anemia (direct Coombs' test positive). Toxicity increases with hepatic enzyme induction. Possible adverse interaction with allopurinol, may prolong succinylcholine action. **RECOMMENDATIONS**: Monitor Na^+ and CBC.
PHENYLALANINE MUSTARD (Alkeran) (Melphalan)	Mild nausea, hypersensitivity reactions.	Severe platelet depression, possible pulmonary fibrosis, interstitial pneumonitis, leukemia. Possible rapid leukopenia with slow recovery (> 42 d). Skin reactions occur with IV adminstration. **RECOMMENDATIONS**: Monitor CBC weekly (discontinue if WBC < 3,000 or platelets < 100,000).
Thio-TEPA (triethylenethiophosphoramide)	Nausea & vomiting, local pain at IV site.	GI ulceration, menstrual dysfunction. Less commonly used agent due to low therapeutic index. **RECOMMENDATIONS**: Monitor CBC weekly and 3 wk post-discontinuance (discontinue if WBC < 3,000 or platelets < 150,000).
BCNU (Bis-chloroethylnitrosourea) (Carmustine)	Nausea & vomiting, local burning, flushing.	Group Remarks, EXCEPT marrow suppression at 4 wks; recovery at 6-8 wks (NADIRS: platelets 4-5 wks, WBCs 5-6 wks). Pulmonary fibrosis and renal failure may develop with prolonged therapy. Hepatotoxicity, usually mild, occurs in 25% patients (reversible). **RECOMMENDATIONS**: Monitor liver enzymes.
CCNU (Cyclohexylchloroethylnitrosourea) (Lomustine)	Nausea & vomiting.	Similar to BCNU. Also, possible neurological reactions. **RECOMMENDATIONS:** Monitor liver enzymes, CBC 6-8 wks after discontinuing therapy.

ALKYLATING AGENTS *Continued*

DRUG	ACUTE TOXICITY	SIDE EFFECTS & REMARKS
PROCARBAZINE (Matulane)	Nausea & vomiting, CNS depression (psychosis & ataxia), alcohol intolerance.	Stomatitis, dermatitis, peripheral neuropathy, hemorrhagic tendencies, ascites, edema, effusion & pulmonary disorders, hyperpigmentation, eosinophilia and RBC inclusions. **RECOMMENDATIONS**: Perform marrow studies before therapy and 2-8 wk after onset. Monitor urine, LFTs, BUN. Discontinue if WBC < 4,000.
DACARBAZINE (DTIC)	Nausea & vomiting, diarrhea, anaphylaxis, pain, flu-like syndrome.	Alopecia, renal impairment, hepatocellular necrosis with hepatic vein thrombosis, flushing, paresthesias, rash & photosensitiviy, CNS effects, extravasation leading to pain and tissue damage. **RECOMMENDATIONS**: Perform frequent CBC.
ESTRAMUSTINE (Emcyt)	Nausea, vomiting, diarrhea.	Group Remarks, EXCEPT marrow suppression uncommon. Mild gynecomastia, fluid retention, estrogen effects, dyspnea. Increased risk of thrombosis and vascular events (including MI). Use cautiously in patients with embolic history. **RECOMMENDATIONS**: Monitor liver enzymes & fluid status.
CISPLATIN (Platinol) (DDP)	Nausea, vomiting, fever, anaphylaxis.	Group Remarks, EXCEPT myelosuppression usually moderate. **NADIRS**: WBC/platelets at 3 wks, recovery at 5 wks. Hematocrit decreases 6% in 25% patients. Renal damage usually 2 wks post-dose (reversible at 2-4 wks)-but NOT if total dose < 700 mg/m^2 or administered over 5 d. Minimize toxicity by: (1) infusion > 6 h, (2) hydration, (3) treatment with Dexamethasone. Ototoxicity in 6% patients, occasional hemolysis, peripheral neuropathy. Mg^{++}, Ca^{++}, K^{+}, phosphorous wasting. Hyperuricemia (peak at 3-5 d). **RECOMMENDATIONS**: Skin test, serum Mg^{++}, Ca^{++}, K^{+}, phosphorous, creatinine, BUN, creatinine clearance, audiometry. During therapy: CBC weekly, repeat creatinine if serum increases > 33%, monitor serum values as above. Hydrate for 24 h after administration.

ANALOGS

GROUP REMARKS: Common delayed toxicity: leukopenia, anemia, thrombocytopenia (bone marrow suppression); alopecia, hepatic damage, oral & intestinal ulceration, hyperuricemia. **RECOMMENDATIONS**: Weekly CBC/differential (discontinue therapy if sudden drop in any cell line count), monitor liver enzyme levels (approximately weekly), monitor serum uric acid level.

DRUG	ACUTE TOXICITY	SIDE EFFECTS & REMARKS
METHOTREXATE (Mexate) (Amethopterin) (MTX)	Nausea & vomiting, diarrhea, fever, anaphylaxis.	Possible cirrhosis, hepatic necrosis, occasional GI perforation, leukoencephalopathy, osteoporosis, infertility, menstrual dysfunction, immunosuppression, nephrotoxicity (azotemia, hematuria, renal failure-avoid with urine alkalination, forced diuresis). Intrathecal use assoc'd with arachnoiditis, paralysis, convulsions and systemic toxicity. **NADIRS**: WBC at 4-7 & 12-21 d; platelets at 5-12 d. Recovery: WBC at 7-13 d and at 15-29 d; platelets at 15-27 d. **RECOMMENDATIONS**: Baseline CBC, urinalysis, BUN, creat. clearance, chest radiograph, coagulation studies, TB skin test. (Liver biopsy recommended if therapy for psoriasis.)
THIOGUANIDINE (6 T-G)	Nausea & vomiting, anorexia.	Group Remarks, EXCEPT alopecia. Stomatitis & diarrhea may require decreasing dose. Nausea/vomiting well tolerated. Marrow depression usually delayed 2-4 wks. **RECOMMENDATIONS**: Group recommendations, bone marrow examination if heme status questionable.
MERCAPTOPURINE (Purinethol)	Nausea & vomiting, diarrhea.	Group Remarks, EXCEPT alopecia. Anorexia. Liver damage, esp. with doses > 2.5 mg/kg/d. Jaundice in 10-40% of leukemic patients, at 1-2 months. **RECOMMENDATIONS**: Weekly liver enzymes & bilirubin: discontinue if signs of hepatic dysfunction.
FLUOROURACIL (Adrucil) (5-FU)	Nausea & vomiting, diarrhea.	Group Remarks, EXCEPT hepatotoxicity. Stomatitis (5-8 d), diarrhea, rash, pigmentation, photosensitivity, acute cerebellar syndrome, amenorrhea, lacrimation, mucocytis. **NADIRS**: WBC at 9-14 d; platelets at 7-17 d. Recovery usually by 30 d. **RECOMMENDATIONS**: Discontinue treatment if WBC < 2,000 platelets < 100,000; intractable vomiting, diarrhea, ulcer or stomatitis.
CYTARABINE (Ara-C) (Cytosar)	Nausea & vomiting, diarrhea, anaphylaxis.	Group Remarks, EXCEPT alopecia. Fever, iritis, pulmonary edema, (high doses), local pain/thrombophlebitis at IV site. **NADIRS**: WBC at 7-9 d; platelets at 12-15 d. Recovery usually 10 d after nadir. **RECOMMENDATIONS**: Periodic renal function tests, daily CBC/differential during therapy.
FLOXURIDINE (FUDR)	Nausea & vomiting, diarrhea.	Pigmentaton. Metabolized rapidly to 5-fluorouracil, therefore similar toxicity. **RECOMMENDATIONS**: Discontinue treatment if WBC < 3,500, platelets < 100,000; intractable vomiting, diarrhea, ulcer or stomatosis.

IMMUNOSUPPRESSANTS AND MISCELLANEOUS ANTICANCER AGENTS

DRUG	ACUTE TOXICITY	SIDE EFFECTS & REMARKS
IMMUNOSUPPRESSANTS		
AZATHIOPRINE (Imuran)	Nausea, vomiting, diarrhea.	Bone marrow depression (dose-related), pancytopenia, hemorrhage due to decreased platelets. Pancreatitis, hepatic jaundice. Oral ulcers, rash. Drug fever, serum sickness. Alopecia. Raynaud's disease. Retinopathy. Prohibitive risk of neoplasia if previous alkylating agent therapy. **RECOMMENDATIONS**: Perform weekly CBC/differential during first month, biweekly for next 2 months, then monthly; also periodic LFTs. Reduce dose or discontinue if hemotologic problems, infection or severe muscle wasting develop. Reduce dose by 30% if concurrent allopurinol.
CYCLOSPORIN-A (Cyclosporin)	Anaphylaxis with IV administration (0.1% patients).	Nephrotoxicity, dose-related (approx. 33% patients): increased BUN, serum creatinine-usually occurs 2-3 months post-transplant, at dosage adjustment. Hepatotoxicity (dose-related): elevated LFTs, may respond to decrease in dose. Hyperkalemia, hypernatremia, decreased serum bicarbonate. Hypertension (13-27%). Tremor (common), seizures, headache, paresthesias. Hirsutism, gingival hyperplasia (common). Nausea, vomiting, diarrhea and abdominal pain. Increased infections. Gynecomastia. Sinusitis, hearing loss. May increase risk of development of lymphoma. Possible adverse interactions with ketoconazole. **RECOMMENDATIONS**: Observe patients over initial 30 min of IV infusion. Avoid using with other nephrotoxic drugs. Reduce dose with concomitant steroid. Periodic BUN, serum creatinine & LFTs. Drug levels: plasma trough = 50-300 ng/ml (monitor 3 times/wk).
ANTIADRENAL AGENTS		
MITOTANE (Lysodren)	Nausea, vomiting, diarrhea.	Adrenal insufficiency, orthostatic hypotension, hypertension. Hemorrhagic cystitis & hematuria, albuminuria. Maculopapular rash (15% patients). Stomatitis. CNS effects (40% patients): lethargy, somnolence, vertigo, depression. Possible brain damage with prolonged treatment. Gynecomastia. Response to therapy may require 3 months. Increased serum cholesterol, hepatic enzyme induction. **RECOMMENDATIONS**: Treat adrenal insufficiency with higher than normal doses corticosteroids. Liver disease may decrease elimination. Avoid tasks requiring alertness. Periodic behavioral & CNS tests if therapy > 2 years. Discontinue if no benefit in 3 months.
AMINOGLUTETHAMIDE (Cytadren)	Rash, drowsiness, nausea, dizziness.	Fluid retention, hypercalcemia, adrenal insufficiency, hypotension. Weakness. Hypothyroidism. Rash. Fever. **RECOMMENDATIONS**: Mandatory mineralocorticoid supplement (hydrocortisone, PO: 20-30 mg/d). Baseline CBC, LFTs. Periodic thyroid function test, CBC & LFTs. Discontinue treatment if rash develops and persists > 5-8 d.

IMMUNOSUPPRESSANTS AND MISCELLANEOUS ANTICANCER AGENTS *Continued*

DRUG	ACUTE TOXICITY	SIDE EFFECTS & REMARKS
		MISCELLANEOUS
TAMOXIFEN (Nolvadex) *ANTIESTROGEN*	Nausea, vomiting, flush, transient increase in bone and tumor pain.	Hypercalcemia, mild decrease in WBCs and platelets. Vaginal bleeding and discharge. Rash, headache, dizziness, leg cramps, edema. With prolonged high dose treatment: retinopathy, corneal opacites, decreased visual acuity. Tumors may redden/increase size. **RECOMMENDATIONS**: Monitor Ca^{++}, CBC.
TESTOLACTONE (Teslac) *ANDROGEN*	Pain at injection site.	Fluid retention, hypercalcemia, masculinization minimal (favored over testosterone). Hypertension, maculopapular erythema, nausea, vomiting, hot flashes, edema, aches, paresthesias, may decrease insulin need. Possible association with hepatoma. **RECOMMENDATIONS**: Monitor serum Ca^{++} levels.
ETOPOSIDE (VP-16) (EPEG)	Nausea, vomiting, diarrhea, transient hypotension (2%), anaphylaxis, bronchospasm, oral pain.	Severe marrow toxicity: leukopenia (60-90% patients), thrombocytopenia (41% patients). **NADIRS**: WBC and platelet at 7-16 d; recovery at 20 d. Anorexia. Stomatitis. Continuous 5 d infusion occasionally assoc'd with MI, CHF. Alopecia (8-20%); reversible. Somnolence, peripheral neuropathy. Impaired hepatic, renal function; may require decreasing dose. **RECOMMENDATIONS**: Infuse slowly over 30-60 min. Discontinue if hypotension occurs. Perform baseline CBC/differential and monitor q2wk. Discontinue if platelets < 50,000 or WBCs < 500-1000.

NATURAL PRODUCTS

GROUP REMARKS: Bone marrow suppression, alopecia, paralytic ileus with constipation, diarrhea, stomatitis, dermatologic effects (including rash). Hyperuricemia with possible uric acid nephropathy. **RECOMMENDATIONS:** Adequate hydration, urine alkalinization & diuresis to counter hyperuricemia.

Treatment of local effects due to extravasation at site of infusion:

- **A**: Cold compresses.
- **B**: Hot compresses & local infiltration of hydrocortisone sodium succinate.
- **C**: 50-100 mg hydrocortisone sodium succinate.
- **D**: Sodium bicarbonate (5 ml of 8.4% solution).
- **E**: Isotonic sodium thiosulfate (4.1% pentahydrate + 2.6% anhydrous salt or 4% solution by mixing 4 ml of 10% injectable + 10 ml water).
- **F**: Ascorbic acid (1 ml of injectable 5% solution).
- **G**: Hyaluronidase.
- **H**: Normal saline for local dilution (25-50 cc).

DRUG	ACUTE TOXICITY	SIDE EFFECTS AND REMARKS
VINBLASTINE (Velban)	Nausea, vomiting; phlebitis, cellulitis & necrosis with extravasation at IV site. Paresthesias at 4-6 h.	Group Remarks (NOT leukopenia), SIADH. CNS effects (depression, convulsions, psychosis and facial pain). ANS effects (urinary retention, sinus tachycardia). **NADIRS**: WBC at 4-10 d with recovery at 10-24 d. **RECOMMENDATIONS**: Pre-existing vascular disease may predispose to local thrombosis. Treat extravasation as per A or B, G, H (above).
VINCRISTINE (Oncovin)	Phlebitis, cellulitis & necrosis with extravasation at IV site.	Bone marrow suppression is mild. Peripheral neuropathy (decreased deep tendon reflexes, paresthesias, weakness, wrist/foot drop) in many patients. Orthostatic hypotension. Ileus; can mimic acute intestinal obstruction Rare SIADH. **RECOMMENDATIONS**: Laxatives, stool softeners, enemas for ileus. Reduce dose in severe neurotoxicity or obstructive jaundice. Treat extravasation as per C, D or H (above).
DACTINOMYCIN (Cosmegan) (Actinomycin D)	Nausea, vomiting; phlebitis, cellulitis & necrosis (extravasation at IV site).	Group Remarks (NOT paralytic ileus), folliculitis, possible GI ulceration. Potentiates side effects of irradiation (esp. dermal). **NADIRS**: WBC and platelets at 14-21 d; recovery at 21-25 d. **RECOMMENDATIONS**: Daily CBC/differential during treatment. Frequent renal and hepatic function tests. Discontinue if stomatitis or diarrhea develop. **CONTRAINDICATIONS**: Smallpox, HZV infection. Treat extravasation as per A, C and/or E (above).
DAUNORUBICIN (Daunomycin) (Cerubidine)	Nausea & vomiting, diarrhea; red urine (1-2 d), severe local necrosis with extravasation, brief EKG changes/arrhythmias.	Group Remarks (NOT paralytic ileus). Cardiotoxicity: rare myo/pericarditis, cardiomyopathy with CHF (1-2% at total dose > 550 mg/m^2); predisposition to CHF with increased dose or previous chest radiation treatment. Anorexia, fever. **RECOMMENDATIONS**: Baseline liver enzymes, BUN, creatinine clearance, CBC, EKG, ejection fraction (not predictive of cardiotoxicity). Discontinue treatment if QRS voltage decreases > 30% or decreased ejection fraction. Decrease dose in hepatic or renal impairment. Total dose dose should NOT exceed 500-600 mg/m^2 (400-450 mg/m^2 if irradiation of chest). Treat extravasation as per A, C/D (above).

NATURAL PRODUCTS *Continued*

DRUG	ACUTE TOXICITY	SIDE EFFECTS AND REMARKS
DOXORUBICIN (Adriamycin)	Nausea, vomiting, diarrhea; red urine (1-2 d), severe local necrosis with extravasation, ventricular arrhythmias, anaphylaxis.	Cardiotoxicity: CHF (responds to digitalis, diuretics, Na^+ restriction); lethal arrhythmias may occur acutely. Pleural effusion (rare with total dose < 550 mg/m^2; < 400 mg/m^2 with chest irradiation, cyclophosphamide). Total dose toxicity additive with Daunorubicin. Urticaria, conjunctivitis, lacrimation, anorexia, fever, chills. **NADIRS**: WBC, platelets & RBC at 10-14 d. Recovery by 21 d. **RECOMMENDATIONS**: Baseline CBC, liver enzymes, EKG, ejection fraction (not predictive of cardiotoxicity). Treat extravasation as per A & C/E or F (above).
MITHRAMYCIN (Mithracin)	Nausea, vomiting, diarrhea, fever.	Group Remarks (NOT paralytic ileus), leukopenia (6% patients), pulmonary fibrosis, hemorrhage (dose-related), anorexia, hypocalcemia, flushing epistasis, prolonged prothrombin time. Transient elevation LFTs, BUN, creatinine clearance. Possible hepatic toxicity, renal toxicity (high doses). Reduces hypercalcemia (esp. if due to tumor) within 24 h, duration 3-15 d. **RECOMMENDATIONS**: Perform baseline renal and liver function tests, with periodic monitoring during therapy (esp. if BUN > 25 mg/dl or SGOT > 600 units/ml), frequent CBC/differential, prothrombin time. Discontinue if WBC < 4,000, platelets < 150,000 or prothrombin time prolonged > 4 sec. Daily dose NOT to exceed 30 µg/kg. Treat extravasation as per B above.
MITOMYCIN (Mutamycin)	Nausea, vomiting, fever; severe local necrosis with extravasation.	Group Remarks (NOT paralytic ileus), pulmonary fibrosis, hemolysis, nephrotoxicity (2% patients), hepatotoxicity (high doses), cumulative marrow suppression. **NADIRS**: WBC at 6-8 wks, platelets at 2-4 wks and 4-6 wks. Recovery at 3 months. **RECOMMENDATIONS**: Monitor CBC/differential & prothrombin time. Discontinue treatment if WBC < 4,000 or platelets < 150,000. **CONTRAINDICATIONS**: Baseline WBC < 3,000, platelets < 75,000, creatinine < 1.7 mg/dl or coagulapathy.
BLEOMYCIN (Blenoxane)	Nausea, vomiting, fever; anaphylaxis, other allergic reactions.	Group Remarks (NOT paralytic ileus), rare marrow suppression. Interstitial pneumonitis (10% patients, LETHAL in 1%), pulmonary fibrosis (increased with dose > 400 units and age > 70 yr); pulmonary function tests NOT helpful. Hyperpigmentation, Raynaud's phenomena, paresthesias, hypotension, anorexia (may be prolonged). **RECOMMENDATIONS**: Monitor chest radiograph q1-2wk, DL_{CO} monthly (discontinue if decreased > 30%).
ASPARAGINASE (Elspar)	Nausea, vomiting, fever; anaphylaxis, hypersensitivity reactions, headache, abdominal pain, hyperglycemia, coma.	Group Remarks (RARE ileus, marrow suppression, stomatitis). CNS depression or excitement. Acute hemorrhagic pancreatitis, azotemia, renal failure. Coagulative effects: increased prothrombin time, thrombin time (rare bleeding). Hepatic toxicity (occasionally fatal) and decreased protein synthesis (including clotting factors). Toxicity cumulative with vincristine. **RECOMMENDATIONS**: Skin test before therapy. Baseline hepatic, renal, pancreatic, CNS and marrow function tests. Frequent serum amylase, BUN, creatinine, glucose.

Section 9: MISCELLANEOUS AGENTS
Table of Contents

ANTITUSSIVES

GROUP REMARKS: Although coughing serves a purpose (clearing secretions or eliminating noxious substances), it can usually be suppressed without endangering the patient. There are two groups of cough suppressants, the narcotics and the nonnarcotics. The narcotics are clearly superior and their effectiveness parallels their analgesic potency as well as their abuse potential. See Narcotics Analgesics for a more detailed discussion. Water and syrups are also useful but are not additionally discussed below.

DRUG	DOSAGE (PO)	REMARKS
CODEINE	**Adult**: 10-20 mg q4-6h (maximum 120 mg/d). **Child (6-12 y.o.)**: 5-10 mg q4-6h (maximum 60 mg/d). **Child (2-6 y.o.)**: 2.5-5 mg q4-6h (maximum 30 mg/d).	Abuse potential at these doses is low. Constipation may occur as a side effect.
DEXTROMETHORPHAN	**Adult**: 10-30 mg q4-8h (maximum 90-120 mg/d). **Child (6-12 y.o.)**: 5-10 mg q4h <u>OR</u> 15 mg q6-8h (maximum 45-60 mg/d). **Child (2-6 y.o.)**: 2.5-5 mg q4h <u>OR</u> 7.5 mg q6-8h (maximum 30 mg/d).	Less effective than codeine, but available without a prescription. May cause slight drowsiness, nausea, dizziness.
HYDROCODONE (in Hycodan)	**Adult**: 5-10 mg q4-6h (maximum 15 mg/dose). **Child (>12 y.o.)**: 0.6 mg/kg/d in 3-4 doses (maximum 10 mg/dose). **Child (2-12 y.o.)**: 0.6 mg/kg/d in 3-4 doses (maximum 5 mg/dose).	May cause slight drowsiness, nausea, dizziness. Causes more sedation than codeine, but not more constipation. Available in many proprietary mixtures: Hycodan contains homatropine in addition to hydrocodone.
BENZONATATE (Tessalon)	**Adult**: 100 mg q8h (maximum 600 mg/d). **Child (>10 y.o.)**: 100 mg q8h (maximum 600 mg/d).	An amide-type local anesthetic, it acts locally to inhibit pulmonary stretch receptors. May cause drowsiness, nausea, nasal congestion, dizziness.

MISCELLANEOUS ANTI-ASTHMATIC AGENT

DRUG	INDICATIONS & DOSAGE	DOSE FORMS	REMARKS
CROMOLYN SODIUM (Disodium Cromoglycate) (Intal) (Nasalcrom)	<u>**Bronchial Asthma**</u>: **Nebulizer**: 20 mg qid. <u>**Exercise-Induced Bronchospasm (Prevention)**</u>: **Nebulizer**: 20 mg ≤ 60 min prior to exercise, repeat PRN during exercise. <u>**Allergic Rhinitis**</u>: **Nasal**: 1 spray/nostril 3-6 times/d.	Nebulizer: 20 mg capsules, 10 mg/ml solution Aerosol Spray: 800 µg/spray Nasal Solution: 5.2 mg/spray	NOT effective in treatment of <u>acute</u> attacks. Capsules for inhalation ONLY. Therapy is most effective when: doses are regularly spaced, administered via a power-operated nebulizer and asthma responds to bronchodilators. Discontinue therapy gradually. **SIDE EFFECTS**: Stinging or sneezing may occur with nasal administration. Others: Tearing, parotid gland swelling, nausea, dizziness, altered urinary frequency, skin reactions, joint swelling/pain.

EXPECTORANT AND MUCOLYTIC AGENTS

GROUP REMARKS: Expectorants increase the clearance of secretions from the respiratory tract by liquifying and increasing their volume. Water is an effective expectorant, especially when inhaled as steam or aerosol. The common expectorants act as gastric irritants to reflexively stimulate formation of respiratory tract secretion.

DRUG	INDICATIONS & DOSAGE	REMARKS
POTASSIUM IODIDE	**Adult**: 300-600 mg q6-8h.	Hypersecretion in the eyes, nose and mouth is common and may resemble the common "cold." Other side effects: brassy taste, skin rash and swelling of the parotid glands.
GUAIFENESIN	**Adult**: 100-400 mg q4 -6h (maximum 2400 mg/d). **Child (6-12 y.o.)**: 50-100 mg q4-6h (maximum 600 mg/d). **Child (2-6 y.o.)**: 5100 mg q4h (maximum 300 mg/d).	Much less effective than iodine agents. Many proprietary mixtures are available with variety of other components.
ACETYLCYSTEINE (Mucomyst)	**<u>Acetaminophen Intoxication</u>**: **PO**: 140 mg/kg once, then 70 mg/kg q4h for 17 doses (repeat if emesis occurs within 1 h of any dose). Dilute to 5% with juice or soft drinks for PO administration <u>OR</u> to 5% in waterfor gastric intubation. **<u>Mucolysis</u>**: **Nebulization**: 3-5 ml of 20% sln (6-10 ml of 10% sln) q6-8h. **Tracheostomy**: 1-2 ml of 10-20% solution q1-4h.	NOT more effective than saline or humidification for mucolysis. Incompatible with rubber and some metals (stainless steel O.K.). **SIDE EFFECTS**: Stomatitis, nausea, vomiting, severe rhinorrhea; may cause bronchospasm.

ANTIHISTAMINES (H_1 ANTAGONISTS)

GROUP REMARKS: The H_1 antagonist antihistamines are used in Type 1 allergic reactions, i.e., in seasonal allergic rhinitis, allergic conjunctivitis and simple urticaria and angioedema. Their relatively slow onset makes them useless in the treatment of anaphylaxis. They are NOT effective against any other allergic reaction. They are widely self-prescribed (OTC) for the common cold with no effectiveness, except possibly to dry secretions. **SIDE EFFECTS**: Antihistamines have anticholinergic side effects (dry mouth, thickened respiratory tract secretions, constipation, urinary retention). A subjectively unpleasant sedation or lassitude is most common and intense with the older drugs, e.g., diphenhydramine or dimenhydrinate; minimal with chlor- or brom- pheniramine. Stimulation occasionally seen. **RECOMMENDATIONS**: In a patient refractory to a single agent, switching to another class occasionally restores the therapeutic effect. **CAUTIONS**: Because of anticholinergic actions, use cautiously in patients predisposed to: urinary retention, bronchial asthma, increased intraocular pressure. **CONTRAINDICATIONS**: Concurrent monoamine oxidase (MAO) inhibitor therapy, nursing mothers.

DRUG	DOSE (PO-Adult)	DOSE FORMS
ETHANOLAMINES	**Antihistaminic Activity:** **Sedative Activity:** **Anticholinergic Activity:**	**LOW- MODERATE** **HIGH** **HIGH**
DIPHENHYDRAMINE (Benadryl) Generics	25-50 mg q4-6h. (maximum 300 mg/d)	Tab's: 25, 50 mg Cap's: 25, 50 mg Liquid
CARBINOXAMINE (Clistin)	4-8 mg q6-8h. (maximum 24 mg/d)	Tab's: 4 mg
CLEMASTINE (Tavist)	1.34-2.68 mg q8-12h. (maximum 8 mg/d)	Tab's: 1.34, 2.68 mg Liquid
ALKYLAMINES	**Antihistaminic Activity:** **Sedative Activity:** **Anticholinergic Activity:**	**MODERATE** **LOW** **MODERATE**
CHLORPHENIRAMINE (Chlor-Trimeton) Generics	4 mg q4-6h. (maximum 24 mg/d)	Tab's: 4 mg Ext'd Release: Tab's: 8, 12 mg Cap's: 8, 12 mg
BROMPHENIRAMINE (Dimetane) (Veltane) Generics	4 mg q4-6h. **Ext'd Release**: 8-12 mg q8-12h. (maximum 24 mg/d)	Tab's: 4 mg Liquid Ext'd Release: Tab's: 8, 12 mg

DRUG	DOSE (PO-Adult)	DOSE FORMS
ETHYLENEDIAMINES	**Antihistaminic Activity:** **Sedative Activity:** **Anticholinergic Activity:**	**LOW-MODERATE** **LOW-MODERATE** **LOW**
PYRILAMINE	25-50 mg q8h.	Tab's: 25 mg
TRIPELENNAMINE (PBZ)	25-50 mg q6-6h. (maximum 600 mg/d)	Tab's: 25, 50 mg Liquid
PIPERIDINES	**Antihistaminic Activity:** **Sedative Activity:** **Anticholinergic Activity:**	**MODERATE** **LOW-MODERATE** **MODERATE**
CYPROHEPTADINE	4 mgtid initially; maintenance 4-20 mg/d. (maximum 0.5 mg/kg).	Tab's: 4 mg Liquid
DIPHENYLPYRALINE (Hispril)	5 mg q12h.	Ext'd Release: Cap's: 5 mg
PHENINDAMINE (Nolahist)	25 mg q4-6h. (maximum 150 mg/d)	Tab's 25 mg

See next page for Miscellaneous Antihistamines.

DRUG	INDICATIONS & DOSAGE	DOSE FORMS	REMARKS
	MISCELLANEOUS ANTIHISTAMINES (H_1 ANTAGONISTS)		
DIMENHYDRINATE (Dramamine)	Allergic Reactions: **PO**: 50-100 mg q4-6h (maximum 400 mg/d).	Tab's: 50 mg Liquid: 12.5 mg/4 ml	**Antihistaminic Activity: LOW to MODERATE** **Sedative Activity: HIGH** **Anticholinergic Activity: HIGH** A combination of diphenhydramine and chlorotheophylline; used often for motion sickness.
TERFENADINE (Seldane)	Allergic Reactions: **PO**: 60 mg q12h.	Tab's: 60 mg	**Antihistaminic Activity: LOW** **Sedative Activity: NONE-LOW** **Anticholinergic Activity: LOW** Sedative acitivity is low to non-existent, but therapeutic effectiveness is also low to non-existent. Available only by prescription in the U.S. Adverse reactions reported: alopecia, angioedema, dermal inflammation, bronchospasm, menstrual irregularities. Cautiously evaluate need in pregnant women; possible associations with fetal malformations have been reported.
PROMETHAZINE [a phenothiazine] (Phenergan)	Allergic Reactions: **PO**: 25 mg at hs (maximum 12.5 mg prior to meals & at hs). **IM, IV**: 25 mg; repeat at 2 h if needed.	Tab's: 12.5, 25, 50 mg Syrup: 6.25, 25 mg/5 ml Injection: 25, 50 mg/ml	**Antihistaminic Activity: HIGH** **Sedative Activity: HIGH** **Anticholinergic Activity: HIGH** See Antipsychotic Tranquilizers for a complete discussion of the general properties of the phenothiazines (including Side Effects, Cautions, Recommendations and Contraindications).

MISCELLANEOUS ANTIRHEUMATIC AGENTS: GOLD COMPOUNDS

GROUP REMARKS: The risk of toxicity increases with increasing dose. Do NOT use if material has darkened; color should not exceed pale yellow. **SIDE EFFECTS**: Thrombocytopenia, aplastic anemia, agranulocytosis, dermatitis, GI disturbances, stomatitis, proctitis, vaginitis, eosinophilia, leukopenia, proteinuria, hematuria, nephrosis, metallic taste, chrysiasis, Guillian-Barré Syndrome, corneal ulcers and gold deposits. Diarrhea is particularly common with auranofin. **CAUTIONS**: Use with care in patients with history of renal or hepatic disease, compromised cardiovascular function, history of impaired cerebrovascular circulation, inflammatory bowel disease, blood dyscrasias, allergy or hypersensitivity to gold medications. **RECOMMENDATIONS**: Monitor: CBC, platelets, eosinophils and urinalysis (at each dose or every other dose). Discontinue at first sign of toxicity, or: if formed elements of blood decrease significantly (WBCs < 4000/cc, granulocytes < 1500/cc, platelets < 100,000-150,000/cc); if 2+ proteinuria, significant hematuria, stomatitis or pruritis occurs or if rash is observed. After a cumulative dose of 1 gm has been given IM without clinical improvement, the drug can be either discontinued, given for an additional 10 wks at 25-50 mg/wk or the dose can be increased by 10 mg increments q1-4wks (with no single injection exceeding 100 mg). Diarrhea due to auranofin can often be managed by decreasing dosage. **CONTRAINDICATIONS**: Gold has been shown to be teratogenic in animals and is generally contraindicated in pregnancy. Others: history of infectious hepatitis, renal or hepatic dysfunction, uncontrolled hypertension, decompensated CHF, SLE, blood dyscrasias, recent radiation treatment, history of severe toxicity from gold or heavy metals, eczema, colitis, poorly controlled diabetes mellitus, pulmonary fibrosis.

DRUG	INDICATIONS & DOSAGE	DOSE FORMS	REMARKS
GOLD SODIUM THIOMALATE (Myochrysine)	**Rheumatoid Arthritis**: **IM**: As single doses: 10 mg in the first wk; 25 mg in the second wk; 25-50 mg in the third wk and weekly thereafter. Continue 1 injection/wk until: 1) significant clinical improvement, 2) major toxicity or 3) cumulative dose reaches 1 gm. After this regimen, maintenance doses of 25-50 mg q2wks for 2-20wks can be given; lengthen interval between injections to q3-4wks and continue indefinitely if clinical course is stable.	Injection: 10, 25 mg/ml (1 ml), 50 mg/ml (1, 10 ml)	Patient should remain prone for 10 min following injection. Gold content = 50%.
AUROTHIOGLUCOSE (Solganal)	**Rheumatoid Arthritis**: **IM**: As single doses: 10 mgin the first wk; 25 mg for the second and third wks; 50 mg in the fourth wk and weekly thereafter. Continue 1 injection/wk until: 1) significant clinical improvement, 2) major toxicity or 3) cumulative dose reaches 0.8-1 gm. After this regimen, maintenance doses of 50 mg q3-4wks can be given indefinitely; reduce this dosage to 25 mg q3-4wks if clinical course is stable.	Injection: 50 mg/ml (10 ml)	Gold content = 50%.
AURANOFIN (Ridaura)	**Rheumatoid Arthritis**: **PO**: 6 mg/d in 1-2 doses. After 6 months, increase to 3 mg tid if response to initial dose is inadequate (maximum dosage). After 3 months at 9 mg/d, discontinue therapy if clinical response is inadequate.	PO (Cap's): 3 mg	Gold content =29%.

MISCELLANEOUS ANTIRHEUMATICS

DRUG	INDICATIONS & DOSAGE	DOSE FORMS	REMARKS
HYDROXYCHLOROQUINE (Plaquenil)	**Rheumatoid Arthritis**: **PO**: 400-600 mg/d (with meals); increase dose after 5-10 d, based on clinical response. After 4-12 wks of optimal response at a given dose level, decrease dose by 50% and continue maintenance dose of 200-400 mg/d. **Lupus Erythematosus**: **PO**: 400 mg q12-24h initially; continue for weeks-months based on clinical response, then decrease dose to 200-400 mg/d; maintain indefinitely.	PO (Tab's): 200 mg (= 155 mg base)	**SIDE EFFECTS**: Side effects rarely require temporary reduction. Corneal epithelial deposits, dose-related retinopathy (including macular edema, atrophy, pigmentary changes), scotomata, bleaching or loss of hair, anorexia, abdominal discomfort, weakness, blood dyscrasias, skin eruptions, lassitude, precipitation of porphyria, immunoblastic lymphadenopathy. Incidence of retinopathy is higher with doses > 400 mg/d. **CAUTIONS**: Use cautiously in conjunction with known hepatotoxic drugs. The risk of dermatologic complications increases if phenylbutazone, gold salts or other sensitizers are used. **RECOMMENDATIONS**: Discontinue therapy if no response after 6 months. If therapeutic response occurs with therapy, taper concomitant steroid use. Perform ophthalmologic examinations at initiation of therapy and q3-4months. Discontinue immediately if retinopathy or keratopathy occurs. **CONTRAINDICATIONS**: Retinal, visual field or other ophthalmologic changes caused by hydroxychloroquine or any other 4-aminoquinoline compound; known hypersensitivity to 4-aminoquinoline compounds; long-term therapy in children.
D-PENICILLAMINE (Cuprimine) (Depen Titratabs)	**Rheumatoid Arthritis**: **PO**: 125-250 mg/d initially, increase dose by 125-250 mg/d q1-3months. After 2-3 months at 500-750 mg/d, increase dose by 250 mg/d q2-3months. Doses > 500 mg/d should be divided. Discontinue therapy if no response after 3-4 months at 1-1.5 gm/d or if significant toxicity develops. Do NOT increase dose beyond a level at which adequate response is obtained. Therapeutic responses may not be seen for 2-3 months after any given dose adjustment. After a remission of 6 or more months, reduce dose by 125-250 mg/d at 3-month intervals. **Cystinuria**: **PO**: 1-4 gm/d in 4 doses; maximum 4 gm/d. **Pediatric PO**: 30 mg/kg/d in 4 doses. **Wilson's Disease**: **PO**: 250 mg qid (30 min before meals and at bedtime), base dose on urinary [copper]; maximum 2 gm/d.	PO (Tab's): 250 mg PO (Cap's): 125, 250 mg	Patients treated for Wilson's disease or cystinuria should be given pyridoxine 25 mg/d. Patients undergoing surgery should have dosage reduced to 250 mg/d until wound healing is complete. Efficacy of penicillamine in juvenile rheumatoid arthritis has not been established. **SIDE EFFECTS**: Severe side effects include fever, rash (early- and late-occurring), nephropathy, obliterative bronchiolitis, leukopenia or leukocytosis, eosinophilia, thrombocytopenia and require discontinuation of drug. Nausea, vomiting, anorexia, loss of taste, renal or hepatic injury, SLE-like syndrome, bleeding diathesis, optic neuritis (responsive to pyridoxine), cataracts, oral ulcerations. **CAUTIONS**: AVOID in patients receiving antimalarial agents, gold therapy, cytotoxic drugs, oxyphenbutazone, or phenylbutazone. Iron salts and antacids decrease gastric absorption. Serum levels of digoxin may be reduced and digoxin dose may need to be increased. Probably fetotoxic or teratogenic in humans. Safe use in the nursing mother has not been established. **RECOMMENDATIONS**: Perform urinalysis, CBC with differential and platelets q3d for 4 wks, weekly for 3 months, then monthly. Perform renal and liver function studies and eye evaluations q6months. Discontinue therapy if hematuria develops, if WBC count < 3500/mm^3, if platelet count < 100,000/mm^3, in unevaluated protenuria or any protenuria exceeding 1 gm/d, hemoptysis, infiltrates on chest X-ray or bullous skin lesions. **CONTRAINDICATIONS**: Pregnancy, renal insufficiency, history of previous reaction to penicillamine.

MISCELLANEOUS ANTIRHEUMATICS *Continued*

DRUG	INDICATIONS & DOSAGE	DOSE FORMS	REMARKS
METHOTREXATE (Folex) (Mexate)	**Severe Psoriasis**: **PO, IM, IV**: 10-25 mg/wk (single dose); maximum 50 mg/wk. **PO**: 2.5 mg q8-12h for 3-4 doses; repeat each week; maximum 30 mg/wk. (*Alternative regimen*: 2.5 mg/d for 5 d followed by no therapy for 2 d; maximum 6.25 mg/d. ***Note***: This regimen may increase risk of serious liver dysfunction.) When clinical respnse reaches optimal level, attempt reduction to lowest effective dose.	PO (Tab's): 2.5 mg Injection: 2.5, 25 mg Powder: 20, 50,100 mg	Use ONLY in patients with severe, disabling psoriasis. **CAUTION**: Use may produce severe or FATAL side effects. See additional information under Cancer Chemotherapeutic Agents.
AZATHIOPRINE (Imuran)	**Rheumatoid Arthritis**: **PO, IM**: 1 mg/kg/d initially, in 1-2 doses (maximum 100 mg/d). After 6-8 wks, increase by 0.5 mg/kg/d q4wks (maximum 2.5 mg/kg/d). Once the effective dosage is found, start maintenance therapy by incrementally decreasing dosage by 0.5 mg/kg/d q4wks; continue until lowest effective dose is found. Discontinue therapy after 12 wks if no response.	PO (Tab's): 50 mg Injection: 100 mg/vial (20 ml vials)	Use ONLY in patients with active, severe disease who are refractory to other, less toxic, agents. See additional information under Cancer Chemotherapeutic Agents.

ANTITHROMBOTIC AND RELATED AGENTS

DRUG	INDICATIONS & DOSAGE	DOSE FORMS	REMARKS
HEPARIN			
HEPARIN (Lipo-Hepin) (Liquaemin Sodium)	***Note***: Doses are recommendations for initiating therapy. Adjust dosage so that APTT is 1.5-2 times control value or when WBCT is 2.5-3 times control value. **Full-Dose Anticoagulation**: **SC**: 10,000-20,000 units initially, then 8,000-10,000 units q8h. (Alternatively, follow initial dose with 15,000-20,000 units q12h.) **IV**: 10,000 units initially, then 5,000-10,000 units q4-6h. **IV Infusion**: 20,000-40,000 units/d in 1000 ml isotonic saline (continuous). **Pediatric IV**: 50 units/kg bolus initially, then 100 units/kg q4h. (Alternatively, follow initial dose with 20,000 units/m^2/d as a continuous IV infusion.) **Low-Dose Prophylaxis Against Thromboembolism**: **SC**: 5,000 units q8-12h for 7 d (postoperatively). Give initial dose 2h prior to surgery. Discontinue and begin protamine sulfate therapy if bleeding continues postoperatively.	Injection: 1,000, 5,000, 10,000, 20,000, 40,000 units/ml (1, 2, 4, 5, 10, 30 ml vials)	Heparin inactivates Factor Xa and inhibits conversion of prothrombin to thrombin (it also inhibits conversion of fibrinogen to fibrin, but is not fibrinolytic). One-stage prothrombin time may be prolonged with heparin for ≥ 5h after IV dose and 24 h after SC dose. SGOT and SGPT elevations may occur without associated liver damage. **SIDE EFFECTS**: Up to 30% of patients receiving heparin therapy develop thrombocytopenia; usually within 2-3 d after initiating therapy, but can be delayed up to 6-12 d. Allergy, thromboembolic complications (assoc'd with thrombocytopenia), hemorrhage (10% of patients) can occur anywhere; primarily significant in adrenal glands, ovaries and in retroperitoneum. Vasoconstrictive reactions may occur 6-10 d after beginning therapy; may last 4-6 h with painful, aschemic or cyanotic limb. **CAUTIONS**: Do NOT administer **IM**. Use with extreme caution whenever there is increased probability of bleeding, as in: threatened abortion; severe liver, renal or gallbladder disease; ulcerative gastrointestinal lesions; hemophilia; following spinal cord, brain, eye or other major surgery; severe hypertension; dissecting aneurysm or subacute bacterial endocarditis. Use of heparin therapy during pregnancy has been associated with complications in ≤ 25% of cases; it is slightly safer than coumarin derivatives (complications in ≤ 33% of cases). **RECOMMENDATIONS**: Discontinue therapy if platelet count < 100,000/mm^3. Monitor via partial thromboplastin time (PTT), activated PTT, whole blood clotting time (WBCT) or activated coagulation time (ACT). **CONTRAINDICATIONS**: Severe thrombocytopenia, uncontrollable bleeding not related to disseminated intravascular coagulation, hypersensitivity to heparin and in patients where tests for blood coagulation cannot be performed for any reason.

DRUG INTERACTIONS:

Drugs which affect platelet aggregation such as ***aspirin, indomethacin, ibuprofen, dipyridamole, hydroxychloroquine, phenylbutazone and high-dose penicillin*** may cause bleeding even with therapeutic levels of **heparin**.

DRUG	INDICATIONS & DOSAGE	DOSE FORMS	REMARKS
COUMARIN DERIVATIVES			

GROUP REMARKS: If prothrombin time is within therapeutic limits and bleeding occurs, investigate for other lesions responsible for bleeding. Patients with genetic resistance to oral anticoagulants are also more likely to have an increased need for vitamin K. **SIDE EFFECTS**: Hemorrhage is the most common complication. Others include: nausea, vomiting, diarrhea, leukopenia, alopecia, hepatitis, jaundice. Hypersensitivity reactions include: agranulocytosis, eosinophilia; and, after 1-3 months of therapy, nephritis, acute tubular necrosis, albuminuria, oliguria and fever. **CAUTIONS**: Risk of complications increased with trauma, infection, antibiotic therapy, dietary deficiencies, significant hypertension, severe diabetes, vasculitis and other factors predisposing to hemorrhage. Decreasing anticoagulant effects include hyperlipemia, hypothyroidism, edema, diabetes mellitus, hereditary resistance to oral anticoagulants. Increasing anticoagulant effects include steatorrhea, carcinoma, infectious hepatitis, vitamin K deficiency, scurvy, collagen disease, hepatic disorders, jaundice, congestive heart failure, scurvy, thyrotoxicosis, infectious hepatitis, diarrhea, renal insufficiency and fever. **RECOMMENDATIONS**: Monitor prothrombin time (PT) daily during initial therapy, decreasing to q4-6wks after stable anticoagulation is achieved (more often with change in medication or status) Note: Dosage is individualized on the basis of the one-stage PT; therapeutic objective is to obtain a value 1.5-2.5 times the control value. **CONTRAINDICATIONS**: Hemorrhagic conditions, thrombocytopenic purpura, recent CNS or spinal cord surgery, threatened abortion, aneurysm, acute nephritis, eclampsia, severe vitamin C deficiency, suspected stroke, uncontrolled hypertension, blood dyscrasias, hemophilia, hepatic insufficiency, major lumbar block anesthesia, subacute bacterial endocarditis, malignant hypertension, pericardial effusion, visceral carcinoma, polyarthritis.

DRUG INTERACTIONS:
A high potential exists for clinically significant drug interactions with the **oral anticoagulants**:
Agents that **increase** their anticoagulant effect include: ***anabolic steroids, chloral hydrate, chloramphenicol, clofibrate, thyroid agents, disulfiram, metronidazole, phenylbutazone, oxyphenbutazone, salicylates, streptokinase, urokinase***. Other agents that **may enhance** anticoagulation include: ***other non-steroidal anti-inflammatory drugs, some antibiotics and some diuretics***.
Agents that **decrease** their anticoagulant effect include: ***barbiturates, glutethimide and oral contraceptives***. Other agents that **may diminish** anticoagulation include: ***other sedative-hypnotics, some anticonvulsants and griseofulvin***.
Variable effects on anticoagulation may occur with ***alcohol*** and ***corticosteroids***.

DRUG	INDICATIONS & DOSAGE	DOSE FORMS	REMARKS
WARFARIN SODIUM (Coumadin) (Panwarfin)	**Full-Dose Anticoagulation**: **PO**: 10-15 mg/d for 2-3d, then use PT response to adjust dosage PRN; maintenance usually 2-10 mg/d. (Alternative (PO, IV, IM): 40-60 mg initially a s a single dose.)	PO (Tab's): 2, 2.5, 5, 7.5, 10 mg Injection: 50 mg/vial, 2 ml diluant	**RECOMMENDATION**:Decrease dosages for elderly or debilitated patients by 1/3-1/2.
WARFARIN POTASSIUM (Athrombin-K)	**Full-Dose Anticoagulation**: **PO**: 40-60 mg/d (single dose), then 2.5-10 mg/d based on the PT. The interval between initial dose and first maintenance dose can be 2-6 d based on PT.	PO (Tab's): 5 mg	**RECOMMENDATION**:Decrease dosages for elderly or debilitated patients by 1/3-1/2.

ANTITHROMBOTIC AND RELATED AGENTS: COUMARIN DERIVATIVES *Continued*

DRUG	INDICATIONS & DOSAGE	DOSE FORMS	REMARKS
DICUMAROL	<u>**Anticoagulation**</u>: **PO**: 200-300 mg for 1 d, then 25-200 mg/d if prothrombin activity is > 25% normal level.	PO (Tab's): 25, 50, 100 mg	
PHENPROCOUMON (Liquamar)	<u>**Anticoagulation**</u>: **PO**: 24 mg/d initially; maintenance 0.75-6 mg/d.	PO (Tab's): 3 mg	
ANISINDIONE (Miradon)	<u>**Anticoagulation**</u>: **PO**: 300 mg on day 1, 200 mg on day 2, 100 mg on day 3; then maintenance 25-250 mg/d.	PO (Tab's): 50 mg	
FIBRINOLYTICS			
STREPTOKINASE (Kabikinase) (Streptase)	<u>**Deep Vein/Arterial Thrombosis, Pulmonary Emboli**</u>: **IV**: 250,000 units over 30 min; then 100,000 units/h for 24-72 h. Follow with heparin IV infusion (delay start until thrombin time has decreased to < 2x normal).	Injection, powder: 250,000, 600,000, 750,000 IU/vial (5, 6.5 ml vials)	Fever reported in ≤ 33% of patients, do NOT treat with aspirin (use acetaminophen).
UROKINASE (Abbokinase)	<u>**Pulmonary Emboli**</u>: **IV**: 4400 units/kg (at 90 ml/h rate for 10 min); then 4400 units/kg/h (at 15 ml/h rate) for 12 h. Should be admixed into 0.9% NaCl or 5% dextrose. Follow with heparin IV infusion (delay start until thrombin time has decreased to < 2x normal)	Injection, powder: 250,000 IU/vial (5 ml vials) Injection, powder for reconstitution: 5,000 IU/ml (1 ml Univials)	
ANTIPLATELET AGENTS			
DIPYRIDAMOLE (Persantine)	**PO**: 50 mg tid, 1 h prior to meals.	PO (Tab's): 25, 50, 75 mg	**SIDE EFFECTS**: Nausea, hypotension, headache, diarrhea. **CAUTIONS**: May worsen migraines or hypotension.
SULFINPYRAZONE (Anturane)	**PO**: 200-400 mg/d in 2 doses; maximum 800mg/d.	PO (Tab's): 100 mg PO (Cap's): 200 mg	**SIDE EFFECTS**: Nausea, vomiting, diarrhea, blood dyscrasias.
ASPIRIN	See section: CNS Agents; Non-Narcotic Analgesics		

PROCOAGULANTS

DRUG	INDICATIONS & DOSAGE	DOSE FORMS	REMARKS
INDICATIONS: Procoagulant indications include: • Prothrombin deficiency secondary to biliary disease. • Prothrombin deficiency secondary to antibiotic/salicylate therapy. • Prothrombin deficiency secondary to anticoagulant therapy. (***Note***: PT = prothrombin time.)			
MENADIONE (VITAMIN K3)	**PO**: 5-10 mg/d.	PO (Tab's): 5 mg	Do NOT administer to infants.
MENADIOL SODIUM DIPHOSPHATE (VITAMIN K4) (Synkayvite)	**PO**: 5-10 mg/d. **IM, IV, SC**: 5-15 mg q12-24h. **Pediatric IM, IV, SC**: 5-10 mg q12-24h.	PO (Tab's): 5 mg Injection: 5, 10, 37.5 mg/ml	
PHYTONADIONE (VITAMIN K1) (Phylloquinone) (Methylphytyl Naptho-quinone) (Mephyton) (AquaMEPHYTON) (Konakion)	**PO**: 2.5-10 mg initially (maximum 50 mg); determine subsequent doses by PT measurements. Repeat in 12-48 h if PT has NOT corrected. **IM, SC**: 2.5-10 mg initially (maximum 50 mg); determine subsequent doses by PT measurements. Repeat in 6-8 h if PT has NOT corrected. **IV (AVOID, if possible)**: Administer < 1 mg/min; 2.5-10 mg initially (maximum 50 mg); determine subsequent doses by PT measurements. Repeat in 6-8 h if PT has NOT corrected. **<u>Hemorrhagic Disease of the Newborn (Prophylaxis)</u>**: **Pediatric IM**: 0.5-2 mg (single dose).	PO (Tab's): 5 mg Injection: 2, 10 mg/ml (0.5, 1, 2.5, 5 ml) IM Injection: 2, 10 mg/ml (0.5, 1 ml)	**CAUTION**: IV administration can produce SEVERE side effects, which can even be FATAL.
PROTAMINE SULFATE	**<u>Treatment of Heparin Overdose</u>**: **IV**: Administer < 50 mg/10min (1 mg protamine sulfate neutralizes approx. 90 USP units heparin).	Injection: 10 mg/ml Powder	

SPECIFIC IONS

GROUP REMARKS: Much of the use of electrolytes depends upon their bulk or osmotic effects when used as "parenteral fluids" or laxatives. Some agents are used as a source of, or to produce, the effects of specific ions.

POTASSIUM

DRUG	INDICATIONS & DOSAGE	DOSE FORMS	REMARKS
POTASSIUM CHLORIDE (K-lor) (Cena-K) (Klorvess)	**Severe Potassium Deficits (K+ < 2.0 mEq/l):** **IV**: ≤ 40 mEq/h (maximum [K+] = 80 mEq/l); maximum 400 mEq/d. **Moderate Potassium Deficits (K+ > 2.5 mEq/l):** **IV**: ≤ 10 mEq/h (maximum [K+] = 40 mEq/l); maximum 200 mEq/d. **Potassium Deficiency**: **PO**: 40-150 mEq/d. **Prevention of Hypokalemia (adjunct to non-potassium-sparing diuretics)**: **PO**: 16-24 mEq/d.	PO (Tab's): 4, 6.7, 8, 10 mEq PO (Liquid): 0.66, 1, 1.33, 2, 2.66, 3 mEq/ml (5, 11.25, 15, 22.5, 30, 120, 480 ml) Powder: 15, 20, 25, 50 mEq/packet Injection: 1, 1.5, 2,4 mEq/ml (5, 10, 12.5,15, 20, 30, 60 ml)	Each 1 mEq/l drop in serum potassium represents a 100-200 mEq deficit of total body potassium stores. **SIDE EFFECTS**: Nausea, vomiting, diarrhea, skin rash, hyperkalemia, gastric ulceration or bleeding. Lethal cardiac arrhythmias with overdosage. In digitalized patients with AV conduction disturbances, use of potassium can precipitate worsening of conduction abnormalities. **RECOMMEND**: Monitor parenteral therapy with frequent EKGs and serum potassium levels. **CAUTIONS**: Extravasation can cause local tissue necrosis. Phlebitis, venospasm and pain at injection site can occur with IV administration, especially at higher concentrations (30-40 mEq/l). **CONTRAINDICATIONS**: Hyperkalemia, dehydration, heat cramps, renal dysfunction with anuria, oliguria or azotemia, adrenocortical insufficiency, adynamia episodica hereditaria, crush syndrome.

PHOSPHATE

POTASSIUM PHOSPHATE	**Phosphate Supplementation During TPN**: **IV**: 10-15 mM/l TPN solution.	Injection: 3 mM phosphate + 4.4 mEq potassium/ml (5, 15, 30, 50 ml)	Injection formulations are composed of monobasic and dibasic forms of potassium salt. Prescribing is in terms of mM (millimoles) of phosphorous. **SIDE EFFECTS**: Hypocalcemic tetany, hyperkalemia. **CAUTIONS**: Overly rapid administration can cause hypocalcemia with consequent tetany. **CONTRAINDICATIONS**: Hyperkalemia, hyperphosphatemia, hypocalcemia.

DRUG	INDICATIONS & DOSAGE	DOSE FORMS	REMARKS
CALCIUM			
CALCIUM SALTS, Parenteral (Calphosan) (Cal-Nor) (Kalcenate)	<u>**Calcium Chloride**</u>: **IV**: 0.5-1 gm q24-72h (rate NOT > 1 ml/min) q1-3d. For cardiac resuscitation, give 0.5-1 gm IV bolus. 1 gm (10 ml) = 272 mg (13.6 mEq) calcium. <u>**Calcium Gluconate**</u>: **IV**: 0.5-2 gm PRN; maximum 15 gm/d (rate NOT > 0.5 ml/min). 1 gm (10 ml) = 90 mg (4.5 mEq) calcium. <u>**Calcium Gluceptate**</u>: **IM**: 0.44-1.1 gm (2-5 ml) into gluteus maximus. **IV**: 1.1-4.4 gm (5-20 ml). 1.1 gm (5 ml) = 90 mg (4.5 mEq) calcium: 1.1-4.4 gm. 1.1 gm (5 ml) = 90 mg (4.5 mEq) calcium.	Calcium chloride: Injection 10% sln (10 ml) Calcium gluconate: Injection 10% sln (10, 20 ml) Calcium gluceptate: Injection 220 mg/ml (5, 50 ml)	Calcium gluconate is less irritating than calcium chloride. **SIDE EFFECTS**: Cardiac syncope with large bolus administrations. Calcium chloride: can cause severe necrosis and sloughing of skin (if extravasation occurs during IV administration), metallic taste, bradycardia, peristhesias, hypercalcemia. Calcium gluceptate can cause local pain with IM injection. **CAUTIONS**: Calcium administration in patients taking digitalis may cause cardiac arrhythmias. Do not mix slns with phosphates, sulfates, carbonates or tartrates. Safe use in pregnancy has not been established. **CONTRAINDICATIONS**: Digitalis toxicity, ventricular fibrillation during cardiac resuscitation.
CALCIUM SALTS, Oral Various	**PO**: 500-2000 mg 1-2 times/d. The Recommended Dietary Allowance is 800 mg/d for children,1200 mg/d for adolescents and 800 mg/d for adults; 1200 mg/d for pregnant/lactating women.	Calcium carbonate (40% Ca++): 260, 500, 600 mg Ca++ Calcium gluconate (9% Ca++): 45, 90 mg Ca++ Calcium lactate (13% Ca++): 42, 84 mg Ca++ Calcium citrate: 250 mg Ca++ (acidified tablets)	Oral calcium salts are used as antacids and as a source of calcium in presence of hypocalcemia, a supplement to treatment of osteoporosis and osteomalacia and in prenatal supplements. Dicalcium phosphate is obsolete. All oral calcium salts are present in many proprietary mixtures with vitamin D, other vitamins and iron.
MISCELLANEOUS			
MAGNESIUM SULFATE *Continued, next page*	<u>**Severe Hypomagnesemia**</u>: **IV**: 5 gm (40 mEq) diluted in 1000 ml D5W; infuse over 3 h. <u>**Mild Magnesium Deficiency**</u>: **IM**: 1 gm (8.12 mEq) q6h for 4 doses; maximum 32.5 mEq/d. *Continued, next page*	Injection: 10, 12.5, 25, 50% slns (0.8, 1, 2, 4 mEq/ml) Vials: 2, 5, 8,10, 20, 30, 50, 150 ml	Normal serum magnesium levels = 1.5-3 mEq/l. Levels of 4-7 mEq/l are associated with successful treatment for preeclampsia, eclampsia, and seizures. Levels > 7 mEq/l are associated with significant toxicity. (1 gm magnesium sulfate = 8.12 mEq magnesium.) **SIDE EFFECTS**: Hypoten- *Continued, next page*

SPECIFIC IONS *Continued*

DRUG	INDICATIONS & DOSAGE	DOSE FORMS	REMARKS
MAGNESIUM SULFATE *Continued*	<u>**Eclampsia, Toxemia of Pregnancy, Nephritis**</u>: **IV**: 1-4 gm of 10-20% sln (rate NOT > 1.5 ml/min for 10% sln, NOT > 0.75 ml/min for 20% sln). **IM**: 1-5 gm of a 25-50% sln q4-6h PRN.	See previous page.	sion, hypothermia, CNS depression, respiratory paralysis, cardiac depression, circulatory collapse. May precipitate hypocalcemia. **CAUTIONS**: With severe renal impairment, may give rapid rise in serum level of magnesium. **RECOMMEND**: Maintain urine output ≥ 600 cc/d. Monitor serum magnesium levels and clinical response; avoid overdosage. **CONTRAINDICATIONS**: Myocardial damage, heart block.
AMMONIUM CHLORIDE	<u>**Metabolic Alkalosis, Hypochloremic States**</u>: **IV**: Multiply total body weight by 0.2 to obtain extracellular fluid volume (ECF). Multiply ECF by the serum chloride deficit (mEq/ml) and SLOWLY give 1/2 of this dose. Then recheck pH and serum chloride deficit (Administer at a rate NOT > 0.9-1.3 ml/min for the 2.14% sln.) <u>**Urine Acidificaton**</u>: **PO**: 500-3000 mg qid. **IV**: 1.5 gm q6h; maximum 6 gm/d.	PO (Tab's): 325, 500 mg PO (enteric-coated Tab's): 0.5, 1 gm Injection: 2.14% sln (0.4 mEq/ml) in 500 ml vials, 26.75% sln (5 mEq/ml) in 20 ml vials.	(1 gm ammonium chloride = 18.7 mEq chloride.) **SIDE EFFECTS**: Metabolic acidosis, hyperreflexia, tremulousness, obtundation. Gastric irritation with oral administration. **RECOMMEND**: Monitor plasma and electrolytes frequently during IV administration. Administer slowly to avoid pain, local irritation and toxicity. **CONTRAINDICATIONS**: Hepatic or renal insufficiency.
SODIUM BICARBONATE (Neut)	<u>**Cardiac Arrest**</u>: **IV**: 1 mEq/kg intially, then 0.5 mEq/kg q10min PRN (based on arterial blood gases). <u>**Metabolic Acidosis**</u>: **IV**: Dosage formula: bicarbonate needed (mEq) = 0.5 x body weight (kg) x base deficit (mEq/l). Give 1/2 of this dose and recheck pH. <u>**Urine Alkalinization**</u>: **PO**: 325-2000 mg 1-4 times/d (maximum 16 gm/d; 8 gm/d if > 60 y.o.).	Injection: 4, 4.2, 5, 7.5, 8.4% slns (0.48, 0.5, 0.595, 0.892, 1 mEq/ml) in 5, 10, 50, 500 ml vials	(1 gm sodium bicarbonate equivalent to 11.9 mEq sodium + 11.9 mEq bicarbonate.) **SIDE EFFECTS**: Alkalosis, edema, hypernatremia, tissue necrosis with local extravasation, sodium overload. **CAUTIONS**: Overly rapid infusion may cause arrhythmias. Sodium load can precipitate CHF in patients with cardiac abnormalities. Overly rapid correction of metabolic acidosis can precipitate LETHAL hypokalemia. If loss of total body chloride has occurred, because of vomiting or nasogastric suction, there is a greater tendency towards developing severe alkalosis when bicarbonate is administered. **RECOMMEND**: Give as small a dose as possible and monitor clinical and laboratory status. **CONTRAINDICATIONS**: Hypochloremic states from any cause, metabolic or respiratory alkalosis and significant hypocalcemia where alkalosis may precipitate tetany.

TREATMENT OF GOUT

GROUP REMARKS: Gout results from the deposition of urate crystals in and around affected joints and the kidneys. Treatment aims: 1) **Relief of acute attacks** of joint pain, 2) **Depletion of excess urate** from the body in order to prevent subsequent joint and kidney damage. Three types of agents are used to treat gout: 1) An anti-inflammatory drug specific for gout, colchicine, 2) A metabolic inhibitor of urate crystal production, allopurinol and 3) Agents increasing excretion of uric acid, the uricosurics.

DRUG	INDICATIONS & DOSAGE	DOSE FORMS	REMARKS
COLCHICINE	**Acute Attacks**: **PO**: 0.5-1.2 mg q1-2h (maximum 4-8 mg/attack). **IV**: 2 mg initially, then 0.5 mg q6h PRN (maximum 4 mg/d); NOT in D5W. **Prophylaxis**: **PO**: 0.5-1.8 (usually 0.5-0.6) mg/d, (3-4 d/wk). **IV**: 0.5-1 mg, 1-2 doses/d. (PO dosing preferred.)	PO (Tab's): 0.5, 0.6 mg Injection: 0.5 mg/ml	Colchicine has anti-inflammatory activity only in gout (diagnostic); it has no other analgesic properties. Used also in familial Mediterranean fever. **SIDE EFFECTS**: Nausea, vomiting, diarrhea (often limit dose). Severe local irritation; do NOT administer SC or IM. **RECOMMEND**: Allow 3 d between courses of acute therapy.
ALLOPURINOL (Zyloprim) (Lopurin)	**Prophylaxis**: **PO**: 100 mg/d initially, then incremental increase = 100 mg/d q1wk; maintenance = 200-300 mg/d in mild cases and 400-600 mg/d in severe cases (maximum 800 mg/d).	PO (Tab's): 100, 300 mg	Allopurinol inhibits the synthesis of uric acid by xanthine oxidase. It is NOT useful in acute attacks; may precipitate attack when treatment begun. Goal is reduction of serum urate ≤ 6 mg/100 ml (then reduce dosage if possible). **SIDE EFFECTS**: Acute gouty attacks initially. Rash (esp. pruritic maculopapular) is the most common and may be delayed ≤ 2 years. Nausea, vomiting, diarrhea. Also peripheral neuritis or necrotizing vasculitis. May alter LFTs. **RECOMMEND**: Use ONLY in gout with one or more of the following: gouty nephropathy or renal urate stones, tophaceous deposits, no response to uricosurics (or inability to use because of impaired renal function). Prophylactic colchicine during initial 3-6 months of therapy. Discontinue at first sign of rash.

URICOSURICS

GROUP NOTES: Uricosurics increase the excretion of uric acid by interfering with its resorption from the renal tubule; as plasma levels decrease, deposition of crystals ceases and resorption of deposits is promoted. Uricosurics therefore prevent arthritis and renal damage, but have NO utility in acute attacks. **NOTES**: Initiate therapy 2-3 weeks after last acute attack. **SIDE EFFECTS**: Initiation of therapy may precipitate acute gouty attacks via mobilization of urate deposites; prophylactic colchicine is recommended for the first 3-6 months of therapy. Elevated uric acid levels in urine may promote formation of renal stones; maintain high output (≥ 2 l/d) of alkaline urine. GI irritation and rashes (hypersensitivity reaction) are common. **CAUTIONS**: Avoid concurrent salicylates (interference with uricosuric action). **CONTRAINDICATIONS**: Renal impairment; creatinine clearance < 50 ml/min.

DRUG	INDICATIONS & DOSAGE	DOSE FORMS	REMARKS
PROBENECID (Benemid)	**PO**: 250 mg bid initially; maintenance = 500-1500 mg bid.	PO (Tab's): 500 mg	Lower incidence of GI irritation than sulfinpyrazone. Use lower doses/incremental imcreases in renal impairment.
SULFINPYRAZONE (Anturane)	**PO**: 200-400 mg bid for 1 week, maintenance = 200-400 mg bid.	PO (Tab's): 100 mg PO (Cap's): 200 mg	Lower incidence of hypersensitivity rashes than probenecid.

LIPID-LOWERING AGENTS

GROUP REMARKS: Must first establish that elevation in plasma lipids represents a primary disorder and is not due to other diseases (e.g., diabetes, hypothyroidism, liver disease, nephrotic syndrome, dysproteinemias).

DRUG	INDICATIONS & DOSAGE	DOSE FORMS	REMARKS
INHIBITORS OF HEPATIC LIPID (CHOLESTEROL) SYNTHESIS			
GROUP NOTES: **RECOMMENDATIONS**: Regularly monitor LFTs, esp. during initial stages of therapy. **CONTRAINDICATIONS**: Pregnancy, lactation, significant hepatic or renal dysfunction, history of hypersensitivity reactions.			
LOVASTATIN (Mevacor)	**Hyperlipidemia**: **PO**: 20 mg/d initially with evening meal; then 20-80 mg/d in single or divided doses. Adjust dose q4wks (maximum: 80 mg/d).	PO (Tab's): 20 mg	Use initial dose = 40 mg/d if serum cholesterol > 300 mg/dl. Indicated as an adjunct to diet for elevated total and LDL cholesterol levels in primary hypercholesterolemia. Less effective in patients with homozygous familial hypercholesterolemia. **SIDE EFFECTS**: 2% of patients have significant increases in serum transaminases; usually reversible by discontinuation and often occurring 3-12 months after starting therapy. Myositis noted in 0.5% of patients in clinical trials. Also: elevated CPK (11% of patients) and myalgias. Others: constipation, diarrhea, abdominal pain, nausea, cramps, flatulence, muscle cramps, dizziness, headache, rash, blurred vision, abnormal taste, lenticular opacities. **CAUTIONS**: React promptly to any elevation of transaminases in patients who consume significant amounts of alcohol.
CLOFIBRATE (Atromid-S)	**Hyperlipidemia**: **PO**: 2 gm/d in divided doses (lower doses may be effective).	PO (Cap's): 500 mg	Particularly useful in type III hyperlipidemia for lowering cholesterol and triglycerides. **SIDE EFFECTS**: Hepatomegaly, increased incidence of gallstones, nausea, vomiting, dyspepsia, flatulence, stomatitis, gastritis, angina, cardiac arrhythmias, thrombophlebitis, rash, pruritus, alopecia, impotence, renal dysfunction, proteinuria, oligouria, leukopenia, myalgia, anemia, fatigue, weakness, polyphagia, weight gain, peptic ulcer, dizziness, headache, gynecomastia, thrombocytopenic purpura, hematuria, increased SGOT & SGPT (usually reversible with discontinuation), increased CPK. **CAUTIONS**: Can potentiate the effect of oral anticoagulants and sulfonylureas. Rifampin may decrease and probenecid may increase the effects of clofibrate. Use with caution in patients with a history of jaundice or hepatic disease, peptic ulcer. **RECOMMENDATIONS**: Regular monitoring of LFTs and CBCs. Take with food or milk if GI upset occurs. Strict birth control procedures MUST be exercised by women of childbearing potential. **CONTRAINDICATIONS**: Pregnancy, lactation, significant hepatic or renal dysfunction, history of hypersensitivity.

LIPID-LOWERING AGENTS: CHOLESTEROL SYNTHESIS INHIBITORS *Continued*

DRUG	INDICATIONS & DOSAGE	DOSE FORMS	REMARKS
GEMFIBROZIL (Lopid)	**Hyperlipidemia**: **PO**: 450-600 mg bid,30 min prior to morning and evening meals (maximum: 1500 mg/d).	PO (Cap's): 300 mg	Indicated in hypertriglyceridemia (type IV hyperlipidemia). Exerts almost no effect on elevated cholesterol levels. Similar to clofibrate; adverse effects of clofibrate may also apply to gemfibrozil. **SIDE EFFECTS**: Hyperglycemia, abdominal pain, diarrhea, nausea, vomiting, rash, urticaria, pruritis, dermatitis, headache, blurred vision, dry mouth, constipation, anemia, leukopenia, eosinophilia, dyspepsia, paresthesias, vertigo, tinnitus, insomnia, arthralgia, myalgia, hypokalemia, fatigue, syncope, cough, urinary tract infections. Increased SGOT, SGPT, CPK, alkaline phosphatase, LDH. **CAUTIONS**: Dizziness, blurred vision may preclude patient from driving or other tasks requiring alertness. May significantly enhance the effect of concurrent oral anticoagulants. **RECOMMENDATIONS**: Carefully monitor blood glucose levels. Closely monitor prothrombin time of patients taking oral anticoagulants concurrently. **CONTRAINDICATIONS**: Gallbladder disease.
PROBUCOL (Lorelco)	**Hyperlipidemia**: **PO**: 500 mg with morning and evening meals.	PO (Tab's): 250 mg	Indicated in patients with primary hypercholesterolemia (elevated LDL). **SIDE EFFECTS**: QT prolongation. 10% of patients have diarrhea or loose stools. Abdominal pain, flatulence, nausea, vomiting, palpitations, syncope, chest pain, headache, paresthesia, peripheral neuritis, pruritis, insomnia, conjunctivitis, blurred vision, anorexia, indigestion, thrombocytopenia, nocturia, angioneurotic edema, goiter. Elevated SGOT, SGPT, BUN, bilirubin, alkaline phosphatase, CPK, uric acid, blood glucose. **CAUTIONS**: QT prolongation may progress to arrhythmias. Effects of other medications or conditions which prolong QT interval may be increased by concurrent use of probucol. **RECOMMENDATIONS**: Take with meals. Manufacturer recommends baseline, 6 month and 1 year EKG.
NIACIN (Nicolar) (Nicotinic Acid)	**Hyperlipidemia**: **PO**: 1-2 gm tid (maximum: 8 gm/d). **Niacin Deficiency**: **PO**: 10-20 mg/d. **Pellagra**: **PO**: Up to 500 mg/d.	PO (Tab's): 25, 50, 100, 500 mg PO (Cap's): 125, 250, 300, 400, 500 mg Elixir: 10 mg/ml (pint, gal) Injection: 50, 100 mg/ml	Recommended daily allowance (adults) = 18 mg in males, 13 mg in females. Adjunct to therapy in patients with significantly elevated cholesterol or triglyceride levels. **SIDE EFFECTS**: Many side effects are transient. Flushing, headache, dizziness, nausea, vomiting, pruritis, postural hypotension. Abnormal glucose tolerance, abnormal LFTs, jaundice, hyperuricemia, toxic amblyopia, hypotension, macular cystoidedema, peptic ulcer, keratosis nigricans. **CAUTIONS**: Safe use in children has not been established in doses that exceed nutritional requirements. Some preparations contain tartrazine. **RECOMMENDATIONS**: Monitor LFTs and blood glucose frequently. Observe diabetic patients for loss of glucose control. Observe patients with gout for elevated uric acid levels. **CONTRAINDICATIONS**: Peptic ulcer, hypotension, hemorrhage.

LIPID-LOWERING AGENTS *Continued*

DRUG	INDICATIONS & DOSAGE	DOSE FORMS	REMARKS
BILE ACID BINDING RESINS			
GROUP NOTES: These resins combine with bile acids in the intestine to increase their fecal excretion, thus decreasing the amounts available for cholesterol synthesis. This mechanism is also shared by natural fibers. **SIDE EFFECTS**: Constipation, bulky stools, hemorrhoids, diarrhea, diverticulitis, obstruction reported only in infants with large doses. Belching, heartburn, nausea, vomiting, anorexia, aggravation of peptic ulcers. Increased serum phosphorus and Cl^-, decreased Na^+ and K^+; may lead to hyperchloremic acidosis. Alleged deficiency of vitamins A, D, E and K.			
CHOLESTYRAMINE (Questran)	<u>**Hyperlipidemia**</u>: **PO**: 4 gm 1-6 times/d.	Packages: 4 gm	Take before meals. Indicated in hyperlipoproteinemia, pruritis associated with partial biliary obstruction. It has also been used to bind to clostridium difficile toxin and in the treatment of chlordecone (Kepone) insecticide poisoning. 4 gm cholestyramine = 5 gm colestipol. **SIDE EFFECTS**: Rash, vertigo, headache, dizziness, paresthesias, femoral nerve pain, tinnitus, syncope, pancreatitis, hematuria, burnt odor of urine, dysuria, uveitis, edema, elevated SGOT, shortness of breath, dysphagia. **CAUTIONS**: Safe use in children and pregnant or lactating women has not been established. **RECOMMENDATIONS**: Take other drugs at least 1 h before or 4-6 h after cholestyramine. **CONTRAINDICATIONS**: Complete biliary obstruction, history of hypersensitivity to resins.
COLESTIPOL (Colestid)	<u>**Hyperlipidemia**</u>: **PO**: 15-30 gm/d in 2-4 doses.	Packets (granules): 5 gm Bottles (granules): 500 gm	Same as for cholestyramine.

NEWER AGENTS/NEWER USES

A number of new agents have become available since the preparation of the individual sections of this book. This section provides information on these newer agents. Practitioners are advised to consult periodical literature for the latest information before using any of these agents.

DRUG	INDICATIONS & DOSAGE	DOSE FORMS	REMARKS
CARDIOVASCULAR AGENT			
TERAZOSIN (Hytrin)	<u>Hypertension</u>: **PO**: 1 mg qhs initially; then 1-5 mg/d in 1-2 doses (maximum 20 mg/d).	PO (Tab's): 1, 2, 5 mg	Terazosin is an *alpha*$_1$-blocker. **SIDE EFFECTS**: Blurred vision, dizziness, peripheral edema, nausea, palpatations, somnolence, nasal congestion, back pain, headache, anxiety, arthralgias, epistaxis, gout, rash, diaphoresis, tinnitus, dyspnea, impotence, nervousness, postural hypotension, tachycardia. Small (but statistically significant) decreases in WBC count, hematocrit, hemoglobin, total protein and albumin have occurred. **CAUTIONS**: High doses in laboratory animals produced benign adrenal medullary tumors, and testicular atrophy. Pregnancy category C. Safety and effectiveness in nursing mothers and in young children have not been established. **RECOMMENDATIONS**: Instruct patient to avoid driving or hazardous tasks for 12h after initial dose or until symptoms of light-headedness have resolved. Monitor blood pressure 2-3 h after dosing and just prior to next dose. If response substantially diminishes at 24 h, consider increased dose or bid regimen. **CONTRAINDICATIONS**: Hypersensitivity.
ANTIBIOTIC AGENTS			
CIPROFLOXACIN (Cipro)	<u>Urinary Tract Infections</u>: **PO**: 250-500 mg q12h. <u>Respiratory Tract, Skin, Bone and Joint Infections</u>: **PO**: 500-750 mg q12h. <u>Infectious Diarrhea</u>: **PO**: 500 mg q12h.	PO (Tab's): 250, 500, 750 mg	**SIDE EFFECTS**: Most common: nausea, vomiting, diarrhea, abdominal pain, headache, rash and restlessness. Occur in < 1% patients (including ciprofloxacin and quinolone cogeners): oral candidiasis, dysphagia, intestinal perforation, gastrointestinal bleeding, vertigo, insomnia, hallucinations, manic reactions, seizures, tremor, ataxia, depression, and other CNS effects. Others: photosensitivity, flushing, fever, chills, facial edema, erythema nodosum, blurred vision, eye pain, myalgias, arthralgias, renal failure, palpitations, hypertension, myocardial infarction, epistaxis, pulmonary edema, bronchospasms, dyspnea, LFT changes (elevated SGPT, SGOT, alkaline phosphatase), elevated serum creatinine & BUN and blood count changes (lowered platelets & WBCs, elevated eosinophils). **RECOMMENDATIONS**: Preferred dosing time is 2 h after meals. Do not take with antacids. Avoid use in children or pregnant women. **CAUTIONS**: May prolong the half-life and elevate plasma concentrations of theophyline. Pregnancy category C; however ciprofloxacin has caused lameness when administered to immature dogs. **CONTRAINDICATIONS**: Hypersensitivity to ciprofloxacin or to other quinolones.

NEWER AGENTS/NEWER USES: ANTIBIOTICS *Continued*

DRUG	INDICATIONS & DOSAGE	DOSE FORMS	REMARKS
NORFLOXACIN (Noroxin)	<u>Urinary Tract Infections</u>: **PO**: 400 mg bid for 7-21 d (maximum 800 mg/d). <u>In Renal Failure</u>: **PO**: 400 mg/d (for 7-21 d) if creat. clearance < 30cc/min.	PO (Tab's): 400 mg	Norfloxacin is similar to the other quinolones cinoxacin and nalidixic acid, see Non-Sulfanamide Urinary Tract Agents. **SIDE EFFECTS**: Occur in 1-3% of patients: dizziness, nausea, headache, elevated LFTs, decreased WBC count, increased BUN or creatinine. Occur in < 1%: rash, abdominal pain, fatigue, depression, somnolence, insomnia, constipation, dry mouth, diarrhea, fever, erythema, lightheadedness, visual disturbances, decreased hematocrit. **CAUTIONS**: Not for use in children or pregnant women. Use with caution in patients predisposed to seizures. **RECOMMENDATIONS**: Drug should be taken 1 h prior to or 2 h after meals. **CONTRAINDICATIONS**: Hypersensitivity to norfloxacin or other quinolones.
HEPATITIS B VACCINE (Heptavax-B) (Recombivax HB)	<u>Prevention of Hepatitis B in High Risk Groups</u>: **IM**: 1 ml initially; then 1 ml at 1 and 6 months. **Pediatric IM (birth-10 y.o.)**: 0.5 ml initially; then 0.5 ml at 1 and 6 months. <u>Prevention of Hepatitis B in Dialysis and Immunocompromised Patients</u>: **IM**: 2 ml initially; then 2 ml at 1 and 6 months. (For Hepatavax-B give each 2 ml dose as two separate 1 ml injections at different sites.) <u>Known/Probable Hepatitis B Exposure</u>: **IM**: 0.06 ml/kg hepatitis B immune globulin ASAP post-exposure; then administ. hepatitis B vaccine: 1 ml initially; then 1 ml at 1 and 6 months. <u>HBV Carrier State in Neonates Born to HBsAG Positive Mothers</u>: **Pediatric IM**: 0.5 ml hepatitis B immune globulin at birth; then administer hepatitis B vaccine: 0.5 ml within 7 d; then 0.5 ml at 1 and 6 months.	Heptavax-B: Vials: 20 μg/ml (0.5, 3 ml) Recombivax HB: Vials: 10 μg/ml (0.5, 3 ml)	**SIDE EFFECTS**: Common: soreness at injection site. Others: local swelling, erythema, chills, fever, adenitis, myalgia, rash, arthralgias, headache, malaise, fatigue, nausea, vomiting, diarrhea, dizziness, paresthesia. **CAUTIONS**: Safe use during pregnancy has not been established. **RECOMMENDATIONS**: Do NOT administer IV or intradermally; inject into deltoid muscle in adults and into anterolateral thigh in pediatric patients. AVOID injection into buttocks. **CONTRAINDICATIONS**: Hypersensitivity.
ZIDOVUDINE (Retrovir) (AZT)	<u>Adjunctive Use in AIDS</u>: **PO**: 200 mg q4h.	PO (Cap's): 100 mg	**SIDE EFFECTS**: Anemia/granulocytopenia seen in up to 30-50% of patients. Others: chills, lymphadenopathy, vasodilation, urticaria, pruritis, chest pain, constipation, bleeding gums, tongue edema, flatulence, arthralgia, tremor, anxiety, depression, syncope, nervousness, vertigo, confusion, acne, cough, pharyngitis, sinusitis, ambloyopia, hearing loss, dysuria, urinary frequency or hesitancy. Adverse hematologic effects directly related to dose and duration of therapy; inversely related to T_4 number, granulocyte count and hemoglobin at beginning of therapy. **CAUTIONS**: Extreme caution indicated when using in patients with compromised bone marrow function or when used in combination with drugs which are bone marrow toxins, nephrotoxic or cytotoxic. Administer during pregnancy ONLY if clearly needed. **RECOMMENDATIONS**: Monitor CBC q2wks; adjust dosage or discontinue if anemia or granulocytopenia occur.

NEWER AGENTS/NEWER USES: *Continued*

DRUG	INDICATIONS & DOSAGE	DOSE FORMS	REMARKS
CENTRAL/AUTONOMIC NERVOUS SYSTEM AGENT			
YOHIMBINE (Yocon)	<u>**Erectile Impotence**</u>: **PC**: 5.4 mg tid, up to 10 wks.	PO (Tab's): 5.4 mg	Blocks *alpha*$_2$ presynaptic receptors. **SIDE EFFECTS**: Nausea, dizziness, nervousness, antidiuresis, elevated blood pressure, elevated heart rate, tremor, vomiting, skin flushing, headache, irritability. **CAUTIONS**: Do NOT co-administer with antidepressants or similar drugs. Extreme caution indicated in patients with gastric or duodenal ulcer and cardiac/renal compromise. **RECOMMENDATIONS**: If side effects occur, reduce dosage by half and gradually restore the full dosage.
DERMATOLOGIC AGENT			
TRETINOIN (Retin-A)	<u>**Acne**</u>: **Topical**: Apply daily at bedtime. Cover entire affected area daily for 2-6 wks. Longer therapy may be required. <u>**Wrinkle Removal**</u> (unlabeled use): **Topical**: Apply 0.025% cream qhs or qod hs PRN.	Cream: 0.25, 0.05%, 1% (20, 45 gm) Gel: 0.025, 0.1% (15, 40 gm) Liquid: 0.05% (28 ml)	**SIDE EFFECTS**: Dermal hyperpigmentation and hypopigmentation. Local redness, blistering, crusting and edema. **CAUTIONS**: Caution indicated in lactating mothers and patients with eczema. Teratogenic when given PO. Use cautiously when co-applying topical peeling agents or other agents with high concentrations of astringents, alcohol or lime. **RECOMMENDATIONS**: Minimize exposure to sunlight/sunlamps during therapy. Consider discontinuation or decreasing frequency of application should adverse effects occur. **CONTRAINDICATIONS**: Hypersensitivity.
MISCELLANEOUS			
IPRATROPIUM BROMIDE (Atrovent)	<u>**Bronchospasm**</u>: **Inhalation**: 2 inhalations q6h (maximum 12 inhalations/d).	Vials: 14 gm (200 inhalations)	Anticholinergic bronchodilator. **SIDE EFFECTS**: Tachycardia, headache, dizziness, tremor, nausea, vomiting, dry mouth, constipation, blurred vision, cough, rash, flushing, urticaria, alopecia. Transient blurred vision may result from aerosol contact with the eye. **CAUTIONS**: NOT appropriate therapy where rapid response is required. Caution in patients with prostatic hypertrophy, narrow-angle glaucoma. Use with caution in pregnant and lactating women. Safe use in children < 12 y.o. and for infants of nursing mothers has not been established. Safety and efficacy in pregnancy have not been established. **CONTRAINDICATIONS**: Hypersensitivity to atropine and its derivatives.

NEWER AGENTS/NEWER USES: *Continued*

DRUG	INDICATIONS & DOSAGE	DOSE FORMS	REMARKS
GASTROINTESTINAL SYSTEM AGENT			
NIZATADINE (Axid)	<u>Duodenal Ulcer (Active)</u>: **PO**: 300 mg qhs <u>OR</u> 150 mg bid. <u>Healed Duodenal Ulcer (Maintenance)</u>: **PO**: 150 mg qhs. <u>In Renal Failure</u>: **PO**: If creat. clearance = 20-50 cc/min, give150 mg qd for active ulcer; 150 mg qod for healed duodenal ulcer maintenance. If creat. clearance < 20 cc/min, then give150 mg qod for active ulcer; 150 mg q3d for healed duodenal ulcer maintenance.	PO (Cap's): 150, 300 mg	Mechanism of action is H_2 receptor blockade. **SIDE EFFECTS**: In 0.5-1% patients: Somnolence, sweating, urticaria. Less common: transaminase elevations (reversible with discontinuation), gynecomastia, rash, exfoliative dermatitis, hyperuricemia. **RECOMMENDATIONS**: Discontinue if elevated transaminases occur. **CAUTIONS**: False-positive urine tests for urobillinogen may occur with Mulitstix™. Safe use in pregnancy, in lactating mothers and children has NOT been established. **CONTRAINDICATIONS**: Hypersensitivity to nizatadine.

Appendix A: ABBREVIATIONS

ACh	acetylcholine
AChE	acetylcholine esterase
ACT	activated coagulation time
adminst	administer/administration
approx	approximately
APTT	activated partial thromboplastin time
ASAP	as soon as possible
b/c	because
bid	two times per day
BW	body weight
cap's	capsules
CBC	complete blood count
cc	cubic centimeters (= milliliters liquid)
clear.	clearance
CNS	central nervous system
CPK	creatine phosphokinase
creat.	creatinine
CVS	cardiovascular system
d	day(s)
d/c	discontinue
esp.	especially
EKG	electrocardiogram
Eq	equivalents
G-6-PD	glucose-6-phosphate dehydrogenase
GI	gastrointestinal
gm	grams
h	hour(s)
Htn	hypertension
HTN	hypertension
hs	bedtime (hour of sleep)
IM	intramuscular administration
IOP	intraocular pressure
IV	intravenous administration
l	liter
lb	pounds
LFTs	liver function tests: AST (SGOT), ALT (SGPT)
maint	maintenance
MAO	monoamine oxidase
max	maximum
mEq	milliequivalents
mg	milligrams
min	minute
ml	milliliters
mM	millimolar
ng	nanograms
NS	normal saline
NSAID	non-steroidal anti-inflammatory drug
oz	ounces
pediat	pediatric
ppm	parts per million
PO	oral administration
PRN	as needed
pt	patient(s)
PT	prothrombin time
PTT	partial thromboplastin time
PVC	premature ventricular contraction
q	every
qid	four times per day
qtt	drops
RBC	red blood cell
s/sx	signs and symptoms
SC	subcutaneous administration
SL	sublingual
SLE	systemic lupus erythematosis
sln	solution
tab's	tablets
TCA	tricyclic antidepressant
tid	three times per day
TPN	total parenteral nutrition
tsp	teaspoon
µg	micrograms
WBC	white blood cell
WBCT	whole blood clotting time
wk	week(s)
X-ref.	cross-reference
y.o.	years old

SYMBOLS

>	greater than
≥	equal to or greater than
<	less than
≤	equal to or less than
[X]	concentration (of substance x)

NOTE: Dosing Terminology:
"increase X mg/d q1wk" means increase daily dose by X mg at weekly intervals.

Appendix B: LIQUID DIETS

	Kcal/l	Electrolytes (mEq/l)						Minerals (mOsm/l)	Caloric Constituents (g/l)			How Supplied
		Na+	K+	Cl-	Ca++	Phos	Iron		Sugar	Fat	Protein	
Ensure	1060	332	32	0	530	530	9	450	145.0	37.2	37.2	8 & 32 oz
Ensure Plus	1500	446	49	5	630	630	13.5	600	200.0	53.3	55.0	8 oz
Vivonex[1]	1000	537	30	2	555	555	10	550	230	1.45	20.4	Powder 80 g
Vivonex HN[1]	1000	533	18	2	333	333	6	810	211	0.9	41.7	Powder 80 g
Vital	1000	117	30	9	670	670	12	450	185.0	10.3	41.7	Powder 78 g
Sustagen[2]	1500	46	72	-	2800	2100	16	-	266	14	94	Powder 1,2 1/2 & 5 lb
Sustacal	1000	41	53	-	1010	930	17	-	140.0	23.4	61.2	8,12 & 32 oz
Flexical	1000	316	34	0	630	530	9	-	152.5	34.0	22.5	Powder 2 & 16 oz
Portagen	1015	220	31	3	950	720	19	-	110.4	45.8	33.6	Powder 16 oz
Osmolyte	1060	223	23	3	530	530	9	300	145.0	38.5	37.2	8 & 32 oz
Isocal	1060	44.4	30	630	530	9	-	132.1	23	34	34.3	8,12 & 32 oz

[1] Full-strength dilution (one 80 g packet diluted with about 255 ml water to a final volume of 300 ml).

[2] Manufacturer's recommended dilution for oral feedings (400 g per 800 ml).

Appendix C: PREGNANCY CATEGORIES

When pregnancy appears as a contraindication or precaution to the use of a drug, it is often qualified by a category. These categories have the same meaning as those in the Code of Federal Regulations.

CATEGORY A
Adequate studies in pregnant women have failed to show a risk to the fetus in the first trimester and there is no evidence of risk in later trimesters.

CATEGORY B
Animal studies have failed to show a risk to fetus and there are no adequate studies in pregnant women; or animal studies have shown an adverse effect but human studies have not in the first trimester, and there is no evidence of risk in later trimesters.

CATEGORY C
Animal studies have shown an adverse effect on the fetus, there are no adequate studies in humans but the benefits outweigh the risks, or there are no animal studies or adequate human studies.

CATEGORY D
Positive evidence of human fetal risk but the benefits outweigh the risks.

CATEGORY X
Animal or human studies have shown fetal abnormalities or toxicity and the risks outweigh the benefits.

Appendix D: CONTROLLED DRUG SCHEDULES

<u>SCHEDULE I</u>: May be used ONLY for RESEARCH.

NARCOTICS: Heroin and numerous synthetic narcotics.

HALLUCINOGENS: LSD, MDA, STP, DMT, DET, mescaline, peyote, bufotenine, ibogaine, psilocybin.

MARIJUANA and **Tetrahydrocannabinols**.

<u>SCHEDULE II</u>: NO REFILLS, NO TELEPHONIC prescriptions.

NARCOTICS: Opium, Opium Alkaloids & derived Phenanthrenes: morphine, codeine,hydromorphone (Dilaudid), oxymorphone (Numorphan), oxycodone (dihydrohydroxycodienone, a component of Percodan). Synthetics: meperiedine (Demerol), alpha-prodine (Nisentil), anileridine (Leritine), methadone, levorphanol (Levo-Dromoran), phenazocine.

STIMULANTS: Cocaine and coca leaves, amphetamine, dextroamphetamine, methamphetamine, phenmetrazine (Preludin), methylphenidate (Ritalin), mixtures of above (such as Dexamyl, Eskatrol).

DEPRESSANTS: Amobarbital, pentobarbital, secobarbital, mixtures of above (such as Tuinal), methaqualone, phencyclidine (PCP).

<u>SCHEDULE III</u>: Prescriptions must be REWRITTEN after 6 MONTHS or 5 REFILLS.

NARCOTICS: Following opiates (in amounts less than indicated) in mixtures: Codeine & hydrocodeine-not to exceed 1800 mg/dl or 90 mg/tablet, dihydrocodeinone (hydrocodone & in Hycodan); not to exceed 300 mg/dl or 15 mg/tablet, opium; not to exceed 500 mg/dl or 25 mg/5ml or other dosage unit (paregoric).

NARCOTIC ANTAGONISTS: Naltrexone (Trexane).

DEPRESSANTS: Schedule II barbiturates in mixtures or in suppository dose form, butabarbital (Butisol), glutethamide (Doriden), methyprylon (Noludar).

STIMULANTS: benzphetamine (Didrex), chlorphentermine (Pre-Sate), diethylpropion (Tenuate), mazindol (Sanorex), phendimetrazine.

<u>SCHEDULE IV</u>: Prescriptions must be REWRITTEN after 6 MONTHS or 5 REFILLS (differ from Schedule III in penalties for illegal possession).

NARCOTICS: pentazocine (Talwin), propoxyphene (Darvon).

STIMULANTS: phentermine, fenfluramine (Pondimin).

DEPRESSANTS: Benzodiazapines: chlordiazepoxide (Librium), clonazepam (Clonopine), clorazepate (Tranxene), diazepam (Valium), flurazepam (Dalmane), lorazepam (Ativan), oxazepam (Serax), prazepam (Verstran), triazolam (Halcion). Choral hydrate, Ethchlorvynol (Placidyl), Meprobamate, Mephobarbital (Mebaral), Paraldehyde, Phenobarbital.

<u>SCHEDULE V</u>: Same as any other (nonnarcotic) prescription drug; may also be dispensed without a prescription unless state regulations apply.

NARCOTICS: Diphenoxylate (not more than 25 mg with not less than 0.025 mg of atropine per dosage unit-(Lomotil), Loperamide (Imodium). Also the following (provided the amount per 100 ml or 100 gm does not exceed that listed) in mixtures: Codeine-200 mg, Dihydrocodeine-100 mg, Ethylmorphine-100 mg.

INDEX

Note: Generic drug names are in CAPITALS